handbook of Cardiac Transplantation

Edited by

Robert W. Emery, M.D.
President, Minneapolis Heart Institute
Director, Cardiothoracic Transplantation
Minneapolis Heart Institute
Department of Cardiovascular Diseases
Abbott Northwestern Hospital
Minneapolis, Minnesota

Leslie W. Miller, M.D.
Professor of Medicine and Surgery
Director, Heart Failure/Heart Transplantation Program
Saint Louis University Health Sciences Center
Saint Louis, Missouri

HANLEY & BELFUS, INC./ Philadelphia
MOSBY/ St. Louis • Baltimore • Berlin • Boston • Carlsbad • Chicago
London • Madrid • Naples • New York • Philadelphia • Sydney • Tokyo • Toronto

Publisher: HANLEY & BELFUS, INC.
210 S. 13th Street
Philadelphia, PA 19107
(215) 546-7293
FAX (215) 790-9330

North American and worldwide sales and distribution:

MOSBY
11830 Westline Industrial Drive
St. Louis, MO 63146

In Canada: Times Mirror Professional Publishing, Ltd.
130 Flaska Drive
Markham, Ontario L6G 1B8
Canada

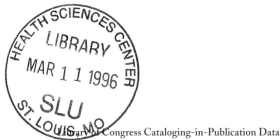

Library of Congress Cataloging-in-Publication Data

Handbook of cardiac transplantation / [edited by] Robert W. Emery, Jr.,
Leslie W. Miller.
        p.   cm.
    Includes bibliographical references and index.
    ISBN 1-56053-157-6 (pbk. : alk. paper)
    1. Heart—Transplantation.   2. Heart—Transplantation—
Complications.   I. Emery, Robert W., 1947–   .   II. Miller,
Leslie W. (Leslie William), 1946–   .
    [DNLM: 1. Heart Transplantation.   WG 169 H2356 1995]
    RD598.35.T7H36   1995
    617.4'120592—dc20
    DNLM/DLC   95-24638
    for Library of Congress   CIP

HANDBOOK OF CARDIAC TRANSPLANTATION   ISBN 1-56053-157-6

Library of Congress catalog card number 95-24638

Last digit is the print number: 9   8   7   6   5   4   3   2   1

Dedication

To the physicians and staff of the
Minneapolis Heart Institute and
Abbott Northwestern Hospital

and

Thomas E. Keller, III
Chairman, Board of Directors
Minneapolis Heart Institute Foundation
1984–1994

Contents

Contributors

Gloria A. Acuña, BSN, RN
Transplant Coordinator, Department of Cardiothoracic Surgery, University Medical Center, Tucson, Arizona

Todd J. Anderson, MD, FRCPC
Assistant Professor, Department of Medicine, University of Calgary Faculty of Medicine, Calgary, Alberta, Canada

Francisco A. Arabia, MD
Assistant Professor of Surgery, Department of Cardiothoracic Surgery, University of Arizona, Tucson, Arizona

Kit V. Arom, MD, PhD
Cardiothoracic Surgeon, Cardiac Surgical Associates, Minneapolis Heart Institute/Abbott Northwestern Hospital, Minneapolis, Minnesota

Mark L. Barr, MD
Associate Professor of Surgery, Director of Cardiothoracic Surgical Research, and Co-Director of Cardiothoracic Transplantation, Division of Cardiothoracic Surgery, University of Southern California School of Medicine, Los Angeles, California

William A. Baumgartner, MD
Professor of Surgery, Division of Cardiothoracic Surgery, Johns Hopkins University School of Medicine, Baltimore; Cardiac Surgeon-in-Charge, The Johns Hopkins Hospital, Baltimore, Maryland

Michel Carrier, MD
Assistant Professor and Chief, Department of Surgery, Montreal Heart Institute, Montreal, Quebec, Canada

Jonathan M. Chen, MD
Department of Surgery, Columbia University College of Physicians and Surgeons, New York, New York

Jack G. Copeland, MD
Michael Drummond Distinguished Professor and Chief of Cardiothoracic Surgery, Department of Surgery, University of Arizona College of Medicine, Tucson, Arizona

Maria Rosa Costanzo, MD
Professor of Medicine, Rush Medical College of Rush University, Rush-Presbyterian-St. Luke's Medical Center, Chicago, Illinois

Catherine Chang Crone, MD
Clinical Assistant Professor, Department of Psychiatry, Georgetown University, Washington, DC

Sandra Cupples, DNSc, RN, CCRN
Heart Transplant Coordinator, Washington Hospital Center, Washington, DC

Stacy F. Davis, MD
Clinical Instructor in Cardiology, Department of Medicine, Cardiovascular Division, Harvard Medical School and Brigham and Women's Hospital, Boston, Massachusetts

Thomas Donohue, MD
Assistant Professor, Department of Internal Medicine, St. Louis University School of Medicine, St. Louis, Missouri

Robert W. Emery, MD
Director, Cardiothoracic Transplantation, Cardiac Surgical Associates, Minneapolis Heart Institute/Abbott Northwestern Hospital, Minneapolis, Minnesota

Pasquale Ferraro, MD
Resident, Department of Surgery, Montreal Heart Institute, Montreal, Quebec, Canada

Kirk J. Fleischer, MD
Senior Resident, Department of Surgery, Division of Cardiac Surgery, The Johns Hopkins Hospital, Baltimore, Maryland

Peter Ganz, MD
Associate Professor, Department of Medicine, Cardiovascular Division, Harvard Medical School, Boston; Associate Director, Cardiac Catheterization Laboratory, Brigham and Women's Hospital, Boston, Massachusetts

Bartley P. Griffith, MD
The Henry T. Bahnson Professor of Surgery, Division of Cardiothoracic Surgery, University of Pittsburgh School of Medicine, Pittsburgh, Pennsylvania

Robert G. Hauser, MD
Cardiologist, Minneapolis Heart Institute, Minneapolis, Minnesota

Frances M. Hoffman, MS, RN, CCTC
Clinical Nurse Manager, Cardiothoracic Transplantation, Abbott Northwestern Hospital, Minneapolis, Minnesota

Sharon A. Hunt, MD
Professor, Department of Cardiovascular Medicine, Stanford University School of Medicine, Palo Alto, California

Linda M. Kallinen, RDCS
Director of Pacemaker/ICD Surveillance Clinic, Minneapolis Heart Institute, Minneapolis, Minnesota

Walter Kao, MD
Assistant Professor of Medicine, Rush Medical College of Rush University, Rush-Presbyterian-St. Luke's Medical Center, Chicago, Illinois

Elizabeth Z. (Lisa) Klein, MSN, RNC
Clinical Nurse Specialist, Women & Children's Outpatient Services, Fairfax Hospital, Falls Church, Virginia

Sudhakar Kosaraju, BA
Management Consultant, American Practitioners Management, New York, New York

Kathleen D. Lake, PharmD, BCPS
Program Director, Division of Cardiothoracic Transplantation and Research, Minneapolis Heart Institute Foundation and Abbott Northwestern Hospital, Minneapolis; Clinical Associate Professor, University of Minnesota College of Pharmacy, Minneapolis, Minnesota

Wendy J. Loken, PhD
Postdoctoral Fellow, Departments of Psychiatry and Psychology, Cleveland Clinic Foundation, Cleveland, Ohio

Kathryn R. Love, MD, FRCP/C)
Abbott Northwestern Hospital, Minneapolis; Assistant Professor of Clinical Medicine, University of Minnesota Medical School, Minneapolis, Minnesota

Michael S. McCarthy
Department of Cardiothoracic Surgery, University of Arizona Health Sciences Center, Tucson, Arizona

Ian T. Meredith, MBBS, PhD
Director, Cardiac Catheterisation Laboratories, and Senior Lecturer, Department of Medicine, Monash University, Clayton, Victoria, Australia

Robert E. Michler, MD
Assistant Professor, Department of Surgery, Columbia University College of Physicians and Surgeons, New York, New York; Director, Cardiac Transplant Service, Columbia-Presbyterian Medical Center, New York, New York

Leslie W. Miller, MD
Professor of Medicine and Surgery, Department of Internal Medicine, St. Louis University School of Medicine, St. Louis; Director, Heart Failure/Heart Transplant Program, St. Louis University Health Sciences Center, St. Louis, Missouri

Randall E. Morris, MD
Research Professor, Department of Cardiothoracic Surgery, Stanford University School of Medicine, Stanford, California

Gilbert H. Mudge, MD
Associate Professor of Medicine, Harvard Medical School, Boston; Director of Cardiac Transplantation and Director of Graduate Medical Education, Brigham and Women's Hospital, Boston, Massachusetts

Linda Ohler, MSN, RN, CCTC, CCRN, CNS
Heart and Lung Transplant Coordinator, Fairfax Hospital, Falls Church, Virginia

Mary Elizabeth O'Kane, BAN, RN, CCTC
Department of Cardiothoracic Transplantation, Abbott Northwestern Hospital, Minneapolis, Minnesota

D. Glenn Pennington, MD
Professor of Surgery, St. Louis University School of Medicine, St. Louis, Missouri

Peter R. Rickenbacher, MD
Senior Registrar, Department of Internal Medicine, University Hospital Basel, Basel, Switzerland

Luis J. Rosado, MD
Assistant Professor of Clinical Surgery, Section of Cardiothoracic Surgery, University of Arizona College of Medicine, Tucson, Arizona

Andrew P. Selwyn, MD
Associate Professor of Medicine, Harvard Medical School, Boston, Massachusetts

Gulshan K. Sethi, MD
Professor of Surgery, and Medical Director, Circulatory Sciences Program, University of Arizona College of Medicine, Tucson, Arizona

Lynne Warner Stevenson, MD
Associate Professor of Medicine, Harvard Medical School, Boston; Clinical Director, Cardiomyopathy and Transplant Center, Brigham and Women's Hospital, Boston, Massachusetts

Timothy V. Votapka, MD
Assistant Professor of Surgery, St. Louis University School of Medicine, St. Louis, Missouri

Elaine Winkel, MD
Assistant Professor of Medicine, Rush Medical College of Rush University, Rush-Presbyterian-St. Luke's Medical Center, Chicago, Illinois

Thomas L. Wolford, MD
Assistant Professor of Medicine, St. Louis University School of Medicine, St. Louis, Missouri

Alan C. Yeung, MD
Assistant Professor, Department of Medicine/Cardiology, Stanford University School of Medicine, Stanford, California

Foreword

Heart Transplantation
Thirty Years Later

Jack G. Copeland, M.D.

In my first year as a medical student, more by chance than by plan, I began working in a heart transplant laboratory in the basement of the Palo Alto Veteran's Administration Hospital. I spent the next 5 years (1964–1969) working in that laboratory under the supervision of a series of brilliant and talented surgeons. Richard Lower, a great surgical technician and a kind and generous man, was my first boss. I met him at 5:30 A.M. each morning to help get the heart transplant operation started. It was a costly and gruesome procedure requiring one liter of fresh blood to prime the disc oxygenator, one donor, and one recipient, necessitating a total of about 7 dogs. In those days, we were concentrating on preserving hearts by refrigeration. We used norepinephrine and pacing at 110–120 to support the animal through the immediate postoperative phase. Then we treated with steroids and azathioprine using a QRS voltage drop as an indication of rejection to be treated with bolus methylprednisolone therapy. Obtaining good or average long-term survival was a rare event. So in 1964–1965, thinking of the next 30 years of developments in cardiac transplantation was a luxury, for those with time to speculate, and a low priority compared with the huge problems we were facing each day. We had little vision of 1995 and the progress that has occurred.

Selection of potential recipients was, at best, an ill-defined art in 1967 when human heart transplants began. Naturally, the sickest patients with the least hope of survival were transplanted and, although technically successful, most died within hours or days because of our lack of understanding of the immune system.

From 1970 until the early 1980s, the belief that the procedure would greatly benefit some patients who were otherwise doomed was the primary driving force which led a few programs in the world to persevere while many imposed a moratorium on heart transplants. Even before cyclosporine became available, survival rates had risen to 65% at 1 year, thanks to improved selection criteria, the cardiac biopsy, and the addition of rabbit antithymocyte globulin to steroids and azathioprine as the method of immunosuppression.

The period between 1981 and 1985 was one of transition, when the use of cyclosporine together with previously used immunosuppressives was learned empirically. This has been followed by a period of "modern" immunosuppression, and survival rates have improved to the point that, if they become any better, we might be accused of being too selective.

As more physicians, surgeons, nurses, and ancillary colleagues have become captivated by transplantation, from the mid-80s to the present time, thousands of new ideas have had an impact on the many facets of the procedure as it relates to strictly medical, as well as many social, psychological, financial, political, and ethical questions. The focus of heart transplantation, which for many years was fixed upon survival, is now directed more toward improvement of quality and quantity of life within our socioeconomic limits. The number of available donors has stabilized enough for us to realize that the impact of heart transplantation on end-stage heart disease will be limited. Spinoff areas, such as bridge to transplantation, which has nurtured a family of implantable blood pumps and xenotransplantation, are receiving attention out of the necessity of finding another long-term solution. Medical therapy has improved the lot of the majority with end-stage heart disease who will not receive transplants. Thus, ACE inhibitors and hydralazine-nitrate therapies combined with digoxin, diuretics, along with new drugs and new uses of old drugs remain the main hope for the majority. We hope that cardiomyoplasty or some other use of stimulated reconditioned skeletal muscle will also help.

This book marks a point in time, summarizing most of what we know of thoracic organ transplantation in 1995. It contains the thoughts of some of our best practitioners and scientists, and is an excellent resource for references. As a participant in the conference from which this text derives, I learned a great deal and was impressed with the depth and breadth of cardiac transplantation 30 years later.

Medical Management Before Cardiac Transplantation

Chapter 1

Lynne Warner Stevenson, MD

REFERRAL FOR TRANSPLANTATION

Most patients referred for cardiac transplantation have persistent symptoms of heart failure. Some patients, however, may be referred primarily because of low left ventricular ejection fractions, malignant ventricular arrhythmias in the setting of reduced ejection fraction, intractable angina, or critical coronary artery anatomy. Functional limitations and risks for potential candidates must be compared with their anticipated restrictions and risks as transplant recipients. These are reflected in the guidelines resulting from the Bethesda Conference on cardiac transplantation (Table 1).[1]

Although left ventricular ejection fraction correlates with the prognosis over a broad population, it does not predict outcome well for any given patient and even when very low may not be considered an adequate indication for transplantation. Many patients with low ejection fractions can enjoy life with minimal symptoms on adequate medical therapy.[2] Symptomatic ventricular arrhythmias should be addressed when possible with amiodarone or potentially with radiofrequency ablation when they are sufficiently frequent to impair patient function and quality of life.[3] Patients at high risk for recurrence of life-threatening arrhythmias may have improved prognosis with an implantable defibrillator, which would not be indicated if refractory hemodynamic compromise threatens to confine the patient within hospital until transplantation. Intractable angina and critical coronary artery anatomy should stimulate a search for major areas of viable myocardium amenable to angioplasty or to revascularization.[4] If this is not possible, transplantation is occasionally performed for relief of intractable chest pain shown to result from ischemia, even in the absence of symptomatic heart failure. As with low ejection fraction and arrhythmia risk, cardiac

1

TABLE I. Selection Criteria for Benefits from Transplantation

Accepted indications for transplantation
  Peak VO_2 < 10 ml/kg/min with achievement of anaerobic metabolism
  Severe ischemia consistently limiting routine activity not amenable to bypass surgery or angioplasty
  Recurrent symptomatic ventricular arrhythmias refractory to all accepted therapeutic modalities
Probable indications for cardiac transplantation
  Peak VO_2 < 14 mg/kg/min and major limitation of the patient's daily activities
  Recurrent unstable ischemia not amenable to bypass or angioplasty
  Instability of fluid balance/renal function not resulting from patient noncompliance with regimen of
    weight monitoring, flexible use of diuretic drugs, and salt restriction
Inadequate indications for transplantation
  Ejection fraction < 20%
  History functional class III or IV symptoms of heart failure
  Previous ventricular arrhythmias
  Maximal VO_2 > 15 m/kg/min without other indications

(Adapted from Hunt SA: Twenty-fourth Bethesda Conference: Cardiac transplantation. J Am Coll Cardiol 22:1–64, 1993.)

transplantation is very rarely considered solely to alleviate a perceived risk or death in a patient with preserved functional capacity.

The vast majority of the remaining 90% of patients are referred with severe symptoms of heart failure. The typical patient is already taking digoxin, diuretics, and an angiotensin-converting enzyme inhibitor, or has been considered "intolerant" of converting enzyme inhibition. Often, repeated hospitalizations for intravenous diuretics and inotropic infusions have been necessary, following which the patient improves briefly only to deteriorate soon after discharge on the previous outpatient regimen. Patients should not, however, be considered "refractory" without further evaluation and intervention.[5] The approach to these patients includes consideration of all potentially reversible factors contributing to decompensation (Table 2); tailoring of therapy under hemodynamic guidance when indicated, as in Table 3; assiduous follow-up with assessment of stability; and reevaluation at 3 to 6 month intervals.

WHEN IS HEART FAILURE REFRACTORY?

The discouraging term "heart failure" has been applied to describe points in the clinical spectrum from cardiogenic shock to the "asymptomatic" population of the Study of Left Ventricular Dysfunction.[6] Both physician and patient need to consider the limitations as potentially reversible even without major improvement in ejection fraction (Table 2). Routine viral illnesses may reversibly depress clinical function in patients with previously stable heart failure, in whom extra vigilance and encouragement may be necessary for the next few months. Atrial fibrillation, in which rate control during activity is rarely achieved, can depress myocardial function further, and can often

TABLE 2. Potentially Reversible Factors in Heart Failure Contributing to Decompensation

Perception and communication of "heart failure"	Poor education about or compliance with:
Recurrent ischemia	Sodium restriction Fluid restriction
Systemic viral infection	Daily weight charts
Tachyarrhythmias, particularly atrial fibrillation	Flexible diuretic regimen Prescribed medications
Heavy alcohol intake	Therapy with negatively inotropic drugs
Endocrine abnormalities	Therapy with prostaglandin inhibitors

TABLE 3.   Indications for Tailored Therapy with Hemodynamic Guidance

Evidence of Impaired Perfusion	Congestion in the Presence of Any of the Following	Persistent Congestion Despite All of the Following
Narrow pulse pressure $\left[\dfrac{(SBP - DBP)}{SBP} = < 25\%\right]$	Angina	Salt and fluid restriction
	Symptomatic ventricular arrhythmias	Multiple adjustments of loop diuretics
Mental obtundation	Baseline renal insufficiency	Addition of metolazone
Worsening renal function in the presence of congestion		

be treated with amiodarone for cardioversion or at least good rate control. Alcohol intake can depress myocardial function regardless of the initial cause of heart failure, and should be prohibited.

The most common cause of recurrent decompensation is failure to recognize fluid overload. Patients with low ejection fractions accompanied by orthopnea or elevated jugular venous distention can be assumed to have excess circulating fluid volume.[7] The majority of patients with chronically elevated filling pressures will have no rales on chest examination despite severe interstitial fluid accumulation, which causes dyspnea. Rehospitalizations frequently occur in patients for whom intravenous therapy has eased symptoms but in whom volume status is only reduced to just below the threshold for pulmonary edema.

Patients with known low ejection fraction should be classified at each examination according to the separate components of congestion and hypoperfusion (Fig. 1). Congestion in a patient on digoxin, diuretics, and an angiotensin-converting enzyme inhibitor without evidence of hypoperfusion, angina, or renal insufficiency may respond well to empiric increases in oral diuretics, perhaps with the intermittent addition of metolazone. Concurrent evidence of congestion and hypoperfusion, however, or refractory congestion despite aggressive outpatient management are indications that empiric adjustment of loading conditions will not be effective and may be dangerous (Table 3). Low serum sodium or an extensive volume reservoir indicated by massive ascites or anasarca are additional clues that empiric therapy will not be adequate. Such patients' conditions are sufficiently tenuous that optimization is usually possible only with simultaneous adjustment of volume status and vasodilation with hemodynamic monitoring.

Therapy for heart failure has historically been restricted by the assumption that normal stroke volumes and filling pressures were neither possible nor desirable. Stroke volume is determined by the product of left ventricular ejection and left ventricular volume, which is often increased three- to fourfold, minus stroke volume lost backward to mitral regurgitation. Ventricular dilation and elevated filling pressures lead to mitral and tricuspid regurgitation, which are pivotal processes in decompensation. It is rare, in fact, to find severe decompensation in their absence. Markedly elevated filling pressures were once assumed to be necessary to maintain cardiac output in heart failure, but have now been recognized to be not only unnecessary but deleterious.[8] Restoration of near-normal filling pressures not only eliminates congestive symptoms, but also reduces

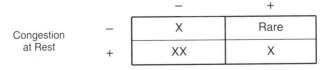

FIGURE 1.   Profiles of symptomatic heart failure.

TABLE 4.   Tailored Therapy for Advanced Heart Failure

Measurement of baseline hemodynamics	Monitored ambulation and diuretic adjustment for 24 to 48 hours
Intravenous nitroprusside and diuretics tailored to hemodynamic goals	Maintenance of digoxin levels 1.0 to 2.0 ng/dl, if no contraindications
Pulmonary capillary wedge pressure ≤ 15 mmHg	
Systemic vascular resistance ≤ 1200 dynes/s/cm^{-5}	Detailed patient education, including sodium/fluid restriction
Right atrial pressure ≤ 7 mmHg	
Systolic blood pressure ≥ 80 mmHg	
Definition of optimal hemodynamics within 24 to 48 hours	Flexible outpatient diuretic regimen, including intermittent metolazone
Titration of high-dose oral vasodilators	Progressive walking or other exercise program
Captopril and isosorbide dinitrate	
Addition of hydralazine, if needed	Vigilant follow-up

valvular regurgitation and allows maximal forward output in the majority of patients with massively dilated hearts.

Hemodynamic goals defined for this population can frequently be achieved by the tailoring of drugs during hemodynamic monitoring (Table 4). Either intravenous nitroprusside, nitroglycerin, or both, are combined with intravenous diuretics to achieve rapid optimization of both volume and systemic vascular resistance.[5] If the initial blood pressure is higher than 80 mmHg, most patients respond well to the initiation of these intravenous vasodilator regimens. Addition of dobutamine may improve hemodynamics quickly but adds an additional step in the process of redesign of the oral regimen, which will not contain any agent equivalent to dobutamine. The results of the intravenous nitrovasodilators, on the other hand, can generally be matched with some combination of oral agents. Dobutamine at 3 to 5 µg/kg/min may occasionally be useful when initial blood pressures are very low or when anasarca necessitates several days of facilitated diuresis before placement of a pulmonary artery catheter.

Of the angiotensin-converting enzyme inhibitors, captopril is easiest to titrate in this setting, but may for some patients be changed to longer-acting agents after stability has been demonstrated for several weeks. Nitrates, once considered to be a passive partner in vasodilator regimens, may have many beneficial effects which render them

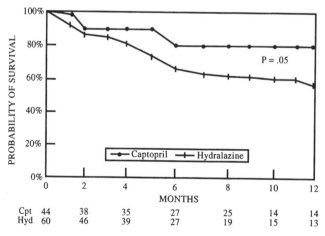

FIGURE 2.   Kaplan-Meier survival curves for the 104 patients discharged on the oral vasodilator regimen of captopril (Cpt) (n = 44) or hydralazine (Hyd) (n = 60) plus isosorbide dinitrate.

Table 5. Hemodynamic Response in 225 Potential Candidates (Left Ventricular Ejection Fraction 17 ± 5%)

	At Referral	On Tailored Therapy
On vasodilators (%)	75	98
Right atrial pressure (mm)	13 ± 7	7 ± 4
Pulmonary artery systolic pressure (mmHg)	53 ± 16	42 ± 12
Pulmonary capillary wedge pressure (mmHg)	16 ± 10	15 ± 7
Cardiac index (L/min/m²)	2.0 ± 0.5	2.7 ± 1.3
Systemic vascular resistance (dynes/s/cm⁵)	1600 ± 500	1150 ± 300
Mean arterial pressure (mmHg)	81 ± 18	72 ± 18
Heart rate (bpm)	92 ± 17	92 ± 13
Serum sodium (mEq/L)	135 ± 6	135 ± 5
Serum creatinine	1.2 ± 0.3	1.3 ± 0.4

central components. For Class III and IV patients, enalapril was not superior to the hydralazine-nitrate combination in the Veterans' Administration Cooperative Trial[9] but the captopril-nitrate combination reduced mortality by 60% compared with the hydralazine-nitrate combination in the Hy-C trial[10] of therapy tailored specifically to hemodynamic goals (Fig. 2). The regimen of tailored therapy was subsequently revised to favor the captopril-nitrate combination, with addition of hydralazine only when necessary because of failure to match the hemodynamic goals.

Early hemodynamic results of tailored therapy in this population are shown in Table 5. This approach to redesign of oral regimen allowed hospital discharge of almost 90% of patients previously considered to require continuous dobutamine infusions. By 4 to 6 weeks after discharge, approximately two-thirds of patients presenting with severe symptoms could meet criteria for stability (Table 6). Stability requires patient understanding and cooperation with not only sodium but also fluid restriction, which is generally 2000 ml/day.

Numerous trials of newer drugs for heart failure exist, which unfortunately do not represent the average transplant candidate (Table 7). There have been no major trials addressing the use of beta blocking agents in patients with heart failure sufficient to warrant consideration for transplantation, although the Metroprolol in Dilated Cardiomyopathy Trial suggested less progression to that level of disease.[11] Preliminary results from the GESICA trial of amiodarone in a population with high mortality rates suggested a benefit in reduction of heart failure hospitalization and mortality.[12] At least part of the benefit of these agents may result from the lower heart rate in the ventricle with impaired ability to release and sequester calcium. The status of current outpatient therapies for potential transplant candidates is shown in Table 8. The overall spectrum of escalating therapies for heart failure from asymptomatic to critical is shown in Figure 3.

TABLE 6. Criteria for Early Stability

Stable blood pressure (SBP ≥ 80 mmHg)	No serious drug side effects
Stable weight on oral diuretic agents	Clinical status unchanged or better than at discharge
Stable creatinine/BUN (BUN ≤ 60 mg/dl)	
Stable serum sodium (usually ≥ 130 mEq/L)	No congestive symptoms at rest
No angina	Can walk for at least half length of a city block

BUN = blood urea nitrogen; SBP = systolic blood pressure.

TABLE 7.   Class IV Heart Failure in Recent Trials

	% Class IV Patients
VHEFT II (enalapril vs. hydralazine/isosorbide)	< 1%
SOLVD Rx (enalapril)	1.7%
Hy-C (captopril/isosorbide vs. hydralazine/isosorbide)	75%
Metoprolol in dilated cardiomyopathy	< 5%
RADIANCE (digoxin)	0%
FACET (flosequinan)	3%
PROMISE (Milrinone)	42%
Enoximone	0%
Vesnarinone	11%

TABLE 8.   Outpatient Therapies for Advanced Heart Failure

Routine Use	Selected Use	Detrimental	Under Clinical Investigation
Angiotensin-converting enzyme inhibitors	Hydralazine	Amrinone, milrinone	Vesnarinone
	Beta blockers	Flosequinan	Carvedilol
Digoxin	Amiodarone	Home prostacyclin infusion	Home dobutamine infusion
Diuretics	Anticoagulation agent		Pimobendan
Nitrates	Magnesium	Diltiazem, nifedipine	Amlodipine
Potassium replacement	Automatic implantable defibrillator	Type I antiarrhythmic agents	Ibopamine
Exercise	Ultrafiltration	Nonsteroidal antiinfammatory agents	Angiotensin II receptor antagonists
	Nocturnal oxygen		Coenzyme Q_{10}
			Levocarnitine

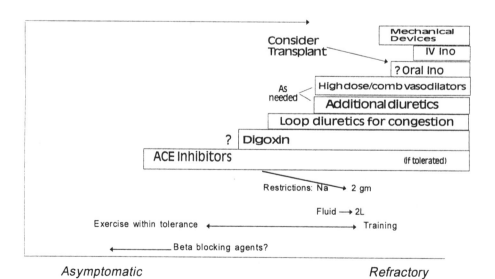

FIGURE 3.   Escalating therapies for heart failure.

TABLE 9. Documented Risk Factors for Potential Transplantation Candidates

Risk of Overall Mortality	Greater Risk of Sudden Death	Greater Risk of Heart Failure Death
Ejection fraction < 20%		
Massive left ventricular dilation	*	larger *
Severe valvular regurgitation		*
Low serum sodium		*
Serum catecholamines		
High pulmonary wedge pressure despite optimal therapy	*	larger *
Low peak exercise oxygen consumption		
Complex ventricular ectopy	Controversial	
History of "secondary" arrest	*	
History of syncope	*	
Atrial fibrillation		
No vasodilator therapy		*
Vasodilator therapy without angiotensin-converting enzyme inhibitors	*	
Type I anti-arrhythmic therapy	*	

* Risk factors that have been associated with a particular mode of death.

REEVALUATION OF POTENTIAL CANDIDATES

Most patients' conditions are deteriorating when referred. Numerous risk factors for sudden death and hemodynamic deterioration have been identified from the profile at initial referral (Table 9). These risk factors may be useful for insight into physiology and for large populations. The dependence of these parameters on therapy, however, limits their usefulness during changing clinical states. In addition to the institution of optimal therapy, resolution of other unrecognized conditions may allow a return of stability. As the waiting list and waiting times lengthen for outpatients (Fig. 4), patients at highest

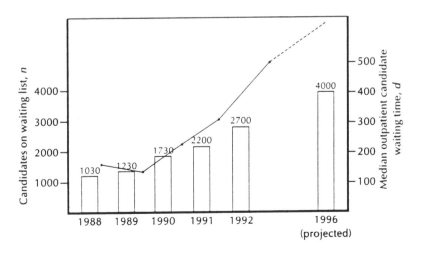

FIGURE 4.   Waiting list length and time. (From Stevenson LW: Selection of candidates for cardiac transplantation. Curr Opin Cardiol 9:315–325, 1994, with permission.)

Outcome After Listing with pkVO$_2$ < 14

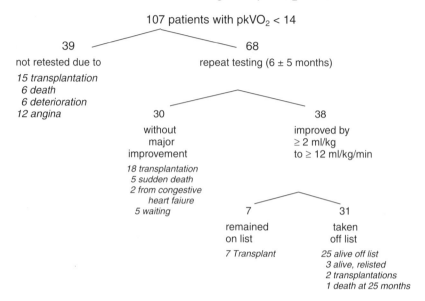

FIGURE 5.   Outcome after listing with pkVO$_2$ < 14.

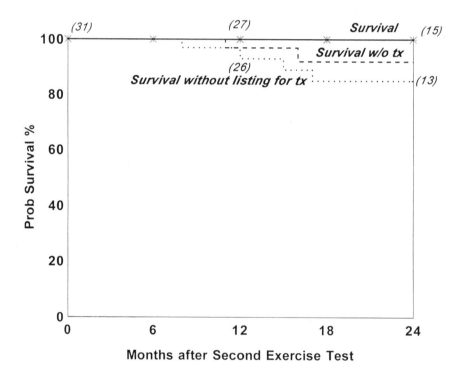

FIGURE 6.

risk may die, whereas others may demonstrate clinical improvement. Reevaluation is essential to identify the patients who continue to meet indications for transplantation.

As discussed, stability on therapy can be defined by simple criteria. Persistently unstable patients should be carefully evaluated for noncompliance with medications and restrictions. Compliant patients who remain unstable should be considered for cardiac transplantation both for quality of life and survival (Table 1).

Patients who demonstrate apparent stability vary greatly in functional capacity. Both activity and prognosis correlate with peak oxygen consumption during exercise. Oxygen consumption and prognosis can improve after initial evaluation.[14] Of 107 ambulatory transplant candidates with peak oxygen consumption lower than 14 mL/kg/min during initial evaluation, 30% improved their clinical status and peak exercise capacity and were removed from the active list, with good 2-year survival rates (Figs. 5 and 6).

As medical management for heart failure at all stages continues to evolve, indications for cardiac transplantation will also undergo revision. Better understanding of different levels of heart failure will allow more focus on appropriate therapy for the individual. Newer drugs and wearable ventricular support devices may change the relative risks and benefits of transplantation in relation to other options. We must maintain vigilance in the consideration of each patient referred to transplantation in order to provide the best current therapy available for both quality and length of life.

REFERENCES

1. Hunt SA (Chairman): Twenty-fourth Bethesda Conference: Cardiac transplantation [review]. J Am Col Cardiol 22:1–64, 1993.
2. Stevenson LW, Sietsema K, Tillisch JH, et al: Exercise capacity for survivors of cardiac transplantation or sustained medical therapy for stable heart failure. Circulation 80:78–85, 1990.
3. Stevenson WG, Stevenson LW, Middlekauff HR, Saxon LA: Sudden death prevention in patients with advanced ventricular dysfunction [review]. Circulation 88:2953–2961, 1993.
4. Louie HW, Laks H, Milgalter E, et al: Ischemic cardiomyopathy: Criteria for coronary revascularization and cardiac transplantation. Circulation (Suppl III):290–295, 1991.
5. Stevenson LW: Tailored therapy before transplantation for treatment of advanced heart failure: Effective use of vasodilators and diuretics. J Heart Lung Transplant 10:468–476, 1991.
6. The SOLVD Investigators: Effect of enalapril on mortality and the development of heart failure in asymptomatic patients with reduced left ventricular ejection fractions. N Engl J Med 327:65–691, 1992.
7. Stevenson LW, Perloff JK: The limited reliability of physical signs for the estimation of hemodynamics in chronic heart failure. JAMA 261:884–888, 1989.
8. Stevenson Lw, Tillisch JH: Maintenance of cardiac output with normal filling pressures in dilated heart failure. Circulation 74:1303–1308, 1986.
9. Cohn JN, Johnson G, Ziesche S, et al: A comparison of enalapril with hydralazine-isosorbide dinitrate in the treatment of chronic congestive heart failure (V-HEFT II). N Engl J Med 325:303–310, 1991.
10. Fonarow GC, Chelimsky-Fallick C, Stevenson LW, et al: Effect of direct vasodilation vs angiotensin-converting enzyme inhibition on mortality in advanced heart failure. The Hy-C trial. J Am Coll Cardiol 19:842_850, 1992.
11. Waagstein F, Bristow MR, Swedberg K, et al: Beneficial effects of metoprolol in idiopathic dilated cardiomyopathy. Lancet 342:1441–1446, 1993.
12. Nul DR, Duval H, et al: Amiodarone reduces mortality in severe heart failure [abstract]. Circulation 88I:603, 1993.
13. Mancini DM, Eisen H, Kussmaul W, et al: Value of peak exercise oxygen consumption for optimal timing of cardiac transplantation in ambulatory patients with heart failure. Circulation 83:778–786, 1991.
14. Stevenson LW, Steimle AE, Fonarow G, et al: Improvement in exercise capacity of candidates awaiting heart transplantation. J Am Coll Cardiol (in press).

Chapter 2

Implantable Cardioverter Defibrillator as a Bridge to Transplantation

Robert G. Hauser, M.D.
Linda M. Kallinen, RDCS

Patients awaiting cardiac transplantation commonly die suddenly as a result of ventricular tachyarrhythmias. Indeed, an annual risk for sudden cardiac death (SCD) was reported to be 20% for patients with underlying ischemic cardiomyopathy who were listed for transplantation at centers around the United States.[1] Other studies have reported the incidence of sudden death among those with advanced heart failure to range from 10 to 50%.[2–4] Predictors of SCD in this population include previous cardiac arrest, history of sustained or nonsustained ventricular tachycardia, recurrent syncope, and an ejection fraction lower than 20%. For patients who have experienced SCD or symptomatic ventricular tachycardia (VT) or ventricular fibrillation (VF), antiarrhythmic drugs or the implantable cardioverter defibrillator (ICD) have been prescribed with favorable results.

However, no randomized controlled clinical trial has compared drug and device therapy or the safety or efficacy of any prophylactic intervention which may prevent SCD in these high-risk patients. Nevertheless, the ICD has been proposed and used as a bridge to transplantation. Until recently, such an approach had serious limitations because implantation of ICDs required thoracotomy. Advances in defibrillation leads and pulse generator technology have, however, allowed physicians to implant these devices transvenously with virtually no mortality. Thus it is timely to review the ICD as a potential bridge therapy and to describe the experience with these devices in patients awaiting transplantation at the Minneapolis Heart Institute.

LEADS AND PULSE GENERATORS

The original ICD required placement of patch defibrillation electrodes on the pericardium or epimyocardium through mid-sternotomy, thoracotomy, or subxiphoid approach. Surgical mortality associated with patch electrode placement ranged from 1.2 to 5%, and morbidity rates were comparable with other open chest procedures. Patch placement is no longer required because transvenous systems are now available.

We have used two transvenous defibrillation lead models, one employing a single (Endotak, Cardiac Pacemakers, Inc., Minneapolis, MN) and the other a multiple lead system (Transvene, Medtronic, Minneapolis, MN). Either transvenous lead model may be combined with a subcutaneous patch electrode to provide an adequate defibrillation threshold (DFT), defined as 10 joules below the maximum shock energy available from the implanted pulse generator.

The leads are inserted through the subclavian vein using standard guidewire and introducer technique. The distal shocking electrode is positioned in the right ventricular apex and the proximal electrode is located in the high right atrium or superior vena cava–innominate vein. The multiple lead system offers an optional coronary sinus lead-electrode which may be used as a third shocking electrode. Pacing and sensing occurs by one or two distal electrodes in contact with the right ventricular endocardium. The leads are tunneled to a subcutaneous pectoral or abdominal pocket where they are connected to the pulse generator.

Perioperative care includes prophylactic antibiotics and ECG monitoring for 24 hours. Most patients can be discharged within 48 hours. Selected patients undergo pre-discharge electrophysiologic evaluation, including initiation and termination of VF by the ICD.

Using this approach, we have attempted transvenous ICD implantation in 120 consecutive nontransplant patients. Satisfactory DFTs were achieved in 112 (93%). Seven patients required thoracotomy for patch placement and one did not receive an ICD because of a high external defibrillation threshold which precluded DFT testing.

Results are summarized in Table 1. There were no deaths within 30 days and no hospital deaths. The most common complication was infection, which developed 19 to 270 days after implantation in six patients (5%). All devices were removed, and four of these patients did not receive reimplantation. Lead complications were rare, with two dislodgements and no mechanical failures. The routine postimplant threshold testing required by various FDA investigative protocols uncovered only one case of high DFT necessitating lead revision.

Long-term results are summarized in Table 2. Two patients died suddenly, most likely as a result of incessant arrhythmia. Over 45% of the patients received shocks and/or antitachycardia pacing, which have been judged to be appropriate based on clinical symptoms or data or ECG documentation stored in the device. The ECG shown in Figure 1 was retrieved from the device of a patient who reported no symptoms. In

TABLE 1.   Surgical Results of ICD Implantation (n = 120)

Mortality (30 day)	0	—
Pneumothorax	1	0.8%
Lead displacement	2	1.6%
Subcutaneous patch erosion	2	1.6%
Pulse generator migration	1	0.8%
Infection	6	5.0%
Loose set screws	4	3.3%

TABLE 2.   Long-term Results of ICD Implantation (n = 120)

Late deaths	7	5.8%
Arrhythmic	2	1.7%
Cardiac	2	1.7%
Noncardiac	3	2.5%
Shock therapy	49	41%
Antitachycardia pacing	19	16%
Antiarrhythmic drug therapy	31	26%
Explant	4	33%
Device failure	0	—

this case ventricular tachycardia was detected quickly and terminated by a single shock before the patient became syncopal.

Major advances in pulse generator technology include the biphasic shock wave form associated with lower DFTs and higher transvenous success rates. Smaller pulse generators are now freely available in Europe but are restricted by the FDA to clinical trial sites in the United States. These pulse generators can be implanted pectorally in most patients.

PATIENTS AWAITING CARDIAC TRANSPLANTATION

We reviewed the records of 296 patients listed for transplantation at our center between January 1986 and January 1993. Twenty-six patients had implantable cardioverter defibrillators which were implanted because of a history of VT or VF. Sixteen

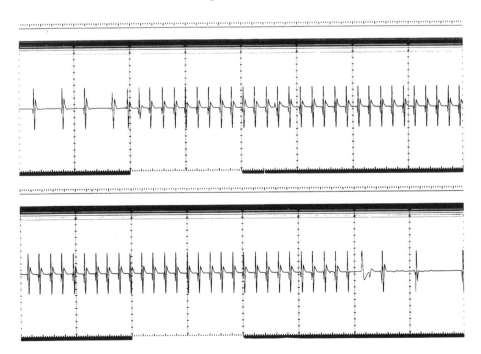

FIGURE I.   Stored electrogram showing ventricular tachycardia terminated with a single ICD shock.

received their ICD before being listed for transplantation, whereas the remaining 10 patients received it after.

These 26 patients with an ICD were predominantly male (88%) and had a mean age of 54, ranging from 38 to 65 years. Seventeen patients (65%) had underlying coronary artery disease with an ischemic cardiomyopathy, whereas the remaining nine had a dilated nonischemic cardiomyopathy. The mean ejection fraction was 21% with a range from 10 to 35%. The presenting arrhythmia was VT in 16 patients and VF in 10. At electrophysiologic testing, VT was induced in 24 of the 26 patients. In two patients, no sustained arrhythmia could be induced. Antiarrhythmic medications wee used concomitantly in 15 patients (58%).

Implantation of the ICD was performed through a thoracotomy using an epicardial lead system in 20 patients, whereas six patients received a transvenous lead system. Tiered therapy (combined defibrillation and pacing) devices were used in nine patients and a standard automatic implantable cardioverter defibrillator (AICD) was used in the remaining 17 patients. Two patients underwent concomitant coronary artery bypass graft surgery. The 30-day mortality rate in these 26 patients was zero.

These 26 ICD patients have been followed for a mean of 24 months over a range of 2 to 60 months. Twenty-five of the 26 patients (96%) have received appropriate therapy from their ICD based on symptoms of syncope or pre-syncope or on ECG documentation or diagnostic data stored within the ICD. In two patients, in addition to receiving appropriate therapy, atrial fibrillation was documented to result in a shock. Only one patient at 14 months postimplantation with inducible ventricular tachycardia and on no antiarrhythmic medications has received no therapy from his device. One patient awaiting transplant required removal of his ICD 5 months post-implant secondary to an infection. He did not have reimplantation of an ICD.

Nine patients have successfully received transplantations with a mean time from ICD implantation to transplantation of 27 months across a range of 10 to 49 months. No operative deaths were related to the transplantation and all patients were discharged from the hospital.

Three patients died despite the presence of an ICD. All three used their devices appropriately to terminate ventricular tachyarrhythmias before death. Only one of these patients was on a concomitant antiarrhythmic medication. Death in all three patients was due to an incessant ventricular tachyarrhythmia with documented appropriate ICD function. Two months after implantation, one patient suffered an unwitnessed sudden death but the diagnostic data within his PRX ICD showed that the ICD detected the occurrence of tachyarrhythmia and appropriately delivered five shocks, although the tachycardia continued. The second patient expired 10 months after implantation while on telemetry in the hospital with appropriate device function as well as complete resuscitation efforts which were not successful. The third patient expired 45 months post implant after being called for transplantation. This death was observed and ICD therapy was given immediately. Further resuscitation efforts in the emergency department failed.

DISCUSSION

These data suggest that the ICD is effective in reducing the incidence of sudden arrhythmic death in patients awaiting cardiac transplantation. The high incidence of appropriate termination of ventricular arrhythmias by the ICD combined with the low incidence of ICD-related complications and a zero surgical mortality rate was also reported by Bolling[5] and Jeevanandam.[6]

Despite the use of a thoracotomy for implantation in the majority of these high-risk patients, surgical complications related to the procedure were minimal. The availability of transvenous leads and the success with implantation using this approach makes this a more acceptable procedure. In addition, use of a transvenous lead system further eases the difficulties encountered in obtaining access to the heart at the time of transplantation in patients with ICD patches.[7]

The incidence of appropriate ICD therapy in this group of patients was significantly higher at 96% (25/26) than our experience with our general ICD patient population, in whom only 45% (99/220) have received appropriate therapy (p < 0.001). This high incidence of ICD therapy has been reported to occur in patients with severely depressed left ventricular function and awaiting transplantation.[8,9]

Despite use of ICDs, these patients have a significant risk for sudden arrhythmic death. In our 26 patients awaiting cardiac transplantation, three of 26 (12%) died as a result of incessant ventricular tachyarrhythmias. This incidence is high compared with our overall experience with ICDs, in which only 7 of 220 patients (3%) experienced sudden cardiac death, and compared with results published indicating a sudden cardiac death survival rate of greater than 95% at one year.[10–13]

Patients with advanced heart failure awaiting transplantation are at significant risk for sudden arrhythmic events and death. We evaluated the cause of death in 71 patients awaiting cardiac transplantation at our center and found that 46% of the deaths were sudden. If one suggests that each appropriate ICD therapy could have prevented a sudden arrhythmic death, incidence of arrhythmic death in our patients had a significant impact from the ICD.

When we consider decreased sudden cardiac death in patients treated with ICDs, the higher incidence of appropriate ICD therapy, and the more significant risk for sudden death in patients awaiting cardiac transplantation, it must be asked whether prophylactic insertion of ICDs in these patients would be of benefit. Randomized clinical trials are needed to further explore this question. Several trials have been proposed and are underway evaluating the prophylactic use of ICDs in various subsets of patients known to be at risk.[14] The significant cost related to the use of ICD technology must be weighed against proposed benefit of prophylactic utilization of this therapy.

CONCLUSIONS

The ICD has ben shown to be an effective therapy as a bridge to transplant for patients with a history of malignant ventricular arrhythmias. Patients awaiting cardiac transplantation will have an increased incidence of appropriate ICD therapy and sudden cardiac death compared with the general ICD population. A randomized clinical trial should be conducted before prophylactic ICD use can become standard practice.

REFERENCES

1. DEFIBRILAT Study Group: Actuarial risk of sudden death while awaiting cardiac transplantation in patients with atherosclerotic heart disease. Am J Cardiol 68:545–546, 1991.
2. Stevenson L, Miller L: Cardiac transplantation as therapy for heart failure. In O'Rourke R (ed): Current Problems in Cardiology. St. Louis, Mosby-Year Book, 1991.
3. Luu M, Stevenson W, Stevenson L, et al: Diverse mechanisms of unexpected cardiac arrest in advanced heart failure. Circulation 80:1675–1680, 1986.
4. Stevenson L, Fowler M, Schroeder J, et al: Poor survival of patients with idiopathic cardiomyopathy considered too well for transplantation. Am J Med 83:871–876, 1987.
5. Bolling S, Deeb GM, Morady F, et al: Automatic internal cardioverter defibrillator: A bridge to heart transplantation. J Heart Lung Transplant 10:562–566, 1991.
6. Jeevanandam V, Bielefeld M, Auteri J, et al: The implantable defibrillator: An electronic bridge to cardiac transplantation. Circulation 86(suppl):II276–II279, 1992.
7. Emery R, Almquist A, Von Rueden T, et al: Implantation of the implantable cardioverter defibrillator in the heart transplant candidate. J Heart Lung Transplant 12:1067–1070, 1993.

8. Vester E, Kuhls S, Winter J, Strauer B: Does therapy with implantable cardioverter/defibrillators really improve the prognosis of patients with highgrade left ventricular dysfunction? (abstract). J Heart Failure 1(suppl):675, 1993.
9. Blakeman B, Calandra D, Sullivan H, et al: Implantable cardioverter/defibrillator as an interval device in the heart transplant patient (abstract). ACCP 765, 1992.
10. Hauser R, Kurschinski D, McVeigh K, et al: Clinical results with nonthoracotomy ICD systems. Pacing Clin Electrophysiol 16:141–148, 1993.
11. Winkle R, Mead R, Ruder M, et al: Long term outcome with the automatic implantable cardioverter defibrillator. j Am Coll Cardiol 13:1353–1361, 1989.
12. Akhtar M, Jazayeri M, Sra J, et al: Implantable cardioverter defibrillator for prevention of sudden cardiac death in patients with ventricular tachycardia and ventricular fibrillation: ICD therapy in sudden cardiac death. Pacing Clin Electrophysiol 16:511–518, 1993.
13. Nisam S, Mower M, Thomas A, Hauser R: Patient survival comparison in three generations of automatic implantable cardioverter defibrillators: Review of 12 years, 25,000 patients. Pacing Clin Electrophysiol 16:174–178, 1993.
14. Nisam S, Thomas A, Mower M, Hauser R: Identifying patients for prophylactic automatic implantable cardioverter defibrillator therapy: Status of prospective studies. Am Heart J 122:607–612, 1991.

Prevention and Prophylaxis of Infection in Thoracic Transplantation

Chapter 3

Kathryn Love, MD, FRCP(C)

Infection, rejection, and malignancy are the most common causes of death in modern thoracic transplant recipients. Many infections are eminently preventable.[1-4] Table 1 provides an overview of organisms with a high propensity for causing infection and disease in thoracic transplant recipients.

Infectious diseases in transplant recipients are acquired exogenously:

1. through nosocomial transmission during periods of maximal immunosuppression, as seen during rejection therapy and viremia with immunomodulating viruses such as cytomegalovirus (CMV), Epstein-Barr virus (EBV), hepatitis viruses (B and C) and human immune deficiency virus (HIV);
2. from the donor organ which may harbor latent organisms whose reactivation causes primary infection in the previously uninfected recipient;[3]
3. in the community;

and endogenously, from reactivation of latent infection in the recipient (i.e., CMV).

Prophylaxis against infection should be comprehensive in the early posttransplant period when immunosuppression is most intense and episodes of rejection are more frequent. The relative benefit of continuing some prophylaxis indefinitely is as yet unstudied, although it is suggested by the late occurrence of some preventable infections such as *Pneumocystis carinii* pneumonia (PCP), toxoplasmosis, and nocardiosis.

A key component of preventing infectious disease in transplant recipients is the management of anti-rejection therapy, and regimens that minimize the intensity and duration of

TABLE I.   Organisms Causing Posttransplant Infections: An Overview

Class of Organism	Organism Name	Usual Disease Causes
Bacteria	Community-acquired bacteria	Various infections
	Nosocomial bacteria	Nosocomial infection
	Legionella species	Pneumonia
	Listeria	Meningoencephalitis
	Mycobacteria	Pulmonary/extrapulmonary infection
	Mycoplasma hominis	Sternal wound infection
	Nocardia species	Pulmonary/extrapulmonary infection
Fungi	*Candida* species	Mucocutaneous candidiasis
		Sternal wound infection
	Cryptococcus neoformans	Meningitis, extraneural infection
	Coccidioides immitis	Disseminated infection/meningitis
	Histoplasma capsulatum	Disseminated infection
Viruses	*Herpesviruses*	
	Herpes simplex (HSV) 1 and 2	Mucocutaneous vesicles
	Varicella-zoster (VZV)	Chickenpox, shingles
	Epstein-Barr virus (EBV)	PTLD*
	Cytomegalovirus (CMV)	CMV syndrome
		Enteritis
		Pneumonitis
		Retinitis
	(?) Human herpesvirus-6	(?) Lymphoma, aplastic anemia
	Jakob-Creutzfeldt virus	Progressive multifocal leukoencephalopathy
	Respiratory viruses	
	Respiratory syncytial (RSV)	Pneumonitis
	Parainfluenza	Pneumonitis
Parasites	*Protozoa*	
	Pneumocystis carinii	Pneumonitis
	Toxoplasma gondii	Myocarditis, pneumonitis, encephalitis
	Trypanosoma cruzi	Disseminated infection
	Nematodes	
	Strongyloides stercoralis	Disseminated infection

* PTLD = Posttransplant lymphoproliferative disorder.

broad-spectrum immunosuppression have greatly reduced the incidence and mortality from infection.

EVALUATION BEFORE TRANSPLANTATION

Determinants of risk for certain infections in transplant candidates include racial or ethnic background, geographic exposure, and history of high risk behaviors and past infectious diseases (Table 2). Antibiotic allergies and intolerances should be documented. Immunization history will dictate pretransplant vaccinations. Occupations and hobbies, such as the keeping of certain pets, may be important. A Mantoux skin test with mumps and *Candida* controls should be carried out, regardless of a history of past positive skin test or vaccination with Bacille Calmette-Guèrin (BCG), unless the reaction was severe. Dental work and surgery (e.g., transurethral resection of the prostate) should be carried out before transplantation as cardiac function allows.

Recipient serology must be obtained before any blood transfusions and may be used to exclude a patient from transplantation (e.g., HIV), or later, either alone (e.g., CMV) or in combination with donor serology (e.g., toxoplasma) to implement prophylaxis. It can also be useful in making the diagnosis of posttransplant infection and disease (e.g., EBV seroconversion).

TABLE 2. Pretransplant infection Work-up: Recipient

Infection Risk	Specifics	Actions
Tuberculosis	Immigration from country with high prevalence Ethnic origin associated with high prevalence High-risk lifestyle/behaviors Exposure to persons with TB History (Hx) of a + Mantoux skin test	Place Mantoux skin test with controls and read at 48–72 hrs. Treat positives according to the CDC guidelines.[13]
Herpes simplex 1,2	Hx of orolabial or genital lesions	
Varicella-zoster	Hx of chickenpox or shingles *or* Hx of children with chickenpox without disease in the patient	Varicella immune status; if negative, varicella vaccine and/or varicella zoster immunoglobulin (VZIG) postexposure prophylaxis is indicated
Epstein-Barr virus	Hx is usually negative though serology shows past infection in at least 90% of adults	Serology is not helpful unless planning to match donor to recipient; can be be done later on stored serum if needed for diagnosis
Cytomegalovirus	Hx of blood transfusions	Positive CMV IgG serology may dictate posttransplant prophylaxis with antivirals +/− CMVIG
Hepatitis	Hx of blood transfusions, high risk behaviors	Hepatitis profile indicated in all candidates. Pos. HBsAg is a contraindication to transplant. Pos. HCV test is not a **proven** contraindication
Toxoplasmosis	Cats, undercooked meat	Toxoplasma IgG test on frozen saved serum if donor is seropositive, mismatch to be treated prophylactically with pyrimethamine or TMP/SMZ
Geographic exposure and history	Southwestern U.S.A. (coccidioides) Third World exposure (any illness?) Risk for Chagas' disease?	Work-up any diarrheal or other illness that seems travel-related; consider empiric thiabendazole for strongyloides Serology for Chagas' disease.
Hx of recurrent infections	Ear/sinus infections, urinary tract infection, skin, dental caries or abscesses	Do any definitive procedures before transplant if possible.
Pets/Hobbies	Cats: who changes litter? Exposure to psittacine birds? Spelunking? Exposure to enclosed bird pens? Aquarium cleaning?	Counseling on avoidance of high risk exposure (i.e., can wear dust mist respirator)
High risk behaviors for HIV: • male to male sexual intercourse • intravenous drug abuse • birth to HIV+ mother • intercourse with HIV+ person	Candidate could be in the antibody negative "window"	HIV-antibody testing indicated for all candidates. In the high-risk seronegative candidate, consider exclusion until repeat test at 3–6 months is negative.
Immunization history All candidates	Tetanus-diphtheria booster in past 10 years? Pneumovax 23 in past 5 yr? Influenza shot? (Oct.–Feb.)	No? Give.
Young adult (up to 20 yr)	Hemophilus vaccine Measles–mumps–rubella booster Hepatitis B vaccine	If not given before If not given, or can test Probably indicated
Pediatric candidates	All childhood immunizations must be up to date, including hepatitis B vaccine	All childhood immunizations must be up to date, including hepatitis B vaccine
Untested prior to transplant	To help diagnose EBV PTLD toxoplasma mismatch, etc. To help with the Dx of EBV-PTLD, toxoplasma mismatch, etc.	Freeze candidate sera for later testing

PTLD = Posttransplant lymphoproliferative disorder.

TABLE 3. Pretransplant Infection work-up: Donor

Infection Risk	Specifics	Actions
Viral	Cytomegalovirus	Serology; prophylaxis of SNR if positive
	Epstein-Barr virus	Serology, to establish the Dx of primary infection in the SNR
	Hepatitis viruses B	Exclude from donation if positive
	C	No consensus on donation if positive
	Retroviruses:	Exclude from donation if positive
	HIV1/2, HTLV-1	Take a careful Hx of risk factors and exclude if positive regardless of serological results
Parasites	*Toxoplasma gondii*	Serology; prophylaxis of the SNR if positive
	Trypanosoma cruzi	Careful Hx for risk factors and exclude from donation if positive or do serology twice and if negative can transplant

SNR = seronegative recipient; Dx = diagnosis; HTLV = human T-cell lymphotropic virus; Hx = history.

Certain active infections in the donor (Table 3) pose contraindications to transplantation and are well outlined in other publications.[2] Nosocomial lower respiratory infection and bacteremia should not preclude transplantation, however. A history of high risk for HIV infection is often more difficult to come by, but efforts to obtain this information should be made and, if there is suspicion, harvesting of donor organs should not be carried out, regardless of serologic results.

PERIOPERATIVE PROPHYLAXIS

For cardiac transplantation, preoperative cephalosporin or vancomycin (in patients with Type I allergy to penicillin) should be given 1 to 2 hours before *incision* to any patient undergoing sternotomy. At our institution, cardiovascular surgical prophylaxis consists of cefuroxime 1.5 gm pre- and 1.5 gm every 8 hours postoperatively for 48 hours. Vancomycin is dosed according to corrected body weight and creatinine clearance so as to arrive at a reasonably accurate mg/kg/min dosage, which avoids the so-called "red man syndrome."

In lung or heart-lung transplants, imipenem-cilastatin (Primaxin) is used, or, for patients with significant penicillin allergy, clindamycin and ceftazidime. Once the results of donor trachea cultures are known, antibiotic choices can be tailored to the organisms isolated while maintaining coverage against *Staphylococcus*. In the absence of any data, we have been continuing prophylactic antibiotics for 5 days and have been using fluconazole for 10 days against *Candida*.

IMMEDIATE POSTOPERATIVE PROPHYLAXIS

After transplantation, patients are cared for in a private room with positive pressure, 90% efficiency air filtration, and at least 10 air exchanges per hour. This air-handling capability, which is monitored on a regular basis, is designed to prevent contact with fungal spores, specifically those of *Aspergillus*. In addition to the special air, therefore, we institute "*Aspergillus* precautions," which include daily damp wiping of all horizontal surfaces, after which the patient wears an 8710 dust-mist respirator mask (3M Corporation) for 30 minutes; this mask is also worn by the patient when out of the room. Visitors must take off their outer garments before entering the room. Patients are not allowed to have flowers or plants, either real or artificial, or plush toys. No pepper is allowed on food (Table 4).

TABLE 4.   Aspergillus Precautions

The patient must be in a private room with positive ventilation and at least 10 air exchanges per hour.

At least 90% of particles over 0.5 microns are filtered from air entering the room.

Not allowed: Plush toys, pepper for food, artificial or real plants or flowers. Visitors must leave overcoats outside the room.

All horizontal and other surfaces capable of gathering dust are damp cleaned daily.

The patient wears an 8710 dust-mist respirator mask (3M) when out of the room, and for 30 minutes after cleaning the room.

All construction projects are reviewed in advance by the Infection Control Department and suitable barriers and removal systems implemented; some projects are postponed until there are no transplant recipients in the area.

These precautions remain in effect for hospitalized patients until the prednisone dose is down to 30 mg/day. Wearing of the mask is encouraged for coming to the hospital (constant renovation), on windy days, or near excavation or construction sites, for 3 months posttransplant.

No literature supports use of barriers such as masks and gowns that were part of traditional "protective isolation." This has been studied in both the neutropenic[5,6] and the transplant patient.[7] The single most important measure to prevent nosocomial transmission of routine bacteria and some viruses is *handwashing*. Gloves and other barriers should be worn as dictated by universal precautions or body substance isolation procedures and for the placement of central lines. Persons must not enter the room when they have a communicable disease unless necessary, and when they do they must wear the appropriate barriers and wash hands properly. All invasive devices are removed as soon as possible. This degree of precaution remains in place until the prednisone dose is down to ≤ 30 mg per day. Often, however patients will be doing well enough to be discharged before that, so they are instructed in the appropriate use of the mask and avoidance of higher risk situations (e.g., visits by ill relatives) until they reach that dose.

PREVENTION OF SPECIFIC INFECTIONS

Bacterial Infection

Full discussion of the prevention of nosocomial bacterial infection as it applies to the intensive care unit (ICU) is beyond the scope of this chapter. Therefore, with the exception of a brief discussion of the management of positive donor trachea cultures in lung transplant recipients above, what follows is a review of prevention and prophylaxis for infections that are more common or more likely to cause clinical disease in the immunosuppressed transplant recipient (Table 1).

Legionella species

Legionella is a gram-negative rod present in many hot and cold water sources,[8,9] although well water appears to be safe. It causes pneumonia and, rarely, extrapulmonary disease[10,11] in transplant recipients. Prevention of this infection requires treatment of contaminated water.

Listeria monocytogenes

Listeria is a gram-positive bacillus found in unpasteurized milk and other dairy products, raw vegetables, and undercooked poultry and meat.[12] It colonizes the gastrointestinal tract and causes bacteremia and meningoencephalitis in persons with compromised cell-mediated immunity (CMI). Although no rigorous studies have been done, it seems likely that the trimethoprim-sulfamethoxazole (TMP-SMZ) prophylaxis given to prevent PCP in transplant recipients also prevents *Listeria* infections because this drug is an effective therapeutic alternative. Patients can be given the following dietary recommendations to minimize the risk of exposure[12a]:

1. Avoid eating raw or partially cooked foods of animal origin.
2. Avoid cross-contamination between raw and cooked foods during food preparation and storage.
3. Reheat leftovers until too hot to touch.
4. Avoid soft cheeses such as feta and Mexican-style cheeses; eat hard cheeses, cottage cheese, and cream cheese.
5. Wash raw vegetables thoroughly before eating.

Mycobacterium tuberculosis

The best time to address the prophylaxis of *Mycobacterium tuberculosis* (M. Tb) is before transplantation (see Table 1), as antituberculosis medications, whether isoniazid (INH) as prophylaxis, or INH + rifampin (RFM) as treatment, interfere significantly with cyclosporine A (CsA) metabolism. Any pretransplant patient with a Mantoux skin test showing induration of ≥ 10 mm in areas of the country with a higher incidence of *M. tuberculosis* and ≥ 15 mm in areas of lower incidence should receive 6 to 12 months of INH at a dose of 5 mg/kg/day (up to 300 mg/day maximum) assuming that active TB is ruled out. If a positive Mantoux result represents a recent conversion, especially through household contact, the cut-off is ≥ 5 mm. This also applies to the patient with stable chest radiographic changes and sputum negative for acid-fast bacilli.[13]

Nocardia

This partially acid-fast filamentous gram-negative organism is most frequently acquired by the respiratory route and usually causes nodular or diffuse pulmonary infiltrates, often with cavitation. It can disseminate causing abscesses in skin, brain, and other tissue. There are two major species, *N. asteroides* and *N. brasiliensis*, the first being more common in clinical infections.

Infection occurs late after transplantation (mean 586 days), and transplant recipients have accounted for 13% of the 500 to 1000 cases reported annually.[14] Incidence in a renal transplant population was 2.6% in patients on azathioprine-prednisone (May 1977 to August 1980) vs. 0.7% in patients on CsA-prednisone (August 1980 to March 1992). In this report routine TMP-SMX prophylaxis, given as one single-strength tablet per day for 1 to 4 months posttransplant, was not started until September 1987. Incidence after this did not change (0.53% vs. 0.87%), and so the authors have concluded that TMP-SMZ prophylaxis has no impact on the incidence. However, because this is usually a late-occurring infection, and because their patients were off TMP-SMZ after 4 months after transplant, it seems possible that longer courses of TMP-SMZ prophylaxis could have some effect. The renal toxicity that results from the interaction between TMP-SMZ and CsA in renal transplant recipients does not seem to occur as frequently or as severely in thoracic transplant recipients so that many thoracic transplant programs have been giving TMP-SMZ prophylaxis for much longer periods.

Fungal Infection

Candida

Topical antifungal agents such as clotrimazole (1 troche t.i.d.) may suppress colonization and/or mucosal invasiveness by *Candida* species and are probably necessary only for the first month posttransplant unless the patient needs prolonged hospitalization. Fluconazole has been studied in neutropenics and in bone marrow transplant recipients.[16,17] I believe fluconazole should not be used for prophylaxis (except in the lung transplant recipient whose donor's trachea has grown *Candida* as already described) because infection with fluconazole-resistant *Candida* species and *Aspergillus* in these populations has been described.[18] Fluconazole should be reserved for the treatment of mucocutaneous candidiasis refractory to clotrimazole or mycostatin, except for esophagitis, where it is the drug of choice. If fluconazole is to be used, the dose should be altered for renal dysfunction and the CsA dose should be halved in anticipation of high levels of CsA resulting from interference with liver metabolism of CsA.

Aspergillus

Pneumonia, with our without dissemination, has been reported in 5 to 10% of CsA-treated patients at University hospitals at Stanford, Minnesota, Houston, and Birmingham.[4] It usually occurs in the 3 months after transplant during the maximal period of polymorphonuclear dysfunction from high doses of prednisone and azathioprine. Prevention focuses on minimizing contact with fungal spores as described in a preceding section; see also Table 3.

Viral Infection

Herpesviruses

Herpes simplex.   Although outbreaks of orolabial or genital herpes are not uncommon posttransplant, they are, in general, not serious and easily treated with acyclovir (ACV). Routine prophylaxis for this indication is not advocated here except for the patient who has more than six recurrences per year, in which case a dose of 400 mg b.i.d. of ACV would be a reasonable place to start.

Varicella-zoster.   A live, attenuated, effective vaccine has been extensively tested. The susceptible transplant candidate would seem to be an ideal target for such active immunization before transplantation, but it must be remembered that vaccines shed virus for ≥ 30 days. Transplantation during that period might precipitate clinical illness and a need for isolation with *negative* ventilation. No long-term studies in transplant recipients look at the incidence of subsequent zoster infection; some questions remain to be answered. Because 85% of people have had chickenpox by age 15 years, the issue is more cogent in the pediatric population of transplant candidates.

After transplantation, passive immunization in the form of hyperimmune globulin (varicella-zoster immune globulin, or VZIG), if given within 72 hours of a significant exposure (same-room contact with a diagnosed case of chickenpox or direct contact with the skin lesions of shingles by a susceptible immunosuppressed host), can prevent or greatly attenuate the disease.[18a]

Pretransplant serology to establish immune status is indicated in pediatric transplant candidates without a positive history of chickenpox. In adults, it is probably not cost-effective in itself; however, the time and effort required to obtain the information needed to decide whether or not an exposed recipient needs VZIG (historic information and serology results) justify the test cost.

Cytomegalovirus.   Of seronegative recipients (SNR) of a CMV-seropositive heart, 83% develop infection with CMV as contrasted with a 0% incidence in SNR of seronegative donor hearts (controlled for CMV-negative blood products).[19] Although prevention of infection can be achieved by matching donor to recipient, this is not practical in thoracic transplantation.[20]

Strategies for prevention and prophylaxis with some track record include:
Seronegative blood products for seronegative recipients (SNR)[21]
Antiviral prophylaxis for SNR and seropositive recipients (SPR)[22-27]
Immunoprophylaxis[28-32]
Preemptive therapy[34-37]

Prophylaxis.   Balfour's group at the University of Minnesota demonstrated a decrease in CMV infection from 29% to 8% in SNR of CMV seropositive kidneys and in seropositive recipients (SPR), in a randomized placebo-controlled trial of acyclovir (ACV) prophylaxis using doses of 800 to 3200 mg/day according to renal function, for 3 months after transplant.[22] Since then a number of other studies suggest a similar benefit in bone marrow, liver, and heart transplantation.[23-25] In addition to decreasing incidence of serious CMV disease, onset of clinical disease was delayed so that it occurred beyond the time of maximal immunosuppression and was therefore less severe. We have not found any statistical difference in ACV-treated vs. non–ACV-treated heart transplant recipients in our program.

Other studies using ganciclovir (GCV) have not shown any benefit over ACV, and the requirement for intravenous administration makes it prohibitively expensive as well as exposes the patient to the risk of intravenous-catheter–associated infection.[24,26,27] Some new agents are on the horizon: an oral GCV is presently being tested in AIDS patients with CMV retinitis; several other promising compounds are in Phase I trials.

Immunoprophylaxis.   Active immunization may be accomplished with a Towne strain of CMV.[28,29] Although severity of CMV disease decreased in vaccinated SNR of SPD, the incidence of infection and disease was no different in the vaccinated vs. the unvaccinated groups. This may be explained by the fact that SNR were infected with a donor strain not represented by the vaccine. Studies are ongoing to identify an effective subunit antigen (e.g., envelope glycoprotein).[30]

Passive immunization has been provided with unselected intravenous immune globulin (IVIG), monoclonal CMV antibodies, and human CMV immune globulin (CMVIG) (high-titer product from patients with naturally occurring antibodies) now marketed as Cytogam. Data on Cytogam show a definite benefit in prophylaxis of SNR of SPD in renal[31] and liver[32] transplantation. Indication for this intervention in heart transplantation is not clear. In our center's experience with over 165 heart transplants, CMV disease has manifested itself as CMV syndrome or enteritis and has been easily treated with GCV without relapse. There is very likely an important role for prophylactic cytomegalovirus (CMVIG) in lung transplantation, however, because CMV pneumonia is much more common in this population and ACV alone has not prevented CMV disease. Multicenter trials are difficult to organize given the wide variation in immunosuppressive regimens used by thoracic transplanters.

There have been no comparative trials of unselected IVIG vs. CMVIG; however, CMVIG has theoretic advantages over IVIG in that it has been shown to be effective in controlled trials, and the titers of CMV antibody are consistent from lot to lot as required by the Food and drug Administration (FDA). Also, because of the high titers of CMV antibody in CMVIG as compared with the variable and lower titers in IVIG, much smaller infusion volumes can be used. The recommended dosage for prophylaxis in high-risk renal transplant recipients is 150 mg/kg within 72 hours of transplant, followed by 100 mg/kg at weeks 2, 4, 6, and 8 after transplant and 50 mg/kg at weeks 12 and 16 after transplant. (High risk = SNR of SPD or SPR).[31]

Recently it has been discovered that one IVIG product has been infected with hepatitis C virus as far back as 1992; it has been taken off the market.[33]

Preemptive therapy.   Another approach to CMV disease prevention is called preemptive therapy. Patients are monitored for CMV infection by culture, antigen detection, or polymerase chain reaction and at the first sign of infection (not disease) they are treated with GCV with or without CMVIG.[34-36] Rubin also advocates starting preemptive GCV with the institution of antilymphocyte therapy for rejection.[37]

Epstein-Barr virus.   Unchecked expansion of the lymphoblastoid cell lines created by EBV infection causes a spectrum of posttransplant lymphoproliferative disorders (PTLD)[2,3] both in SNR of SPD and in SPR, with disease tending to be more severe in the previously uninfected patient. The issue is more of a concern in pediatric transplantation, where at least 50% of recipients are SNR, contrasted with 10% of adults. The only certain way to prevent these conditions is to match the SND to the SNR, but this is not practical. It has also been suggested that SNR of SPD not get prophylactic OKT3 after transplantation, as some studied have shown a high rate of PTLD in patients thus treated.[4,38]

This has not been our experience,[39] nor that of others.[40,41] Cosimi and Rubin maintain that it is the "net state of immunosuppression" induced, rather than the role of any one agent, that is important. They cite a multi-institutional study of liver allograft recipients and their own renal transplant experience, with CsA not started until 3 days before the end of OKT3 therapy: the rates of PTLD were 0% and 1.5%, respectively; and in renal transplant recipients, the rate of PTLD not receiving OKT3 at all was 1.1%.

Recently data suggest that elevated interleukin-6 (IL-6) levels play an important role in the pathogenesis of PTLD.[42] Perhaps through a better understanding of this and other mechanisms we can explore new ways to prevent this usually fatal complication.

Hepatitis Viruses

Hepatitis B (HBV).   Inadvertent transplantation of hepatitis B surface-antigen–positive organs into SNR has been described. It seems possible to prevent infection of the recipient through the administration of hepatitis B immune globulin (HBIG) and hepatitis B vaccine in the same way as infection of the neonate born to the seropositive mother is accomplished. Though promising work is in progress with new therapeutic approaches to suppress viral replication in the infected recipient, in many centers hepatitis B seropositivity, especially with positive HBV DNA, is a contraindication to transplantation.

Hepatitis C (HCV).   No effective prophylaxis is known against HCV, but transmission in transplantation seems infrequent and the resulting infection relatively inconsequential in one study.[43] Some centers have advocated excluding HCV-positive donors,[1,45] but policies regarding transplanting seropositive thoracic organs are inconsistent across a wide range of centers responding to a survey published by Milfred and co-workers.[45] The controversy has been made more difficult by the insensitivity of available serologic techniques. It would now appear that second-generation ELISA (ELA2) serology cannot be relied upon to make decisions about liver transplantation;[46] the presence of HCV RNA in the serum of the donor is most highly predictive of transmission because 100% of recipients of these livers have HCV infection by polymerase chain reaction (PCR). There is a much lower prevalence of HCV infection and clinical liver disease in the recipient of an EIA2 positive/HCV–RNA-negative donor liver, suggesting that such organs can be used for transplantation, especially in the case of urgent need. Reactivated infection in the SPR appears to cause mild disease but the long-term sequelae are not yet known.

At present, our program reserves HCV SPD for HCV SPR. We are conducting a serologic survey of all our living recipients to gather more data.

HIV and Other Retroviruses

Careful historical and serologic screening has made posttransplant infection with HIV extremely rare. Inadvertent transplantation of seropositive organs has occurred, and rapid progression to the acquired immunodeficiency syndrome (AIDS) with fatal outcome has been universal. As in many cases of postexposure prophylaxis for health care workers and others, immediate administration of azidothymidine (AZT) has not altered the course of the infection.

Human lymphotropic virus 1 and 2 (HTLV-1, HTLV-2) and HIV-2 have similar modes of transmission to HIV-1.[47] HTLV-1 is endemic in Japan, the Caribbean, Africa, the southeastern U.S., and South America[48] and causes T-cell lymphoma/leukemia and spastic paraparesis in a small percentage of infected individuals. A case of rapidly progressive myelopathy resuting from transmission of HTLV-1 from a blood transfuion during cardiac transplantation has been reported.[49] HTLV-2 has been linked to hairy cell leukemia[50] and HIV-2 causes AIDS.[51] Screening for these viruses needs to be part of the work-up for donors.

Parasitic Infection

Pneumocystis carinii

Pneumocystis carinii pneumonia (PCP) is said to be the most common late infection after cardiac transplantation, occurring in 3% of recipients. The best-controlled data on the efficacy of prophylaxis with TMP-SMZ come from Hughes' studies of leukemic children[52] and from the AIDS literature.[53,54]

For patients unable to take TMP-SMZ, alternatives include aerosolized pentamidine (AP) and dapsone. The low frequency of disease makes the inconvenience of AP unappealing; dapsone seems a better choice for this population of patients. The optimal dosing regimen is not known; dapsone has a long half-life but a variable one. Data on its pharmacokinetics in transplant recipients would be enlightening.[55,56]

Toxoplasma gondii

The infective oocysts of this protozoan are excreted in the feces of cats; the organism also lies encysted in the skeletal muscle of animals so that the ingestion of raw or undercooked meat is another source of infection. In cardiac and heart-lung transplant recipients, primary infection with toxoplasma occurs in about 45% of SNR of SPD and can cause myocarditis with a presentation which is indistinguishable from rejection. Disseminated infection, pneumonitis, and encephalitis occur much less frequently. Disease rarely, if ever, results from reactivation in an SPR in the CsA-treated patient.[57] Prophylaxis of the SNR of the SPD with pyrimethamine 25 mg/day for 6 weeks posttransplant has been shown to be effective.[58] Extrapolating from the AIDS literature, prophylaxis with TMP-SMZ should also be effective and makes more sense because patients are already receiving TMP-SMZ prophylaxis for PCP. In our program, toxoplasma serology is done on the recipient only if the donor serology is positive; the SNR is then followed closely for evidence of disease while on routine TMP-SMZ prophylaxis. SNR should also be counseled to avoid contact with cat feces and undercooked meat.

Trypanosoma cruzi

This protozoan parasite, transmitted by the bite of reduviid bugs, causes American trypanosomiasis, or Chagas' disease. It is endemic in all Latin American countries, including Mexico. Although many insects and wild mammals of the Southwestern and Southern United States are infected with the parasite, the density of infected bugs is low and only three cases of vector transmission have been reported in the United States. In the past 20 years, there have been six cases of acute trypanosomiasis resulting from laboratory accidents and nine imported cases, none in returning tourists. Two transfusion related cases have been reported in the United States and one

TABLE 5.   Summary of Recommendations for Prevention and Prophylaxis of Infection after Thoracic Transplantation

Organism/Infection	Prevention/Prophylaxis
Sternal wound infection	Cephalosporin or vancomycin
Anastomotic infection in LuTR	Treat donor trachea isolates
Legionella species	Water treatment to control nosocomial transmission
Listeria monocytogenes	Dietary precautions TMP-SMZ probably prevents*
Mycobacterium tuberculosis	Testing and treatment before therapy
Nocardia species	TMP-SMZ probably prevents*
Candida species	Clotrimazole troches × 1 month 14 days of fluconazole for positive donor trachea culture in LuTR
Aspergillus species	See Table 4
Herpes simplex I and II	Acyclovir 400 mg b.i.d. for patients with ≥ 6 recurrences/yr
Varicella zoster virus (VZG)	Active immunization if available Postexposure varicella zoster immune globulin (VZIG)
Cytomegalovirus (CMV)	CMV negative blood products for SNR High-dose p.o. ACV for SNR of SPD, or SPR, × 3 months Plus CMV IVIG for lung transplant recipients (LuTR) Preemptive treatment with GCV for LuTR
Epstein-Barr virus (EBV)	Optimal immunosuppression, ?ACV/GCV, ?CMVIG
Hepatitis B virus (HBV)	(?) ACV
HIV	HBV vaccine + HBIG ASAP Azidothymidine
Pneumocystis carinii	TMP-SMZ × 1 year†
Toxoplasma gondii	TMP-SMZ probably works* or can give pyrimethamine 25 mg/day × 6 weeks for SNR of SPD
Trypanosoma cruzi	History/serology/exclusion of positive
Strongyloides stercoralis	Serology and/or treatment with thiabendazole for candidates with geographic exposure

* As for Pneumocystis prophylaxis.
† Optimum duration of prophylaxis has never been established.
SNR = seronegative recipient. SPR = seropositive recipient. SPD = seropositive donor. ACV = acyclovir.
GCV = ganciclovir. LuTR = lung transplant recipients.

from Canada. Several reports from endemic areas describe the transmission by kidney transplantation.[59]

The prevalence of infection in a group of Salvadoran and Nicaraguan immigrants living in the Washington, D.C. area was 5%; extrapolating this to the number of immigrants from endemic areas yields a possible 50,000 to 100,000 cases of chronic trypanosomiasis in the United States today. Because the infection is lifelong and asymptomatic in most, the risk to recipients of blood and organs will persist, and at present no prospect exists for routine screening serology because the overall prevalence of the infection is so low. The only test that is licensed by the FDA (Chagas' IgG ELISA, Gull Laboratories, Salt Lake City) needs further testing to determine its sensitivity and specificity; the latter is the major limitation of the tests used in Latin America.

One group found that eliminating donors in the Los Angeles area by questionnaire reduced the blood supply by only 2.1%. At present, therefore, transplantation of organs from a donor deemed at risk for trypanosomiasis is contraindicated unless two consecutive serologic determinations are negative.

Because immunosuppression can reactivate quiescent trypanosomiasis, cardiac transplantation in persons with end-stage Chagas' cardiomyopathy is probably contraindicated.

Strongyloides stercoralis

Travel to endemic areas of the world (Latin America, Mexico, southern United States, and all other countries outside of western Europe) may expose patients to *Strongyloides stercoralis*, which can remain in the gastrointestinal tract for many years without causing symptoms. After transplantation the recipient may experience active disease, which consists of fever, diarrhea, and manifestations of dissemination to the lung, liver, and other vital organs. Transplant candidates with a significant travel history or geographic origin should therefore be screened with three stools for ova and parasites or empirically given a 2–3 day course of thiabendazole.[60,61]

CONCLUSION

Despite improved survival in thoracic transplant recipients, infection remains a leading cause of morbidity and mortality. In addition to minimizing the net state of immunosuppresion, we believe that the strategies for prevention and prophylaxis of infection developed for the Minneapolis Heart Institute Thoracic Transplant Program, as shown in Table 5, provide maximum benefit to our patients.

REFERENCES

1. Keating MR, Wilhelm MP, Walker RC: Strategies for prevention of infection after cardiac transplantation. Mayo Clinic Proc 67:676–684, 1992.
2. Love KR: Nonbacterial infections in thoracic transplantation. In Cardiac Surgery: State of the Art Reviews 2:657–658, 1988.
3. Love KR: Donor transmitted infections. In Cardiac Surgery: State of the Art Reviews 3:639–652, 1989.
4. Petri WA Jr: Infections in heart transplant recipients. Clin Infect Dis 18:141–148, 1994.
5. Verhoef J: Prevention of infections in the neutropenic patient. Clin Infect Dis Supp. 2:S359–367, 1993.
6. Armstrong D: Protected environments are discomforting and expensive and do not offer meaningful protection. In Brown AE, Armstrong D (eds): Infectious Complications of Neoplastic Diseases: Controversies in Management. New York, York Medical Books, 1985, pp 395–407.
7. Wash TR, Guttendorf J, Dummer S: The value of protective isolation procedures in cardiac allograft recipients. Ann Thorac Surg 47:539–545, 1989
8. Edelstein PH: Legionnaire's disease. Clin Infect Dis 16:741–749, 1993.
9. Yu VL: Legionnaire's disease: New understanding of community acquired pneumonia. Hosp Prac 63–70, 1993.
10. Kilborn JA, Manz LA, O'Brien M, et al: Necrotizing cellulitis caused by *Legionella micdadei*. Am J Med 92:104–106, 1992.
11. Ampel NM, Ruben FL, Norden CW: Cutaneous abscess caused by *Legionella micdadei* in an immunosuppressed patient. An Intern Med 102:630–632, 1985.
12. Anaissie E, Kontoyianis DP, Kantarjan H, et al: Listeriosis in patients with CLL who were treated with fludarabine and prednisone. Ann Intern Med 117:466–468, 1985.
12a. Schuchat A, Deaver KA, Wenger JD, et al: Role of foods in sporadic listeriosis. 1: Case-control study of dietary risk factors. JAMA 267:2041–2045, 1992.
13. The use of preventive therapy for tuberculous infection in the United States Recommendations of the Advisory Committee for Elimination of Tuberculosis. MMWR 39:9–12, 1990.
14. Bearman BL, Burnside J, Edwards B, Causey W: Nocardial infections in the United States, 1972–1974. J Infect Dis 134:286–289, 1976.
15. Arduino RC, Johnson PC, Miranda AG: Nocardiosis in renal transplantation recipients undergoing immunosuppression with cyclosporine. Clin Infect Dis 16:505–512, 1993.
16. Samonis G, Rolston K, Karl C: Prophylaxis of oropharyngeal candiasis with fluconazole. Rev Infect Dis 12(Suppl 3):S369-373, 1990.
17. Goodman JL, Winston DJ, Greenfield RA, et al: A controlled trial of fluconazole to prevent fungal infections in patients undergoing bone marrow transplantation. N Engl J Med 326:845–851, 1992.

18. Wingard JR, Merz WG, Rinaldi MG, et al: Increase in *Candida krusei* infection among patients with bone marrow transplantation and neutropenia treated prophylactically with fluconazole. N Engl J Med 325:1274–1277, 1991.

18a. Varicella-zoster immune globulin for the prevention of chickenpox. MMWR 33:84–96, 1984.

19. Bowden RA. Cytomegalovirus infections in transplant patients: Methods of prevention of primary cytomegalovirus. Transplant Proc 23(Suppl 3):136–138, 1991.

20. Ludwin D, White N, Tsai S, et al: Results of prospective matching for cytomegalovirus status in renal transplant recipients. Transplant Proc 19:3433–3434, 1987.

21. Bowden RA, Ayers M, Flournoy N, et al: Cytomegalovirus immunoglobulin and seronegative blood products to prevent primary CMV infection after bone marrow transplant. N Engl J Med 314:1006–1010, 1986.

22. Bafour HH, Chace BA, Stapleton JT, et al: A randomized, placebo controlled trial of oral acyclovir for the prevention of cytomegalovirus disease in recipients of renal allografts. N Engl J Med 320:1381–1387, 1989.

23. Meyers JD, Reed EC, Shepp DH, et al: Acyclovir for the prevention of cytomegalovirus infection and disease after allogeneic bone marrow transplantation. N Engl J Med 318:70–75, 1988.

24. Freise CE, Pons V, Lake J, et al: Comparison of three regimens for cytomegalovirus prophylaxis in 147 liver transplant recipients. Transplant Proc 23:1498–500, 1991.

25. Elkins CC, Frist WH, Dummer JS, et al: Cytomegalovirus disease after heart transplantation: Is acyclovir prophylaxis indicated? Ann Thorac Surg 56:1267–1273, 1993.

26. Merigan TC, Renlund DG, Keay S, et al: A controlled trial of ganciclovir to prevent cytomegalovirus disease after heart transplantation. N Engl J Med 326:1182–1186, 1992.

27. Martin M: Antiviral prophylaxis for CMV infection in liver transplantation. Transplant Proc 25(Suppl 4):10–14, 1993.

28. Plotkin SA, Starr SE, Friedman HM, et al: Effect of towne live virus vaccine on cytomegalovirus disease after renal transplant: A controlled trial. Ann Intern Med 114:525–531, 1991.

29. Brayman KL, Dafoe DC, Smythe WR, et al: Prophylaxis of serious CMV infection in renal transplant candidates using live human cytomegalovirus vaccine. Arch Surg 123:1502–1508, 1988.

30. Starr SE, Friedman HM, Plotkin SA, et al: The status of cytomegalovirus vaccine. Rev Infect Dis 13(Suppl 11):S964–S965, 1991.

31. Snydman DR: Review of the efficacy of cytomegalovirus immune globulin in the prophylaxis of CMV disease in renal transplant recipients. Transplant Proc 25(Suppl 4):25–26, 1993.

32. Snydman DR, Werner BG, Dougherty NN, et al: Cytomegalovirus immune globulin prophylaxis in liver transplantation: A randomized, double-bind, placebo-controlled trial. Ann Intern Med 119:984–991, 1993.

33. Outbreak of hepatitis C associated with intravenous immunoglobulin administration—United States October 1993–June 1994. MMWR 43:505–509, 1994.

34. Farrugia E: Management and prevention of cytomegalovirus infection after renal transplantation. Mayo Clinic Proc 67:879–890, 1992.

35. Goodrich JM, Mori M, Gleaves CA: Early treatment with ganciclovir to prevent cytomegalovirus disease after allogeneic bone marrow transplantation. N Engl J Med 325:1601–1607, 1991.

36. Rubin R: Preemptive therapy in immunocompromised hosts [editorial]. N engl J Med 324:1057–1059, 1991.

37. Rubin R: First North American Transplant Infectious Disease Symposium, Boston, 1993.

38. Swinnen LJ, Costanzo-Nordin MR, Fischer SG: Increased incidence of lymphoproliferative disorder after immunosuppression with monoclonal antibody OKT3 in cardiac-transplant recipients. N Engl J Med 323:1723–1728, 1990.

39. Emery RW, Lake KD: Post-transplantation lymphoproliferative disorder and OKT3. N Engl J Med 324:1437, 1991.

40. Brouwer RML, Balk AHMM, Weimar W: Post-transplantation lymphoproliferative disorder and OKT3. N Engl J Med 324:1437, 1991.

41. Cosimi AB, Rubin R: Post-transplantation lymphoproliferative disorder and OKT3. N Engl J Med 324:1438, 1991.

42. Strauss S, Cohen JI, Tosato G, Meier J: NIH Conference: Epstein-Barr virus infections: Biology, pathogenesis, and management. Ann Intern Med 118:45–58, 1993.

43. Roth D, Fernandez JA, Babischkin S: Detection of hepatitis C virus infection among cadaveric organ donors: Evidence for low transmission of disease. Ann Intern Med 117:470–475, 1992.

44. Pereira BJG, Milford EL, Kirkman RL: Transmission of hepatitis C virus by organ transplantation. N Engl J Med 325:454–460, 1991.

45. Milfred SK, Lake KD, Anderson DJ, et al: Practices of cardiothoracic transplant centers regarding hepatitis C seropositive candidates and donors. Transplantation 57:568–572, 1994.

46. Wright TL: Hepatitis C and other NANB forms of hepatitis in transplantation. North American Transplant Infectious Disease Symposium, Boston, 1993.

47. Larson CJ, Taswell HF: Human T-cell leukemia virus type 1 (HTLV-1) and blood transfusion. Mayo Clin Proc 63:869–875, 1988.
48. Minamoto GY, Gold JWM, Scheinberg DA, et al: Infection with human T-cell leukemia virus type-1 in patients with leukemia. N Engl J Med 318:219–222, 1988.
49. Gout O, Baulac M, Gessain A, et al: Rapid development of myelopathy after HTLV-1 infection acquired by transfusion during cardiac transplantation. N Engl J Med 322:383–388, 1990.
50. Rosenblatt JD, Golde DW, Wachsman W, et al: A second isolate of HTLV-II associated with atypical hairy-cell leukemia. N Engl J Med 315:372–377, 1986.
51. Khabbaz RF, Onorato IM, Cannon RO, et al: Seroprevalence of HTLV-1 and HTLV-2 among intravenous drug users and persons in clinics for sexually transmitted diseases. N Engl J Med 326:375–379, 1992.
52. Hughes WT, Rivera GK, Schell MJ, et al: Successful intermittent chemoprophylaxis for *Pneumocystis carinii* pneumonitis. N Engl J Med 316:1627–1632, 1987.
53. Fischl MA, Dickinson GM, La Voie L: Safety and efficacy of sulfamethoxazole and trimethoprim chemoprophylaxis for *Pneumocystis carinii* pneumonia in AIDS. JAMA 259:1185–1189, 1988.
54. Wormser GP, Horowitz HW, Duncan son FP, et al: Low-dose intermittent trimethoprim-deficiency virus infection. Arch Intern Med 151:688–692, 1991.
55. Lucas CR, Sandland M, Mjich A, et al: Primary dapsone chemoprophylaxis for pneumocystis carinii pneumonia in immunocompromised patients infected with the human immunodeficiency virus. Med J Aust 15:30–33, 1989.
56. Pieters FAJM, Quidema J: The pharmacokinetics of dapsone after oral administration to healthy volunteers. Br J Clin Pharmacol 22:491–494, 1986.
57. Luft BJ, Naot Y, Araujo FG, Stinson EG, et al: Primary and reactivated toxoplasma infection in patients with cardiac transplants: Clinical spectrum and problems in diagnosis in a defined population. Ann Intern Med 99:27–31, 1983.
58. Wreghitt TG, Hakim M, Gray JJ, et al: Toxoplasmosis in heart and heart and lung transplant recipients. J Clin Pathol 42:194–199, 1989.
59. Kirchoff LV: American trypanosomiasis (Chagas' disease)—A tropical disease now in the United States. N Engl J Med 329:639–640, 1993.
60. White MJ: Prevention of infections in patients with neoplastic disease: use of a historical model for developmental strategies. Clin Infect Dis 17(Suppl 2):S359–S367, 1993.
61. Genta RM: Global prevalence of strongyloidiasis: Critical review with epidemiologic insights into the prevention of disseminated disease. Rev Infect Dis 11:755–767, 1989.

Pulmonary Hypertension and Cardiac Transplantation

Chapter 4

Elaine Winkel, MD
Walter Kao, MD
Maria Rosa Costanzo, MD

HEART FAILURE AND PULMONARY HYPERTENSION

Patients with long-standing heart failure who are referred for orthotopic heart transplantation (OHT) commonly have significant pulmonary hypertension.[1] Potential mechanisms for its development include elevated left ventricular filling pressure due to impaired systolic function, neurohormonal activation with increased circulating levels of vasoactive substances, structural changes in the pulmonary vasculature, and pulmonary parenchymal factors such as alveolar hypoventilation and interstitial edema. Depending on the severity and duration of heart failure, pulmonary hypertension may be reactive and reversible, fixed and permanent as a result of morphologic abnormalities of the pulmonary vasculature, or, more commonly, a combination of both. The reactive component is thought, at least in part, to result from elevated left atrial pressure, similar to the setting of isolated mitral valvular stenosis. Although elevated left atrial pressure is a stimulus for reactive pulmonary hypertension, other factors can trigger the reactive component. Intermittent pulmonary hypertension and consequent right heart failure have been seen after OHT despite having a reactive pulmonary vasculature preoperatively and normal left atrial pressure after OHT.[2] Nevertheless, the greatest challenge facing heart transplant clinicians in this regard lies in (1) the determination of whether or not to consider patients with certain degrees of fixed pulmonary hypertension for OHT; and (2) the pre- and postoperative management of such individuals.

MEASUREMENT OF PULMONARY VASCULAR RESISTANCE (PVR)

Calculated PVR has traditionally been used as a measure of impedance to right ventricular ejection in the absence of pulmonary valve disease. Resistance to flow through a distensible system is directly related to the pressure difference across the system and inversely related to flow. Therefore, PVR can be calculated by dividing the transpulmonary gradient by cardiac output:

$$TPG = MPAP - MPCWP$$

$$PVR = \frac{TPG}{CO}$$

where TPG = transpulmonary gradient (mmHg); PVR = pulmonary vascular resistance (Wood units); MPAP = mean pulmonary artery pressure (mmHg); MPCWP = mean pulmonary capillary wedge pressure (mmHg); and CO = cardiac output (liters/ minute).

Because, however, the resistance across the pulmonary bed varies in relation to such factors as vascular compliance, alveolar pressure, recruitment of parallel pulmonary vascular pathways with increasing flow and pressure, the critical opening pressure for microvascular flow, and the potential reactivity of the pulmonary microvasculature, the calculated PVR may not accurately represent all forces opposing flow through the system. Therefore, controversy exists over the optimal measurement of resistance of the pulmonary circuit. Some investigators have favored a modification of the standard PVR to allow for body size, particularly in the pediatric age group: the PVR "index," represented by the absolute PVR multiplied by body surface area (m^2)[3] Others suggest that TPG, which is flow independent, is a truer prepresentation of the pulmonary vascular tone than PVR because the latter is derived from and thus depends on pulmonary blood flow or cardiac output.[4,5] When pulmonary blood flow is artificially increased, TPG does not change, although calculated PVR decreases. In addition, standard thermodilution techniques may be imprecise in patients with severely impaired cardiac performance as a result of the presence of tricuspid regurgitation, thereby adding to uncertainty in the calculation of PVR. Clinical use of PVR is thus limited by the difficulty of its accurate measurement as well as the inability to distinguish clearly between the reactive and the fixed components of pulmonary hypertension in patients with end-stage heart failure.

PULMONARY VASCULAR RESPONSE TO CARDIAC TRANSPLANTATION

Orthotopic heart transplantation has become standard therapy for patients with severe chronic heart failure. Unfortunately, candidates for OHT, by virtue of the advanced state of their heart disease, frequently suffer from concomitant pulmonary vascular disease. Bourge et al. examined the phenomenon of PVR after OHT using frequent right heart catheterizations beginning 1 week postoperatively.[2] They found that OHT patients, as a group, had a normal PVR, TPG, and pulmonary artery systolic pressure within 1 week postoperatively. Patients with reversible elevation of PVR preoperatively typically had both reactive and fixed components. Transplantation relieved the reactive but not the fixed component, so that, in these patients, both early and late after OHT, PVR had fallen but had not completely normalized. Some patients continued to have variability in PVR suggesting persistence of pulmonary vascular reactivity. In this cohort, preoperative PVR was the strongest predictor of PVR early after OHT, and PVR 1 week after OHT was the major predictor of subsequent PVR. Bhatia et al. examined the effects of elevated PVR on posttransplant right ventricular function by echocardiography.[6] They reported right ventricular dilatation and tricuspid regurgitation in the majority of patients on the first postoperative day. This increase in right ventricular size was maintained whereas incidence of tricuspid regurgitation decreased over the subsequent year, indicating remodeling of the right ventricle.

ELEVATED PULMONARY AND POSTTRANSPLANT MORBIDITY AND MORTALITY

The right ventricle of the typical transplanted heart functions in a normal hemodynamic milieu before OHT as a predominantly volume-driven pump. It therefore may respond poorly when subjected to the abrupt increase in afterload associated with OHT into a recipient with preoperative pulmonary hypertension. The risk of post-OHT right ventricular failure further increases when primary right ventricular dysfunction is induced in the donor heart by prolonged ischemic time, preservation injury, body size mismatch, prolonged cardiopulmonary bypass time, and rapid rewarming. Donor-related complications such as hypotension, administration of exogenous catecholamines, and thyroxine depletion may contribute further to early post-OHT right ventricular dysfunction.

Early reports noted that patients with severe pre-OHT pulmonary hypertension were at risk for right heart failure and death early after OHT.[7] Griepp observed that, of the first 26 consecutive patients undergoing OHT at Stanford University, the 3 early (< 72 hours postoperative) deaths, all from right ventricular failure, occurred in patients with severe pulmonary hypertension (MPAP = 55 mmHg, PVR = 11.5 Wood units). In the subsequent 10 years (1969–1979), when a MPAP > 40 mmHg and a PVR > 5 Wood units were contraindications to OHT, there was only one death attributable to post-OHT right ventricular failure.[8] Although the marked improvement in survival and the decreased incidence of rejection and infection after the introduction of cyclosporine have made prior contraindications for OHT less restrictive, severe pulmonary hypertension has been demonstrated consistently to be a major risk factor affecting both early and late post-OHT survival in both children and adults.[9,10]

Because severe pre-OHT pulmonary hypertension is associated with a high risk of immediate postoperative right ventricular failure and increased 6- and 12-month all-cause mortality, it is important to determine accurately the pulmonary vascular resistance in all heart-failure patients being considered for OHT. Some investigators have suggested that demonstration of *reactivity* in the pulmonary vasculature is the more important consideration in predicting early post-OHT mortality. A significant reduction in TPG or the calculated PVR during vasodilator and/or inotropic infusion without systemic hypotension is evidence for reactive pulmonary hypertension. Because patients may remain on the OHT waiting list for long periods, serial determinations are generally necessary to determine if the pulmonary hypertension has become fixed.

METHODS OF RISK STRATIFICATION USING PULMONARY VASCULAR RESISTANCE

Many transplant groups cite a specific PVR value as an absolute contraindication to OHT. However, the exact level of pulmonary vascular resistance in heart failure patients beyond which the risk of post-OHT right ventricular failure is excessive remains unclear. The relationship between preoperative pulmonary hemodynamics on both early and late post-OHT mortality has been systematically analyzed only recently. Addonizio et al. retrospectively analyzed the postoperative outcome of 82 patients undergoing OHT, comparing preoperative PVR with the incidence of post-OHT right

TABLE 1. Pulmonary Vascular Resistance Index (PVRI) and the Incidence of Right Ventricular (RV) Failure and Death

PVRI	n	RV Failure	Death
> 6 units	33	11*	5*
< 6 units	48	0	0

* p < 0.001

heart failure and death.[3] They found that the PVR index (PVRI) better reflected the risk of right heart failure post-OHT than the absolute PVR, which does not correct for body size. A PVRI threshold of 6 Wood units/m[2] identified all 11 patients who developed significant right heart failure in the early post-OHT. Patients with PVRI greater than 6 had a significantly higher incidence of right ventricular failure and death than patients with a PVRI below 6 (Table 1).

When pulmonary resistance was calculated in Wood units, PVR identified only 4 of the 11 patients with post-OHT right ventricular failure. Of the remaining 73 patients with PVR less than 6, 25 had resistance less than 6 Wood units but greater than 6 indexed-resistance units. Seven of these 25 had right ventricular failure and 4 died (Table 2).

Kirklin demonstrated that elevated preoperative PVR and the risk of post-OHT death varied continuously rather than showing a steep increase in mortality at a specific PVR, although the preoperative PVRI was a more accurate predictor of survival than PVR.[11] However, other hemodynamic variables, such as the TPG or the response of PVR to vasodilator therapy, were not evaluated. Subsequent observations have shown that TPG has greater prognostic value for early mortality after OHT than PVR. Kormos and colleagues reported that TPG and not PVR or PAP correlated with 7- and 30-day post-OHT mortality, considering both all-cause mortality as well as mortality from right ventricular failure.[4] (Table 3). There was a significant increase in mortality noted if preoperative TPG exceeded 15 mmHg.

This was confirmed by Murali et al., who demonstrated in 425 patients that baseline preoperative TPG, but not PVR, was a significant independent predictor of early post-OHT mortality.[12] Although both TPG and PVR were sensitive predictors of increased 0- to 2-day post-OHT mortality, only TPG was a significant predictor of 3- to 7-day and 8- to 30-day mortality. When TPG and PVR were considered together, they could be used to further stratify patients by risk before OHT (Table 4).

In this study group, female patients had significantly higher 0- to 2-day and 8- to 30-day mortality compared with male recipients (p < 0.001), independent of the level of pulmonary hypertension. The 3- to 7-day mortality also tended to be higher in women. Females with severe preoperative pulmonary hypertension had significantly higher immediate (0 to 2 days) mortality than those without serious pulmonary hypertension,

TABLE 2. Pulmonary Vascular Resistance (PVR) and the Incidence of Right Ventricular (RV) Failure and Death

	n	RV Failure	Death
PVR			
> 6 Wood units	8	4	1
< 6 Wood units	73	7	4
PVRI			
> 6 units	25	7	4
< 6 units	45	0	0

TABLE 3. Relationship of Transpulmonary Gradient and Pulmonary Vascular Resistance (PVR) to Posttransplant Survival

	Survival (%)	
	7 Day	30 day
PVR < 6	88	85
PVR ≥ 6	92	85
TPG < 10	95	92
TPG 10–15	84	81
TPG > 15*	79*	71*

* ($p < 0.05$) when compared with TPG < 10. TPG = transpulmonary gradient (mmHg).

whether defined by TPG ($p < 0.01$) or PVR ($p < 0.05$). Most interestingly, there was no significant difference in mortality among men with or without pulmonary hypertension. There was also no difference in the prevalence of preoperative pulmonary hypertension or in recipient or donor ages between men and women. More deaths attributed to primary graft failure occurred among female recipients compared with men (62.5% vs. 44.8%). Perhaps the higher overall mortality in women made it easier to demonstrate individual predictive factors because the incidence of death in men was too low to show any difference. The correlation between sex of recipient, PVR, and post-OHT mortality has not been shown by other investigators.

The TPG has also been shown to predict late post-OHT mortality. Erickson reviewed baseline pre-OHT TPG, pulmonary artery systolic (PAS) pressure, PVR, and PVRI in 109 OHT patients.[5] Elevated TPG had a prognostic value greater than PAS, PVR, or PVRI. Mortality at 6 and 12 months after OHT was significantly greater in patients with preoperative TPG ≥ 12 mmHg than in patients with preoperative TPG < 12 mmHg.

ROLE OF HEMODYNAMIC VASODILATOR RESPONSE IN ESTIMATING RISK OF CARDIAC TRANSPLANTATION

The previously cited studies have examined the relationship of baseline pulmonary hemodynamics to post-OHT right ventricular failure and death. There are reports suggesting that the hemodynamic response of pulmonary pressures to vasodilators may be useful prognostically.[13] The potential of sodium nitroprusside (SNP) to reduce pulmonary hypertension has long been recognized.[14,15] It has been suggested that the hemodynamic response to SNP can be used to differentiate between reversible and fixed pulmonary hypertension. Because of conflicting data regarding the optimal measurement of pulmonary vascular resistance and because certain patients with moderate to severe pulmonary hypertension have been successfully transplanted,[3] investigators

TABLE 4. Preoperative Hemodynamics and Posttransplant Morbidity and Mortality

Hemodynamic Subset	No. of Patients	No. of Deaths—All-Cause (%)	No of Deaths—Primary Graft Failure (%)
A. TPG < 15 and PVR < 5	332	33 (9.9)	14 (4.2)
B. TPG < 15 and PVR ≥ 5	15	2 (13)	1 (6.7)
C. TPG ≥ 15 and PVR < 5	45	10 (21.7)*	7 (15.2)
D. TPG ≥ 15 and PVR ≥ 5	32	8 (25)*	6 (18.8)

* $p < 0.05$ when compared with A. TPG = transpulmonary gradient.

TABLE 5.   Preoperative Pulmonary Hypertension–Reactivity to Sodium Nitroprusside (SNP)

Group	PVR	SNP	PVR-SNP	SAP	N	90-Day Mortality
A	≤ 2.5	No	—	—	140	7.1%
B	> 2.5	Yes	≤ 2.5	≥ 85	78	3.8%
C	> 2.5	Yes	≤ 2.5	< 85	40	27.5%
D	> 2.5	Yes	> 2.5	—	32	40.6%

sought to further define the relationship of preoperative right-sided hemodynamic status to the risk of post-OHT right heart failure and death. Costard-Jäckle examined pulmonary vasodilatory response in heart-failure candidates and its correlation with post-OHT outcome.[16] Multivariate analysis of 301 patients undergoing OHT revealed that response of pulmonary pressures to SNP challenge in the preoperative period was a stronger predictor of right ventricular failure and death than baseline preoperative pulmonary hemodynamics. Four risk groups were differentiated by hemodynamic criteria (Table 5).

Patients in whom elevated baseline PVR could be reduced to less than 2.5 Wood units with SNP while maintaining a systolic blood pressure ≥ 85 mmHg had a 3-month mortality rate comparable with the patients with normal baseline PVR and were considered "low risk." In contrast, patients whose pulmonary vascular resistance could not be lowered below 2.5 Wood units with SNP as well as those patients in whom this could only be achieved at the expense of significant systemic hypotension (systolic blood pressure less than 85 mmHg) had a six-fold higher 3-month postoperative, all-cause mortality compared with the low-risk groups ($p < 0.0001$). The hemodynamic response to SNP not only identified patients at high risk of dying early after OHT, but also identified those patients at risk for developing and/or dying from right heart failure early after operation. These data demonstrate that the response of right heart hemodynamics to vasodilator challenge is a better predictor of early mortality after OHT than baseline PVR but underscores that valid risk stratification based on this response requires consideration of the concomitant change in systemic pressure.

Although earlier studies have suggested that PVRI or TPG better identified patients at risk for early post-OHT right heart failure and/or death than PVR, these authors found that PVR ≥ 2.5 identified patients at high risk of early postoperative death with similar accuracy to that of other measures of resistance but was superior in specifically identifying those at risk of death from right heart failure, suggesting that PVR should be used specifically for that purpose.

ACCURACY OF OTHER VASODILATORS IN IDENTIFYING THE HIGH-RISK PATIENT

Newer agents to assess reactivity of the pulmonary vascular bed include prostaglandin E_1 (PGE_1), prostacyclin (PGI_2), adenosine, and inhaled nitric oxide. PGE_1 is a potent vasodilator that is 85 to 90% cleared by a single pass through the lungs. This makes it useful as a relatively selective pulmonary vasodilator because its systemic effects are minimized by this first pass effect. Armitage reported that PGE_1 was effective in the perioperative treatment of pulmonary hypertension after OHT and suggested its use to test pulmonary vascular reactivity in OHT candidates with pulmonary hypertension.[17] Similar results were obtained by other investigators.[18] Murali retrospectively analyzed data comparing the hemodynamic effects of comparable doses of PGE_1, nitroglycerin, SNP, dobutamine, and enoximone in 66 heart-failure patients undergoing OHT evaluation to determine which agent was most effective in reversing pulmonary hypertension.[19] The magnitude of decline of PVR was greatest with PGE_1, which was the only agent that also significantly lowered TPG. This was later confirmed in a prospective study.[20] Although higher doses can potentially result in systemic vasodilatation and hypotension, effective pulmonary vasodilatation can usually be achieved with a 2 to 10 µg/kg/min infusion without significant risk of concomitant systemic hypotension.

Prostacyclin, unlike PGE_1 is a nonselective vasodilator which has been shown to reduce PVR effectively in patients with primary pulmonary hypertension.[21] Prostacyclin has been recently shown to be useful for the treatment of post-OHT pulmonary hypertension and right heart failure. However, it had no greater pulmonary selectivity than equipotent doses of SNP.[22] Prostacyclin is still an investigational drug and is thus limited in availability.

Adenosine has been shown to possess selective pulmonary vasodilatory activity in normal subjects and in patients with primary pulmonary hypertension, but has only recently been evaluated in patients with heart failure. Haywood examined acute pulmonary vascular reactivity in 29 patients referred for OHT using adenosine and SNP.[23] Administration of adenosine (100 µg/kg/min) or SNP resulted in similar decreases in PVR (approximately 40%) but adenosine lowered TPG more than SNP (35% vs. 9%, $p < 0.02$) while increasing left atrial pressure. Because of its adverse effect on left atrial pressure, adenosine appears poorly suited as a maintenance therapy in patients with left ventricular failure; however, it may be useful in acutely testing pulmonary vascular reactivity. Adenosine is also expensive and produces dysphoric effects in some patients.

Emerging reports state that inhaled nitric oxide (NO) may be useful in determining pulmonary vascular reactivity in OHT candidates. Inhaled NO selectively dilates ventilated lung areas but does not cause systemic vasodilation because of the inhalation strategy and the rapid inactivation of NO in blood by its combination with hemoglobin. Case reports describe the efficacy of inhaled NO in treating pulmonary hypertension after cardiac surgery and OHT.[24,25] Semigran and others used inhaled NO to evaluate pulmonary vascular reactivity before OHT.[26] When compared with SNP, inhaled NO was as effective in reducing PVR and TPG without the limitation of systemic hypotension. Kieler-Jensen compared the hemodynamic effects of increasing concentrations of inhaled NO to SNP and PGI_2 in OHT candidates with elevated PVR.[27] Nitric oxide at 20 ppm significantly lowered TPG and PVR with no further effect at higher doses. All three agents lowered PVR to a similar degree but only NO significantly lowered TPG. In this study of patients with severe heart failure, NO inhalation did not decrease the mean PAP as seen when given to patients with chronic pulmonary hypertension. The beneficial vasodilating effects of NO inhalation must be weighed against the potentially toxic effects of NO and its byproducts, as well as possible cytotoxic effects and inhibitory effects on platelet aggregation.[28] At present, the role of NO in the setting of heart failure patients with elevated PVR is unclear. Because the long-term effects of inhaled NO are not well studied, it appears prudent to restrict NO therapy to short-term use, employing the minimum effective concentration in the smallest possible amount of oxygen and avoiding prolonged mixing before administration.

LONG-TERM VASODILATOR THERAPY FOR PULMONARY HYPERTENSION

Although vasodilator agents are useful to test pulmonary vascular reactivity, many heart-failure patients do not respond to a single vasodilator challenge or vasodilators used without inotropic agents. Amrinone, a phosphodiesterase inhibitor with vasodilator and inotropic actions, primarily reduces right ventricular afterload and is effective in the treatment of severe right heart failure.[29] Bolling reported that sustained infusions of amrinone lowered both TPG and PVR in patients awaiting OHT who were refractory to SNP.[30] Patients received an 0.75 mg/kg loading dose of amrinone followed by continuous infusion, titrated to a TPG < 15 or PVR < 3, until the time of OHT (range 0.5 to 7 days, mean 3 days) with an average dose of 9 µg/kg/min (range 5 to 20 µg/kg/min). Twenty-four of 27 patients had significant decreases in TPG and PVR with amrinone therapy, as well as an increase in cardiac output ($p < 0.001$). There was no significant change in SVR, right atrial pressure, or mean arterial pressure. Twenty-one patients went on to OHT with 20 surviving to discharge (perioperative mortality 5%). One patient who responded to amrinone and had acceptable pulmonary pressures at the time of OHT died from severe right heart failure in the early postoperative period. Of note is that he had been switched to oral milrinone before OHT. The only adverse side effects were two instances of thrombocytopenia that responded to platelet transfusions.

Deeb compared prolonged amrinone infusion with conventional heart failure therapy (digitalis, diuretics, and captopril) in OHT candidates refractory to vasodilator challenge with SNP.[31] Both regimens were effective in lowering pulmonary hemodynamic values to a suitable range for OHT. A similar number of patients in each group responded to therapy, but the response time of pulmonary pressures to therapy was significantly less in the amrinone group (3.5 days vs. 8.2 days, $p < 0.05$). Time to OHT was shorter (27 days vs. 8.5 months) and pre-OHT survival was significantly higher in the amrinone group (91% vs. 63%, $p < 0.05$). There were no perioperative deaths in either group. Amrinone achieved a more effective rate of response but required continuous infusion to maintain that effect. None of the patients in Bolling's or Deeb's studies responded to the loading dose of amrinone, rather it was only after prolonged infusion (0.5–7 days, mean 3.5 days) that improvement in pulmonary hypertension was seen. This suggests that amrinone is not helpful in the setting of acute vasodilatory challenge to determine pulmonary reactivity. No data exist on the use of milrinone in acute or chronic vasodilator challenge in heart transplant candidates with pulmonary hypertension.

Iberer and Wasler also reported improved pulmonary hemodynamics after a 6- to 8-day infusion of PGE$_1$ in combination with catecholamines in OHT candidates with elevated PVR.[32] In this cohort, the pulmonary hemodynamic benefit *persisted up to 4 months* after PGE$_1$ infusion was discontinued. Unfortunately, all patients had severe side effects at the mean maintenance dose of 35 ng/kg/min (range 25 to 60 ng/kg/min), requiring concomitant intravenous analgesics, diuretics, and catecholamines to ameliorate systemic hypotension, tachycardia, digital edema, joint pain, headache, and abdominal pain. Patients with pulmonary hypertension treated with PGE$_1$ actually had *better* pre-OHT survival ($p < 0.005$) when compared with candidates without pulmonary hypertension despite similar waiting times. Post-OHT survival was similar. It should be noted that, although prostaglandins acutely lower pulmonary pressures in a variety of conditions, administration of prostaglandins without catecholamines yields no long-lasting benefits.[33]

Short-term manipulation of pulmonary hypertension may appear more important than its long-term reduction because the risk of post-OHT right ventricular failure is particularly high intraoperatively and in the first few hours after surgery.[2] As waiting times for donor organs increase, however, long-term reduction of pulmonary pressures may become necessary to ensure better pre-OHT survival in candidates with elevated PVR.

ERA OF TRANSPLANTATION AND POSTTRANSPANT MORTALITY

As the worldwide experience in OHT has evolved, there have been significant modifications in recipient and donor selection, immunosuppressive protocols, and postoperative management. With the resultant improved survival and the increasingly sophisticated preoperative screening of OHT candidates, PVR may have lost some predictive value as OHT candidates become a more homogeneous group. Murali stratified post-OHT mortality data by pre-OHT pulmonary hemodynamics with respect to the era of OHT in 425 OHT patients between 1980 and 1991.[12]

Before 1988, the 0–2-day mortality rate was significantly higher in patients with TPG ≥ 15 or PVR ≥ 5 but this difference was no longer present in patients who had transplants after 1988. A multivariate analysis of data from the Cardiac Transplant Research Database (CTRD) identified risk factors for death after OHT by analyzing the total primary OHT experience (n = 911) among 25 institutions from January 1, 1990 through June 30, 1991.[34] Risk factors for death during the study period included extremes of age, ventilator support at the time of OHT, abnormal renal function, lower pre-OHT cardiac output, longer donor ischemic time, older donor age, and donor/recipient blood type not being 0. Elevated pre-OHT PVR was only a risk factor for death in recipients younger than age 16.

TREATMENT OPTIONS IN PATIENTS WITH ELEVATED PULMONARY PERFUSION PRESSURES

Heterotopic Heart Transplantation

Heterotopic heart transplantation (HHT), developed a few years after OHT, was initially reported to be advantageous for patients with severe pulmonary hypertension. The rationale for HHT was that the recipient's hypertrophied right ventricle would support the pulmonary circulation, thus avoiding acute afterload increase in the heterotopically grafted right ventricle. Because, however, there is prompt improvement in pulmonary hemodynamics postoperatively, the native right ventricle is not necessary to support the pulmonary circulation. Additionally, subsequent reports have shown that patients undergoing HHT have decreased postoperative survival when compared with OHT. In a study of patients with PVR ≥ 4 undergoing either OHT or HHT, HHT was associated with higher risk of death than OHT.[35] OHT patients were smaller and received larger donor hearts with shorter ischemic times than HHT patients, reflecting patient selection and surgical complexity. Comparison between hospital survivors and nonsurvivors identified the selection of HHT and graft ischemic time in excess of 150 minutes as potent risk factors for death after transplantation. The incidence of graft failure was similar between groups, but HHT recipients frequently developed pulmonary complications and infection, resulting in a 30% hospital survival in contrast to a 71% survival in OHT recipients (p < 0.05).

Multiple factors underlie this increased mortality. HHT is technically more difficult to perform than OHT. In HHT, the failing ventricles are not removed, often contract poorly, often do not eject, and may chronically fibrillate. They represent a source both of infection and emboli. Preservation of the original heart can result in continuing angina. The position of the heterotopic transplant can cause significant obstruction of the right and middle lobes of the lung, leading to atelectasis and pulmonary insufficiency, further limiting survival.

Preoperative pulmonary hypertension has been found to be a potent risk factor among HHT as well as OHT recipients.[35] HHT in patients with preoperative pulmonary hypertension carries much higher risks than in other patients undergoing HHT or in OHT recipients with comparable pretransplant pulmonary hypertension. Therefore, preoperative pulmonary hypertension is no longer considered a good indication for HHT, further restricting its use. Many centers now use OHT of an oversized donor heart for patients with preoperative pulmonary hypertension.

Oversized Donor Hearts in Patients with Elevated Pulmonary Vascular Resistance

It is commonplace to use donors whose body weight is equal to or greater than that of the recipient for OHT candidates with significant preoperative pulmonary hypertension. It is believed that the larger donor heart has a greater ability to adapt to the recipients' elevated PVR without right-ventricular dilatation and failure. It is also hoped that this early adaptation will improve long-term allograft function and survival and prevent the development of restrictive physiology.

Some investigators have recently challenged this practice, suggesting that the use of oversized hearts is unnecessary. To determine the effects of donor/recipient weight mismatch on allograft function and survival, Costanzo-Nordin retrospectively compared the clinical and hemodynamic features of OHT recipients weighing more than their donor (undersized) with those weighing less than their donor (oversized).[36] They were further divided by preoperative TPG ≥ 12 or < 12 mmHg during SNP infusion. Patients with donor weight greater than recipient ideal weight (DW > RW) had a significantly greater risk of death compared with patients with DW < RW (relative risk = 2.19, $p < 0.05$). The risk of death remained greater in oversized than in undersized OHT recipients after adjustments were made for age, gender, and preoperative TPG. These data suggest that oversizing of donor hearts does not improve the outcome of OHT recipients with preoperative pulmonary hypertension that can be partially or completely reversed with SNP infusion. They also suggest that undersizing of donor hearts does not predict a poor outcome after OHT. Increased risk of death in recipients of oversized hearts than in recipients of undersized hearts may result from poorer myocardial preservation of larger hearts than smaller ones.

Yeoh analyzed OHT patients in whom there was donor:recipient size mismatching and found no significant correlation between PVR or heart allograft size and mortality.[37] Interestingly, their group evaluated long-term cardiopulmonary function by measuring both resting and exercise hemodynamics and oxygen uptake 1 year after OHT. In patients with moderate preoperative pulmonary hypertension (PVR ≥ 3) exercise capacity was better in recipients of sized-matched (D:R = 0.75 to 1.25) than oversized hearts (donor:recipient weight ratio > 1.25). In the absence of pulmonary hypertension, undersized allografts (D:R < 0.75) had adapted to their hosts, maintaining normal cardiac output, and the recipients had exercise profiles similar to that of patients with size-matched allografts. These data support that of Costanzo-Nordin and suggest that undersized allografts continue to accommodate to their hosts more than 3 months after OHT.

Domino Heart Transplantation (DHT)

Some patients undergoing heart-lung transplantation (HLT) have irreversible cardiac dysfunction, whereas others have well-preserved cardiac function. This latter group can, in turn, serve as donors of cardiac allografts at the time of HLT, the so-called "domino procedure."[38] Some HLT recipients have elevated pulmonary vascular resistance resulting in a "conditioned," hypertrophied right ventricle. Some authors have suggested that the use of such hearts for OHT has theoretic appeal for heart failure patients with elevated pulmonary vascular resistance. However, the use of domino hearts in these circumstances remains unproved.

Papworth Hospital in Cambridge, England, has a large experience with domino heart transplantation (DHT). Oaks reviewed the Papworth experience from 1988 to 1992, comparing 32 DHT recipients with 166 non-domino (OHT) recipients.[38] Pretransplant recipient characteristics, including PVR, were similar between groups. There was no difference in 3-month (85% vs. 83%) or 1-year (74% vs. 76%) survival between domino and non-domino recipients. Advantages of the domino procedure are a shorter ischemic time (if the organ is used in the same institution), the ability to perform a more complete pretransplant evaluation of the donor heart; including HLA matching, the absence of adverse neural, endocrine, and metabolic changes associated with brain death and the absence of physical trauma that may occur in cadaveric donors from motor vehicle accidents. The disadvantages of DHT are the necessity of separate superior and inferior venal caval anastomoses during the heart-lung procedure rather than the simpler right atrial anastomosis. Whether DHT will be beneficial in the setting of heart transplant candidates with pulmonary hypertension is unknown and awaits further investigation.

SUMMARY

Preoperative pulmonary hypertension, whether reflected by PVR, PVRI, or TPG, clearly increases the risk of post-OHT right heart failure and death. This risk has been shown to vary continuously, rather than sharply increasing at some specific value. Therefore, there is no support in the data presented for establishing a precise level of PVR beyond which OHT is contraindicated. The level of preoperative TPG appears to be a more reliable predictor of early postoperative mortality than PVR, whereas the PVR appears to be a more reliable predictor of postoperative right-ventricular failure, necessitating the use of both values to assess risk. The response of pulmonary hemodynamics to vasodilator challenge is more sensitive and specific than baseline values in estimating risk. Therefore, all OHT candidates should undergo preoperative right heart catheterization with measurement of TPG and PVR, and, if elevated, should receive a vasodilator challenge. If the acute response is unsatisfactory, then a longer trial with phosphodiesterase inhibitors or PGE_1 may be considered. The use of HHT, DHT, or oversized donor hearts has not yet been demonstrated to provide additional benefit in the setting of heart transplant candidates with pulmonary hypertension.

Figure 1 shows the vasodilator protocol used by the Rush-Presbyterian St. Luke's Heart Failure and Transplant Program for heart transplant candidates with pulmonary hypertension. If, on initial right heart catheterization, the PVR is ≥ 2.5 Wood units and the TPG is ≥ 12, nitroprusside 50 mg in 250 ml 5% D/W is started at 0.25 µg/kg/min and increased every 3 to 5 minutes by the following regimen until hemodynamic goals are achieved or until systolic B/P ≤ 85 mmHg. PGE_1 500 µg in 250 ml 5% DW infusion is used if the patient is refractory to the SNP challenge and the systolic B/P is > 90 mmHg.

Nitroprusside regimen	PGE1 regimen
0.5 µg/kg/min × 3–5 min	Start at 0.01 µg/kg/min and increase 0.0025 µg/kg/min
1.0 µg/kg/min × 3–5 min	every 15 min until a maximum of 0.05–0.10 µg/kg/min
1.5 µg/kg/min × 3–5 min	or hemodynamic goals are met or B/P < 85 mmHg.
2.0 µg/kg/min × 3–5 min	Taper off over 30 minutes.
2.5 µg/kg/min × 3–5 min	
3.0 µg/kg/min × 3–5 min	

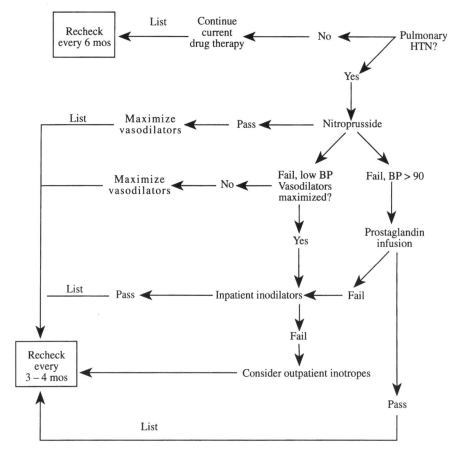

Key: Pulmonary HTN = PVR ≥ 2.5 Wood units and TPG ≥ 12
Pass = PVR < 2.5 Wood units and TPG < 12
Fail = PVR ≥ 2.5 Wood units and TPG ≥ 12
List = list for orthotopic heart transplantation (OHT)
HTN = hypertension; PVR = pulmonary vascular resistance; TPG = transplulmonary gradient.

FIGURE 1. Rush heart failure and transplant program: algorithm for protocol for pulmonary hypertension.

Because of present day preemptive elimination of OHT candidates with high PVR, clinicians are faced with an extremely narrow spectrum of PVR (or TPG) values in their potential candidates. Whether indices of pulmonary vascular status retain the same degree of predictive power within this narrow spectrum that they formerly possessed when applied to the broader range of values in years past is, as yet, uncertain. Additionally, with the recent, marked improvement in overall OHT survival, it has become increasingly difficult to demonstrate meaningful mortality correlations with traditional risk factors. PVR may retain predictive value when considering younger (< 16) and female patients for OHT. The predictive value of PVR may be further confounded by manipulations of PVR with long-term pre-OHT vasodilator therapy with amrinone or the preemptive use of prophylactic prostaglandin therapy perioperatively. Further studies treating PVR as a continuous variable with relation to risk of death are necessary. Better ways to establish the case of death post-OHT will separate allograft failure from right ventricular dysfunction secondary to preoperative pulmonary hypertension as compared with dysfunction from preservation injury or hyperacute rejection.

REFERENCES

1. Grossman W, Braunwald E: Pulmonary hypertension. In Braunwald E: Heart Disease: A Textbook of Cardiovascular Medicine, 4th ed. Philadelphia, W.B. Saunders, 1992, pp 790–816.
2. Bourge RC, Kirklin JK, Naftel DC, et al: Analysis and predictors of pulmonary vascular resistance after cardiac transplantation. J Thorac Cardiovasc Surg 101:432–435, 1991.
3. Addonizio J, Gersony WM, Robbins RC, et al: Elevated pulmonary vascular resistance and cardiac transplantation. Circulation 76(Supp V):V-52–55, 1976.
4. Kormos RL, Thompson M, Hardesty RL, et al: Utility of preoperative right heart catheterization data as a predictor of survival after heart transplantation. J Heart Transplant 5:391, 1986.
5. Erickson KW, Costanzo-Nordin MR, O'Sullivan EJ, et al: Influence of preoperative transpulmonary gradient on late mortality after cardiac transplantation. J Heart Transplant 9:526–537, 1990.
6. Bhatia SJ, Kirshenbaum JM, Shemin RJ, et al: Time course of resolution of pulmonary hypertension and right ventricular remodeling after orthotopic cardiac transplantation. Circulation 76:819–826, 1987.
7. Griepp RB, Stinson EB, Dong E, et al: Determinants of operative risk in human heart transplantation. Am J Surg 122:192–197, 1971.
8. Baumgartner WA, Reitz BA, Oyer PE, et al: Cardiac homotransplantation. In Current Problems in Surgery. Chicago, Year-Book Medical Publishers Inc., 1979, pp 1–61.
9. O'Connell JB, Bourge RC, Costanzo-Nordin MR, et al: Cardiac transplantation: Recipient selection, donor procurement and medical follow-up. Circulation 86:1061–1079, 1992.
10. Copeland JC, Emery RW, Levinson MM, et al: Selection of patients for cardiac transplantation. Circulation 75:1–9, 1987.
11. Kirklin JK, Naftel DC, Kirklin JW, et al: Pulmonary vascular resistance and the risk of heart transplantation. J Heart Transplant 7:331–336, 1988.
12. Murali S, Kormos RL, Uretsky BF, et al: Preoperative pulmonary hemodynamics and early mortality after orthotopic cardiac transplantation: The Pittsburgh experience. Am Heart J 126:896–904, 1993.
13. Costard-Jäckle A, Hill I, Schroeder JS, et al: The influence of preoperative patient characteristics on early and late survival following cardiac transplantation. Circulation 84(Suppl III):III-329–III-337, 1991.
14. Simonsen S, Molstad P, Geiran O, et al: Heart transplantation in patients with severe pulmonary hypertension and increased pulmonary vascular resistance. Scand J Thor Cardiovasc Surg 24:161–164, 1990.
15. Bixler TJ, Gott VL, Gardner TJ, et al: Reversal of experimental pulmonary hypertension with sodium nitroprusside. J Thorac Cardiovasc Surg 81:537–545, 1981.
16. Costard-Jäckle A, Fowler MB: Influence of preoperative pulmonary artery pressure on mortality after heart transplantation: Testing of potential reversibility of pulmonary hypertension with nitroprusside is useful in defining a high risk group. J Am Coll Card 19:48–54, 1992.
17. Armitage JM, Hardesty RL, Griffith BP: Prostaglandin E1: An effective treatment of right heart failure after orthotopic heart transplantation. J Heart Transplant 6:348–351, 1987.
18. Weiss CI, Park JV, Bolman RM: Prostaglandin E1 for treatment of elevated pulmonary vascular resistance in patients undergoing cardiac transplantation. Transplant Proc 21:2555–2256, 1989.
19. Murali S, Uretsky BF, Reddy S, et al: Reversibility of pulmonary hypertension in congestive heart failure patients evaluated for cardiac transplantation: Comparative effects of various pharmacologic agents. Am Heart J 122:1375–1381, 1991.
20. Murali S, Uretsky BF, Armitage JM, et al: Utility of prostaglandin E1 in the pretransplantation evaluation of heart failure patients with significant pulmonary hypertension. J Heart Lung Transplant 11:716–723, 1992.
21. Palevsky HI, Long W, Crow J, et al: Prostacyclin and acetylcholine as screening agents for acute pulmonary vasodilator responsiveness in primary hypertension. Circulation 82:2018–2026, 1990.
22. Kieler-Jensen N, Milocco I, Ricksten S: Pulmonary vasodilation after heart transplantation. A comparison among prostacyclin, sodium nitroprusside, and nitroglycerin on right ventricular function and pulmonary selectivity. J Heart Lung Transplant 12:179–184, 1993.
23. Haywood GA, Sneddon JF, Bashir Y, et al: Adenosine infusion for the reversal of pulmonary vasoconstriction in biventricular failure. A good test but a poor therapy. Circulation 86:896–902, 1992.
24. Tibbals J: Clinical applications of gaseous nitric oxide. Anaesth Intensive Care 21:866–871, 1993.
25. Foubert L, Latimer R, Oduro A, et al: Use of inhaled nitric oxide to reduce pulmonary hypertension after heart transplantation [letter, comment]. J Cardiothorac Vasc Anesth 7:640–641, 1993.
26. Semigran MJ, Cockrill BA, Kacmarek R, et al: Nitric oxide is an effective pulmonary vasodilator in cardiac transplant candidates with pulmonary hypertension. J Heart Lung Transplant 12:S67, 1993.

27. Kieler-Jensen N, Ricksten S, Stenquist O, et al: Inhaled nitric oxide in the evaluation of heart transplant candidates with elevated pulmonary resistance. J Heart Lung Transplant 13:366–375, 1994.
28. Rossaint R, Pison U, Gerlach H, et al: Inhaled nitric oxide: Its effects on pulmonary circulation and airway smooth muscle cells. Eur Heart J 14(Suppl I):133–140, 1993.
29. Konstam MA, Cohen SR, Salem DN, et al: Effect of amrinone on right ventricular function: Predominance of afterload reduction. Circulation 74:359–366, 1986.
30. Bolling SF, Deeb GM, Crowley DC, et al: Prolonged amrinone therapy prior to orthotopic cardiac transplantation in patients with pulmonary hypertension. Transplant Proc 20:753–756, 1988.
31. Deeb GM, Bolling SF, et al: Amrinone versus conventional therapy in pulmonary hypertensive patients awaiting cardiac transplantation. Ann Thorac Surg 48:665–669, 1989.
32. Iberer F, Wasler A, Tscheliessnigg K, et al: Prostaglandin E1-induced moderation of elevated pulmonary resistance. Survival on waiting list and results of orthotopic heart transplantation. J Heart Lung Transplant 12:173–178, 1993.
33. Higgenbottam T, Wheeldon D, Wells F, et al: Long term treatment of primary pulmonary hypertension with continuous epoprostenol (prostacyclin). Lancet 1:1046–1047, 1984.
34. Bourge RC, Naftel DC, Costanzo-Nordin MR, et al: Pretransplantation risk factors for death after heart transplantation: A multiinstitutional study. J Heart Lung Transplant 12:549–562, 1993.
35. Kawaguchi A, Gandjbakhch I, Pavie A, et al: Cardiac transplant recipients with preoperative pulmonary hypertension. Circulation 80(Suppl III):III-90–III-96, 1989.
36. Costanzo-Nordin MR, Liao Y, Grusk BB, et al: Oversizing of donor hearts: Beneficial or detrimental? J Heart Lung Transplant 10:717–730, 1991.
37. Yeoh T, Frist WH, Lagerstrom C, et al: Relationship of cardiac allograft size and pulmonary vascular resistance to long-term cardiopulmonary function. J Heart Lung Transplant 11:1168–1176, 1992.
38. Oaks TE, Aravot D, Dennis C, et al: Domino heart transplantation: The Papworth experience. J Heart Lung Transplant 13:433–437, 1994.

Chapter 5

Surgical Alternatives to Transplantation: High-Risk Cardiac Repair Procedures— Cardiomyoplasty and Permanent VAD

Timothy V. Votapka, MD
D. Glenn Pennington, MD

As transplant centers have become increasingly disillusioned with long waiting lists and chronic complications of transplantation such as rejection, infection, and graft atherosclerosis, a general proclivity is developing to pursue conventional forms of treatment for certain subsets of patients referred for transplant evaluation. Although these patients certainly represent a high-risk cohort, it is becoming increasingly clear that reparative procedures, whether valvular or revascularization, can be performed at acceptable mortality rates. If patients are to be exposed to the risks of conventional surgery, then it is important that the operative mortality rates, long-term survival, and functional recovery be comparable to transplantation. This is especially true if this is considered an endpoint procedure. Because the ten-year actuarial survival rate for heart transplantation is approximately 50%, some younger patients may prefer, and be better served by, a reparative procedure which would provide them with several years of quality life before cardiac transplantation. This staging technique could extend total survival time by a significant percentage. As with any procedure, the quality of life provided would have to be evaluated. In addition, in the current climate of health care cost control, it is also necessary that the chosen treatment option have an acceptable cost-benefit ratio.

It is not surprising that the definition of a "high risk" cardiac surgical candidate has changed over time. Early reports of high-risk patients or patients with severely dysfunctional hearts focused on patients with ejection fractions less than 0.35.[1,2] Many, if not most, patients considered for transplantation have ejection fractions of less than 0.20, a degree of dysfunction earlier felt to be incompatible with operative survival. Although it is the most common parameter used to identify this cohort of patients, the use of ejection fraction as a risk factory may be questioned. It is not unusual even in a patient in overt heart failure to find a rather acceptable ejection fraction. The ejection fraction provides only a *snapshot* view of cardiac performance in a certain environment, with certain treatment modalities present and with a certain state of patient anxiety.[3] As such it may not provide an accurate assessment of a given patient's routine cardiac performance. Tests such as exercise-induced oxygen consumption and coronary artery flow reserve may better identify this high-risk subgroup and perhaps should be more universally reported when analyzing surgical results.

Identifying which patients have such dysfunctional myocardium that they are truly *inoperable* is clearly the most important and difficult analysis to make. Several authors have suggested that patients who present with angina are better candidates than those who present primarily with heart failure.[3-5] Not only does the presence of angina suggest that there is at least some viable *hibernating* myocardium, but those with symptoms of heart failure almost invariably have some degree of end organ dysfunction, thus making postoperative recovery problematic. Patients who have had previous revascularization or valvular procedures tend to respond particularly poorly and probably represent at least a relative contraindication to high-risk cardiac surgery.[6] Louie and co-workers attempted to correlate successful outcome with preoperative measurements of left ventricular end diastolic dimension (LVEDD) and found that the mean LVEDD for survivors was 68 mm vs. 81 mm for nonsurvivors.[7] Most current attempts at identifying patients who can be expected to have reasonable outcomes involve imaging viable myocardium, either through thallium studies or positron emission tomography (PET).[3,7] Although volumes of information regarding these techniques are available, reliably predicting which patients will survive operation still is not possible.

Despite their significant debilities, survival rates in reporting series of such patients are surprisingly good. Kron and colleagues[3] reported on a series of patients who had ejection fractions of less than 0.20 and all of whom underwent revascularization. In that series, the operative mortality rate was only 2.6%. By life-table analysis, that series of patients had a three-year survival rate of 83%. Blakeman's series of patients,[6] with a mean ejection fraction of 18%, included patients who underwent revascularization alone or revascularization and valve replacement, and also included 10 patients who had had previous cardiac surgery. In this series, the operative mortality rate was 15%. At a mean of 1 year follow-up, nine of the original 20 patients in the series had either died or had required heart transplantation. Sanchez and coworkers[8] presented a series of patients requiring either bypass grafting, valve replacement, or both, with a mean ejection fraction of 0.28 for the entire group. The operative mortality rate in this group was 9%. With a mean follow-up of 25 months, the 1- and 2-year actuarial survival rates were 82% and 76%, respectively.

As of September 1994, at Saint Louis University we have performed high-risk reparative cardiac procedures on 32 patients. All of these patients were either referred to our center for transplant evaluation or developed hemodynamic compromise while in-patients and were considered for transplant. All procedures but one were done electively. There were 26 males and 6 females aged 40 to 61 years (mean 52 years). Left ventricular ejection fractions ranged from 10 to 40% (mean 25%) with 23 having only ischemic disease, four with only valve disease and five with ischemic and valve disease.

Eight of these 32 had previous cardiac surgery, five had intra-aortic balloon pumps pre-operatively, and seven were receiving inotropic drugs preoperatively. All patients were operated on with ventricular assist device on standby with the understanding that they would be bridged to transplant if appropriate. There were four operative deaths (12%), one of whom died in the operating room of bleeding and biventricular failure, one of whom received a left ventricular assist device (LVAD) and died of arrhythmias 9 days postoperatively (7 days after LVAD was removed), and two of whom died of sudden cardiac arrest 3 and 23 days postoperatively. After a mean follow-up time of 19 months, there were 3 late deaths at 6, 8, and 14 months; the actuarial 1-year survival postopera-tive was 81%. Of the seven total patient deaths, four patients had coronary bypass only, two had coronary bypass grafts plus valve replacement, and one had mitral valve re-placement alone. One patient was transplanted 8 months postoperatively.

In carefully selected series of patient subsets, it can be seen that operative mortal-ity rates can be compared with the operative mortality rates in transplantation. It is not yet clear how the long-term survival will compare between these two treatment strate-gies and even less clear how the functional results will compare. Although some studies have looked at postbypass ventricular function by gated blood pool studies or echocar-diography, little is known about these patients' necessity for frequent medical follow-up and their satisfaction with lifestyle. An equally important question, but because of the inherent complexities involved in data acquisition heretofore unanswered, is which of the two strategies is the most cost effective. Although conventional surgery ostensibly appears to be the least expensive, if such patients require repeated hospitalizations and admissions to intensive care and if a significant number eventually require transplanta-tion, then *a priori* transplantation may be more economically sound.

CARDIOMYOPLASTY

In 1984, when Carpentier described the first clinical use of stimulated muscle to augment myocardial function, he established a new mentality for the treatment of re-fractory heart failure.[9] Previous modalities for treating dysfunctional myocardium that no longer responded to medical regimens involved either removing the failing heart or attempting revascularization in the hope of restoring function to hibernating my-ocardium. From a very crude viewpoint, cardiomyoplasty attempts to *force* normal he-modynamic function from the failing heart by skeletal muscle actuation. From the mid-1980s until the present, well over 200 patients in the United States and Europe have undergone dynamic cardiomyoplasty procedures.[10] Only recently have good clini-cal follow-up studies become available, and although issues of indications for surgery and patient selection are still controversial, certain observations have been established.

The technique for wrapping the heart with latissimus dorsi has been well de-scribed.[11–13] Basically the latissimus dorsi is mobilized from the chest wall while its neu-rovascular bundle is preserved. In a separate procedure, several days later in a two-stage procedure, it is is first placed in the pleural space through a second or third rib space and then, through a median sternotomy, it is wrapped around the heart. After a 2-week recovery period, a 2-week muscle conditioning program is begun during which time the skeletal muscle is exposed to a progressive series of programmed electrical stimula-tions that are synchronized with ventricular contractions. At the end of this 6-week conditioning program, the muscle fibers have been transformed from the *fast-twitch* morphology to the nonfatigable *slow-twitch* morphology.

Early studies on laboratory animals revealed marked improvement in hemody-namic parameters, ventricular geometry, and cardiac performance.[11,14] Most of the stud-ies, however, were performed on animals with otherwise normal hearts and the validity of improved performance has been questioned. Clearly the results of clinical studies in which the muscle wraps have been performed in grossly abnormal hearts have been less conclusive and reproducible.

Most clinical studies suggest that the operative mortality for this procedure is between 10 and 30%.[12,15,16] One-year survival has been reported up to 65%.[15] Although these results are clearly disappointing, as with many such new procedures, most of the earliest patients operated on were the most compromised and the most desperate. As experience is gained in patient selection and operative technique, mortality rates will improve. Magovern et al. point out that although operative mortality rates have declined 6% as their group has gained experience with this procedure, the one-year survival has not improved.[15]

In contrast to survival studies, functional studies are encouraging. Most patients who survive the operation experience at least transient improvements in well-being. In comparing pre- and postoperative functional status, most studies have reported improvement by at least one NYHA functional class in patients who survive at least one year.[12,17,18] In their recent report, Magovern et al. found survivors improving from a mean NYHA class 3.3 to 1.9[15] Whether functional status improved as a result of the muscle wrap or whether the patients who survive a year are a selected group who have undergone myocardial recovery is not clear. A recent study by Bocchi et al. demonstrated significantly improved ejected fractions in survivors of cardiomyoplasty when their myostimulators were turned off.[16]

Studies of ventricular mechanics and hemodynamics are often confusing and equivocal. Although some studies document significant improvements in ventricular performance parameters, such as regional wall motion, end-diastolic pressure, systolic wall stress, and maximal elastance,[16,19] studies of more conventional end-points, such as cardiac output and ejection fraction, are more varied. Some researchers found no significant improvement in these basic parameters, although their patients may have an improved functional status.[15]

Improving patient selection criteria would seem to be the key to improving the results of this new modality. It has become clear that Class IV patients are poor candidates for this procedure.[12,18,20,21] Best results have been obtained in Class II and III patients; however, many question whether it is appropriate to expose patients doing this well to an operation with such significant mortality rates.[18] It is also becoming clear that only patients with left ventricular failure are reasonable candidates, as patients with even minimal degrees of right-sided failure have done poorly.[12,18,20]

PERMANENT VENTRICULAR ASSIST DEVICES

High-risk revascularization and dynamic cardiomyoplasty seem to be relatively conservative alternative procedures to heart transplantation and certainly represent currently available clinical procedures. These starkly contrast with the implantation of permanent ventricular assist devices (VAD). Although VADs have been used clinically for more than 15 years, and although long-term *wearable* VADS are available, they are approved only for use as a bridge to transplantation. Currently no federally funded trials of permanent VADS are under way in the United States; however, the shortage of organ donors fuels ongoing research at several centers. The complex proclivities of FDA regulations and the generalized limitations of available funding have significantly limited the number and size of active research programs.

Although it is the goal of most researchers in this field to one day have available a safe and reliable heart replacement device, it is probably more realistic to pursue initially a permanent heart assist device. Several reports suggest univentricular support is sufficient to reverse heart failure in the majority of patients.[22–24] Current incidence of right-heart failure following left ventricular assist (LVA) device placement is around 20% and should continue to decline with improvements in chemotherapeutic manipulations and patient selection.[22] In addition, many of the complications of mechanical circulatory support, such as thromboembolism and device-related infection can be expected to be lower with univentricular support versus total heart replacement. Patients requiring univentricular support also have superior survival rates compared with patients requiring biventricular support.[25,26] Obviously most data come from patient populations being bridged to transplantation; however, it seems reasonable to extrapolate this data to help predict expected outcome in the permanent VAD population.

There are currently two assist devices being utilized as a bridge to transplant that seem most likely to be revised for permanent implantation.[27] Thermocardiosystems Inc.'s (Woburn, MA) HeartMate and Novacor's (Novacor Division, Baxter Healthcare, Oakland, CA) LVAs are both electrically powered pulsatile implantable ventricular assist devices. Both these devices have undergone significant clinical trials of transient implantation with similar and encouraging results. Developers of these two devices, as well as developers of several other prototypes of mechanical pumps, are attempting to revise various biomechanical design features to make them compatible for permanent use. Clinical trials of the Novacor wearable vented system[28] as a permanent device have been initiated at Cambridge University in England. At this writing, the first patient had undergone implantation and was doing well. Thermocardiosystems and several of its clinical investigators plan to design and implement a similar study in the United States using the vented electrical HeartMate. By using a transcutaneous energy transfer system and compliance chamber, Novacor hopes to develop a totally implanted device without cables or cannulas traversing the abdominal or thoracic wall.

From a purely technologic standpoint, biomedical engineering expertise is available to produce these permanent devices. The major obstacles to their development are primarily financial. The cost of producing a device that can meet stringent FDA requirements and the testing involved to prove its safety and efficacy is a tremendous disincentive to its production. Current focus on health care costs and the national attention on the public cost-benefit ratio for public health care dollars has undoubtedly added further constraint to the rapid development of these much needed circulatory support systems.

REFERENCES

1. Killip T, Passamani E, Davis K: Coronary artery study (CASS): A randomized trial of coronary bypass surgery. Circulation 72(Suppl I):V102–V9, 1986.
2. Coles JG, Del Campo C, Ahmed SN, et al: Improved long-term survival following myocardial revascularization in patients with severe left ventricular dysfunction. J Thorac Cardiovasc Surg 1:846–850, 1981.
3. Kron IL, Flanagan TL, Blackbourne LH, et al: Coronary revascularization rather than cardiac transplantation for chronic ischemic cardiomyopathy. Ann Surg 210:348–354, 1989.
4. Hoehnberg MS, Parsonnet V, Gielchmsky I, Hossain SM: Coronary artery bypass grafting in patients with ejection fractions below forty percent. J Thorac Cardiovasc Surg 86:519–527, 1983.
5. Luciani GB, Faggian G, Razzolini R, et al: Severe ischemic left ventricular failure: Coronary operation or heart transplantation? Ann Thorac Surg 55:719–723, 1993.
6. Blakeman BM, Pifarre R, Sullivan H, et al: High-risk heart surgery in the heart transplant candidate. J Heart Transplant 9:468–72, 1990.
7. Louie HW, Laks H, Milgalter E, et al: Ischemic cardiomyopathy criteria for coronary revascularization and cardiac transplantation. Circulation 84(Suppl III):III290–III295, 1991.
8. Sanchez JA, Smith CR, Drusin RE, et al: High-risk reparative surgery: A neglected alternative to heart transplantation. Circulation 82(Suppl IV):IV302–IV305, 1990.
9. Carpentier A, Chacques JC: Myocardal substitution with a stimulated skeletal muscle: First successful clinical case. Lancet 1:1267, 1985.

10. Oakley RM: Current expectations in cardiomyoplasty [letter]. Ann Thorac Surg 56:1214, 1993.
11. Park SE, Cmolik BL, Lazzare RR, et al: Right latissimus dorsi cardiomyoplasty augments left ventricular systolic performance. Ann Thorac Surg 56:1290–1295, 1993.
12. Furnary AP, Magovern JA, Christlieb IY, et al: Clinical cardiomyoplasty: Preoperative factors associated with outcome. Ann Thorac Surg 54:1139–1143, 1992.
13. McGovern GJ, Heckler FR, Park SB: Paced skeletal muscle for dynamic cardiomyoplasty. Ann Thorac Surg 45:614–619, 1988.
14. Cheng W, Justicz AG, Soberman MS, et al: Effects of dynamic cardiomyoplasty on indices of left ventricular systolic and diastolic function in a canine model of chronic heart failure. J Thorac Cardiovasc Surg 103:1207–1213, 1992.
15. Macgovern JA, Magovern GJ, Maher TD, et al: Operation for congestive heart failure: Transplantation, coronary artery bypass and cardiomyoplasty. Ann Thorac Surg 56:418–425, 1993.
16. Bocchi EA, Moreira LFP, de Moraes AV, et al: Effects of dynamic cardiomyoplasty on regional wall motion, election fraction, and geometry of left ventricle. Circulation 86(Suppl II):II231–II235, 1992.
17. Almada H, Molteni L, Ferreira R, Ortega D: Clinical experience with dynamic cardiomyoplasty. J Cardiac Surg 5:193–198, 1990.
18. Magovern JA, Magovern GJ Jr, Magovern GJ, et al: Surgical therapy for congestive heart failure: Indications for transplantation versus cardiomyoplasty. J Heart Lung Transplant 11:538–544, 1992.
19. Bellotti G, Moraes A, Bocchi E, et al: Late effects of cardiomyoplasty on left ventricular mechanics and diastolic filling. Circulation 88(p. 2):304–308, 1993.
20. Jegaden O, Delahaye F, Montagna P, et al: Cardiomyoplasty does not preclude heart transplantation. Ann Thorac Surg 53:875–881, 1992.
21. Moreira LFP, Stolf NAG, Bocchi EA, et al: Latissimus dorsi cardiomyoplasty in the treatment of patients with dilated cardiomyopathy. Circulation 82(Suppl 4):257–263, 1990.
22. Oz MC, Levin HR, Rose EA: Wearable left ventricular assist device for long-term mechanical circulatory assistance. Cardiac Chronicle 7:1–7, 1993.
23. Frazier OH, Rose EA, Macmanus Q, et al: Multicenter clinical evaluation of the HeartMate 1000 IP left ventricular assist device. Ann Thorac Surg 53:1080–1090, 1992.
24. Estrada-Quintero T, Vestsry BF, Morali S, et al: Amelioration of the heart failure state with left ventricular assist system support. J Am Coll Card 19:254A, 1992.
25. Pennington DG, McBride LR, Peigh PS, et al: Eight years' experience with bridging to cardiac transplantation. J Thorac Cardiovasc Surg 107:472–481, 1994.
26. Farrar DJ, Hill JD: Univentricular and biventricular Thoratec VAD support as a bridge to transplantation. Ann Thorac Surg 55:276–282, 1993.
27. Saperstein JS, Pae WE Jr, Rosenberg G, Pierce WS: The development of permanent circulatory support systems. Semin Thorac Cardiovasc Surg 6:188–194, 1994.
28. Loisance DY, Deleuze PH, Mazzucotelli JP, et al: Clinical implantation of the wearable Baxter Novacor ventricular assist system. Ann Thorac Surg 58:551–554, 1994.

Strategies of Organ Preservation: Current and Future

Chapter **6**

Kirk J. Fleischer, MD
William A. Baumgartner, MD

Availability of donor organs remains the major limiting factor to heart transplantation. Fewer than 20% of potential recipients undergo transplantation each year because of the critical donor shortage. This scarcity of organs is compounded by the relatively short acceptable ischemic time of cardiac allografts.

Current clinical preservation techniques generally permit a "safe" ischemic period of 4 to 6 hours. Although numerous experimental studies have demonstrated significantly longer periods of storage without functional myocardial impairment, this has not been translated into safe extension of preservation times in humans. Two fundamental factors may explain why attempts to prolong ischemic times of the heart have not met with the same dramatic clinical success as seen with abdominal organs. First, it is imperative that transplanted cardiac allografts function immediately upon implantation. Although myocardial performance can be augmented to some degree with inotropic support, no convenient alternatives (e.g., dialysis) exist to support the severely failing heart through a period of delayed recovery. Second, unlike the kidney and liver, the heart poorly tolerates depletion of adenosine triphosphate (ATP) resulting in the development of ischemic contracture and ventricular dysfunction.

The status of the human donor heart at explanation is an additional factor not accounted for in laboratory preservation studies. Significant injury can result during management of the donor before heart procurement. Furthermore, in an attempt to increase the number of available organs, the profile of the donor pool has changed to accommodate a greater percentage of older donors and with it an unavoidable increase in baseline coronary artery disease in these allografts.[1]

The great importance of myocardial function in the early postoperative period cannot be overemphasized. Primary organ failure remains the leading cause of perioperative mortality and accounts for more than 25% of early recipient deaths. Moreover, 30-day, 1-year, and 5-year mortalities correlate with the duration of allograft ischemia even within the current clinically accepted time limits.[2,3] Therefore, in addition to rigorous selection criteria for donor hearts, optimal hypothermic preservation techniques are necessary to minimize early and late morbidity and mortality.

DONOR ORGAN INJURY

The donor heart is vulnerable to injury at all stages of transplantation. Factors contributing to the severity of postoperative myocardial dysfunction include insults associated with suboptimal donor management, hypothermia, ischemic-reperfusion injury, and depletion of energy stores.

Suboptimal Donor Management

Donor organ preservation begins long before procurement of the heart. Hemodynamic instability, loss of thermal regulation, and metabolic derangements accompanying brain death complicate management of these patients. Microinfarctions result from hypo- and hypertensive episodes. Electrolyte imbalances result in myocardial edema and predispose the donor to dysrhythmias. If aggressive efforts are not taken to minimize these inevitable events of brain death, one not only jeopardizes the potential suitability of the heart for transplantation, but more importantly, also increase likelihood of significant early and late dysfunction of the cardiac allograft.

Hypothermia

Hypothermia is the cornerstone of current organ preservation. Unfortunately, it also contributes to untoward cellular changes characteristic of ex vivo organ storage.[4] Tissue edema occurs as deep hypothermia inactivates membrane-bound enzymes and alters the permeability of lipid bilayers. Cell volume regulation is lost as the Na^+-K^+ ATPase pump is inhibited, permitting entry of sodium. To equalize the resultant osmotic gradient, water passively crosses the sarcolemma. The intracellular milieu is further altered by the sequestration of calcium due in part to hypothermic-inactivation of the Ca^+ ATPase pump.

Ischemic-Reperfusion Injury

The complex pathophysiology of myocardial ischemic-reperfusion injury involves many interrelated mechanisms still under intense investigation. Increasing evidence suggests the vast majority of damage is sustained during reperfusion, whereas longer ischemic times predispose to more extensive cellular injury at the restoration of coronary blood flow.

Oxygen Free Radicals

Oxygen-derived free radicals are highly reactive molecules that exert their cytotoxic effects through direct attack on cells or initiation of chain reactions leading to the formation of other harmful radicals.[5] Although their role in ischemia-reperfusion injury of the myocardium remains controversial because of their transient nature, convincing evidence is accumulating that these toxic oxygen species are intimately involved in this destructive phenomenon.

The endothelial xanthine oxidase pathway appears to be the primary source of oxygen radicals in postischemic tissue. Hypoxanthine, the purine substrate for this enzyme, accumulates in ischemic myocardium as ATP is catabolized. On reperfusion with oxygen-rich blood, a burst of superoxide and peroxide is synthesized. Additional concurrent biochemical pathways yield other oxygen radicals including singlet oxygen, hydroxyl radical, and peroxynitrite.

Cellular damage caused by reactive oxygen intermediates is often widespread. Peroxidation of membrane lipids and denaturation of proteins results in disruption of homeostatic mechanisms in myocytes and endothelial cells. Increased permeability of the cell membrane contributes to intracellular edema characteristic of the donor heart. Oxidative damage of the sarcoplasmic reticulum hinders calcium transport, whereas mitochondrial injury manifests as impaired oxidative phosphorylation. Ultrastructural injury from oxygen free radicals is amplified by the by-products of arachidonic acid oxidation, which act as chemotactic factors for the sequestration of leukocytes in the injured tissue.

Natural intracellular scavengers (e.g., superoxide dismutase, catalase, and peroxidase) protect against the normal accumulation of oxygen radicals. Under pathologic conditions such as ischemic-reperfusion, however, excess reactive oxygen intermediates overwhelm these endogenous antioxidant defense mechanisms leading to irreversible myocardial damage.

Leukocytes

Leukocytes also play an important role in myocardial reperfusion injury after ischemic storage of the donor heart. Expression of neutrophil adhesion molecules on the coronary vascular endothelium after hypoxic-ischemic insults results in binding of the leukocytes at reperfusion. In addition to causing mechanical obstruction of the capillaries, bound leukocytes synergistically release cytotoxic molecules including oxygen and halide radicals, granule proteases, as well as metabolites of arachidonic acid. Not only do these substances directly mediate tissue injury and local vasoconstriction, they also initiate the activation cascades of complement, platelets, and other neutrophils. This inflammatory response of cascade activation is magnified by the contact of the recipient's blood with the synthetic surfaces of the extracorporeal cardiopulmonary bypass circuit during transplantation.

Depletion of Energy Stores

Static cold storage inevitably results in exhaustion of high energy phosphate stores. Unlike the liver or kidney, which readily tolerate extended storage despite depletion of ATP, the heart must maintain sufficient ATP levels to prevent formation of ischemic contracture. Without exogenous substrates for energy metabolism, the allograft must resort to finite glycogen and lipid stores limiting the safe duration of storage.

MANIFESTATIONS OF PRESERVATION INJURY

Myocardial edema and ischemic contracture bands are the predominant histologic changes associated with heart preservation. The resultant postoperative myocardial dysfunction often manifests as diastolic stunning and reduced ventricular compliance. Donor electrolyte imbalances, hypothermia of storage, and ischemic-reperfusion injury are etiologies of tissue edema, which may affect both systolic and diastolic function. Development of contractures results from energy depletion and oxygen free radical-mediated injury to intracellular organelles with subsequent disturbance in calcium homeostasis. Mitochrondrial damage exacerbates the progressive depletion of energy stores associated with ischemia by further reduction of ATP availability. Altered membrane permeability and a reduction of Ca^{2+} ATPase activity in the sarcoplasmic reticulum in conjunction with this decrease in high-energy phosphates results in sluggish resequestration of calcium and in turn prolongation of diastolic relaxation. Cytosolic free calcium accumulates and binds with tropomyosin creating a high affinity state between actin and myosin. With depleted ATP, the actinomyosin cross-bridges are unable to be broken, and irreversible myocardial contracture and myocardial dysfunction occur in the transplanted heart.

Endothelial cell injury accompanying the global parenchymal insult may result in coronary vascular dysfunction. Depositions of activated leukocytes and platelets in capillary beds of the donor heart contribute to the development of the "low reflow" phenomenon occasionally observed at reperfusion.

DONOR MANAGEMENT

Medical management of donors must be considered an integral part of organ preservation. Optimal care requires that the donor be treated as any other ICU patient with invasive hemodynamic monitoring, ventilatory support, and meticulous attention to intravascular volume status, electrolytes and acid-base balance.[6] Some transplant centers have already established mobile intensive care teams that are dispatched to ensure appropriate management of these highly labile patients.

Hemodynamic instability may result from hypovolemia, vasomotor instability, or dysrhythmias. Maintenance of a mean arterial pressure near 80 mmHg involves volume therapy, inotropes (dopamine, dobutamine), afterload reduction (sodium nitroprusside, esmolol), or afterload augmentation (dopamine, Neosynephrine). Warming IV fluids as well as using warming lights and blankets reduces the incidence of hypothermia-induced dysrhythmias. Diabetes insipidus commonly develops and is managed with vasopressin, whereas volume and diuretics (furosemide, mannitol) treat episodes of oliguria. Myocardial benefits of donor pretreatment with triiodothyronine and insulin have been demonstrated in several series, but hormone replacement therapy continues to remain controversial.[7]

Brain death is a complex physiologic phenomenon. Better understanding its hemodynamic and metabolic effects will surely permit significant advancements in donor care. These refinements have an immediate impact on the quantity and quality of allografts harvested.

PRESERVATION STRATEGIES

Despite two decades of investigation, no single preservation regimen of the heart has yielded consistent, clinically significant improvement in allograft function. Controversy abounds regarding storage temperature, composition of cardioplegic and storage solutions, techniques of solution delivery, additives, and reperfusion modification.

Hypothermia

Hypothermia is the most important component of cardiac preservation and the only factor universally considered essential. The primary protective effect of hypothermia is a dramatic reduction of myocardial oxygen consumption and metabolic demands. Cold, arrested allografts have metabolic rates less than 2% of normal. Despite the reduction in temperature, anaerobic pathways of metabolism are sufficiently conserved to permit maintenance of ATP levels in the myocyte for at least 6 hours of ischemia. Metabolism is still ongoing, albeit at a slower rate, and thus hypothermia can provide only a finite amount of protection as energy stores are eventually depleted and toxic metabolites accumulate. Additional benefits of hypothermia include suppression of the activity of hydrolytic enzymes as well as microbial growth in the allograft.

Target temperature depends on the institution and generally ranges between 0 and 7°C. Experimental evidence suggests that 4°C, the temperature of melting ice, provides the best protection. Although the majority of centers report using this as their goal, few actually monitor the temperature of the storage solution.

Cardioplegic Solutions

Perfusion of the donor heart with a cardioplegic solution to achieve electromechanical arrest is an invaluable adjunct to topical hypothermia. Crystalloid solutions of widely differing compositions are currently available. They are classified as either *intracellular* or *extracellular* depending on their ionic composition.

Intracellular solutions are characterized by low concentrations of sodium. They also contain moderate to high concentrations of potassium and little or no calcium. By mimicking the normal intracellular environment, these solutions reduce the electrochemical gradients of ions across the cell membrane. The primary potential benefit of such a composition is reduction of hypothermia-induced cellular edema. Sodium influx and osmotic reequilibration with obligatory passive entry of water is minimized. Furthermore, energy is conserved as the activity of the Na^+-K^+ ATPase pump is limited. Commonly used intracellular solutions in cardiac transplantation are University of Wisconsin, Euro-Collins, and, in Europe, Bretschneider (HTK).

Extracellular solutions are characterized by high sodium and low to moderate potassium concentrations. Proponents point to the theoretic potential for cellular damage and increased coronary vascular resistance associated with some hyperkalemic solutions. Stanford, Johns Hopkins, and St. Thomas Hospital solutions are the representative extracellular cardioplegic examples.

In the recent Papworth heart donor survey, cardioplegic solution was not an independent predictor of mortality in a multivariant analysis.[8]

Storage Solutions

Cold saline is the most frequently used storage medium. In the aforementioned survey, storage in any nonsaline solution is correlated with a greater than twofold increase in mortality.[8] Controlled studies will be necessary to confirm this finding.

Potassium and Calcium

Of electrolytes included in cardioplegic-storage solutions, the optimal concentration of potassium and calcium has stimulated the most controversy. In selected situations, high concentrations of potassium have been associated with cellular injury, particularly to the coronary endothelium. Nevertheless, most investigators agree that convincing evidence demonstrating significant injury to the hypothermic cardiac allograft secondary to exposure to the currently available hyperkalemic solutions is lacking. Supporters of the addition of calcium warn of the possibility of the *calcium paradox* with acalemic solutions particularly in the setting of a low sodium-preservation medium.

Calcium overload, however, is intimately involved in the development of ischemic contractures in the myocyte, and recent experimental evidence suggests only micromolar amounts are necessary to prevent the rare calcium paradox phenomenon.

Perhaps, as some investigators have theorized, if allograft ischemic periods are significantly extended in the future, electrolyte composition and concentrations will become increasingly more important. However, despite the vehement claims of investigators worldwide, *no* compelling clinical evidence exists at this time that any solution is clearly superior to the others when used within the current 6-hour limit of ischemia.

Solution Additives

Inclusion of pharmacologic additives is another area of active research and controversy in cardiac preservation. Although a plethora of substances have been added to cardioplegic-storage solutions, the greatest potential for future routine use may lie with impermeants, substrates, and antioxidants.

Impermeants.   The majority of currently used impermeants (mannitol, lactobionate, raffinose, and histidine) are osmotic agents. They purportedly reduce hypothermia-induced cellular edema in the allograft by counteracting the intracellular osmotic pressure imparted by protein and other cytosol-confined molecules. Other impermeants act as oncotic agents to offset development of myocardial interstitial edema (hydroxyethyl starch). Although reports suggest these substances are potentially essential in continuous perfusion storage systems, including impermeants in static solutions remains debatable.

Substrates.   Preservation of myocardial high-energy phosphates during ischemia (to prevent contracture bands) and their rapid regeneration at reperfusion (to fuel the newly contracting heart) are the primary objectives for the use of substrate-enhanced media. Adenosine, L-pyruvate, and L-glutamate have been most intensely studied. ATP can be repleted from adenosine through the purine salvage pathway and from these amino acids through the citric acid cycle. The biochemical rationale for provision of substrates in cardioplegic-storage solutions appears theoretically sound. Yet, it remains unclear whether exogenous substrates can be taken up and utilized by the quiescent myocytes, and moreover whether their addition significantly improves outcome.

Antioxidants.   Recognizing that oxygen-derived free radicals are likely the critical mediators of myocardial reperfusion injury, pharmacologic interventions to neutralize these toxic molecules were a natural extension of preservation research. A principle common to all antioxidant strategies is that the myocardium be prepared with these drugs before reperfusion.

Administration of exogenous free-radical scavengers is believed by some investigators to assist the recipient's intrinsic antioxidant defenses in the metabolism of the oxygen intermediates to benign molecules. Examples of these agents include allopurinol, glutathione, superoxide dismutase, catalase, mannitol, and histidine. Because the transition metals copper and iron have been implicated as catalysts in Haber-Weiss and Fenton reactions of oxygen radical synthesis, metal chelators (deferoxamine, TPEN, and neocuproine) are another class of drugs proposed to combat reperfusion injury. As with the other additives, use of scavengers and chelators is controversial because of conflicting experimental and clinical results.

PRESERVATION TECHNIQUE

A single flush of cardioplegic solution followed by a static hypothermic storage is the method employed by more than 90% of transplant centers. At the time of organ procurement, a bolus of cardioplegia is administered in standard fashion with 14-gauge

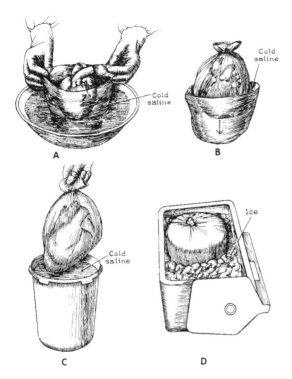

FIGURE 1.   Preparation of the donor heart for transport. (From Baumgartner WA, Reitz BA, Acuff SC [eds]: Heart and Heart-Lung Transplantation. Philadelphia, W.B. Saunders, 1990, with permission.)

catheter proximal to the aortic crossclamp. Rapid topical cooling of the heart is achieved with cold saline poured into the pericardial well. After explantation is complete, the allograft is sequentially placed in two sterile bowel bags, each filled with cold saline, a saline-filled air-tight container, and finally a standard cooler of ice for transport (Fig. 1). This technique is simple and provides excellent short-term myocardial protection.

To extend preservation times, efforts have been directed toward developing a strategy for continuous perfusion of the explanted heart. The advantages of this technique over static storage are the presence of a constant supply of oxygen and substrate for basal metabolic demands and washout of toxic by-products of metabolism. Unfortunately, these potential benefits are currently overshadowed by exacerbation of extracellular cardiac edema and the logistic problems inherent to a complex perfusion apparatus. Hence, clinical experience with continuous perfusion has been disappointing. Consensus among transplant surgeons is that with current perfusion techniques, these allografts would be sufficiently impaired that they would not be able to sustain the recipient if transplanted orthotopically.

The concept of *microperfusion* was recently proposed to reduce interstitial edema and associated diastolic dysfunction accompanying continuous perfusion techniques.[9] It is characterized by perfusion at low pressures to attenuate the intravascular hydrostatic component of the Fick equation and thus reduce fluid extravasation. Perfusate oncotic pressure can be augmented with the addition of impermeants to the solution to further minimize edema.

A compromise between single flush and continuous perfusion cardioplegic delivery is a multiple flush technique extended over the course of the ischemic interval. Although experimental evidence suggests improved results with this intermittent perfusion, clinical application has been limited.

PRESERVATION DURING IMPLANTATION

The time necessary to perform cardiac implantation may account for a significant proportion of the total ischemic time of the heart. During this period, the allograft may be warmed by blood from the pulmonary venous system as well as direct thermal transfer from adjacent thoracic structures.

Several methods are used to maintain allograft hypothermia at implantation. At our institution, continuous aspiration of pulmonary venous return is achieved by insertion of a vent into the left atrium through the right superior pulmonary vein or left atrial appendage (Figure 2). After completion of the posterior left atrial suture line, topical cold is initiated, and the patient is oriented in a "left side down–head up" position to allow drainage of the cold saline away from the operative field and maximal exposure to the left and right ventricles.

To shorten the allograft ischemia period, some centers perform the aortic anastomosis before that of the pulmonary artery and then complete implantation with the crossclamp removed. We believe, however, that the additional 10 minutes of ischemia necessary to perform the pulmonary anastomosis is relatively short in exchange for greatly facilitating this important anastomosis.

REPERFUSION MODIFICATION

Underscoring the recurrent theme of leukocyte- and oxygen radical-mediated allograft injury, a considerable investigative effort has been undertaken to modify the untoward events of ischemia-reperfusion. In addition to the antioxidant agents proposed as solution additives, various pharmacologic and mechanical strategies of leukocyte inhibition and depletion are currently being explored. The goal is to dramatically reduce or inhibit the number of potent leukocytes circulating at reperfusion.

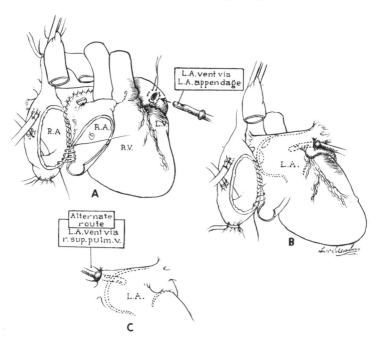

FIGURE 2.   Left atrial vent placement via the right superior pulmonary vein or left atrial appendage.

Adhesion to myocytes and endothelial cells is critical for the release of free radicals and proteases by the activated neutrophil. Monoclonal antibodies to the integrin adhesion molecules block this intercellular contact thereby presumably attenuating leukocyte-mediated myocardial injury.[10,11] Mechanical neutrophil depletion can be safely and easily achieved with filters placed in the cardiopulmonary bypass circuit or during the initial reperfusion using filtered warm blood cardioplegia.[12]

Evidence to date demonstrates no significant improvement in postoperative myocardial function with leukocyte depletion-inhibition techniques if ischemic times are less than 3 hours.[13] It is uncertain if the additional immunosuppression significantly increases risk of infection in transplant recipients. Prospective, randomized clinical trials are ongoing to better elucidate the benefits and potential drawbacks of these innovative additions to the repertoire of cardiac preservation techniques.

CONCLUSIONS

Injury to the cardiac allograft may result during donor management and organ preservation. Resultant myocardial dysfunction complicates postoperative care and contributes to decreased early and late survival.

Medical management of the heart donor is evolving into a vital component of allograft preservation. With better understanding of the physiologic changes of brain death will come needed refinements in the care of these patients. Further clinical studies will determine if poorly functioning donor hearts might be resuscitated with hormonal pretreatment before explantation. Development of objective tests to evaluate the extent of allograft injury will facilitate selection of donors.

The current strategy of single cardioplegic flush followed by static hypothermic storage is satisfactory for relatively short ischemic times. Extension of storage times may provide a modest increase in the donor pool as well as permit human leukocyte antigen matching. Improved techniques of the future not only will prolong the duration of safe organ preservation, but, more importantly, also will ensure consistent reliable function of hearts preserved within the 4 to 6 hour limits. Because hemodynamic and age criteria are now less strict because of the great demand for cardiac allografts, improved short-term preservation has become even more important with increasing numbers of marginal donors.

The controversy surrounding the wide variety of cardioplegic-storage solutions bespeaks the fact no ideal solution currently exists. Attempts to formulate a universal solution for multiorgan preservation have met with variable success. As clinical experience has clearly demonstrated, preservation of the heart has unique requirements, and thus a cardiospecific solution will likely yield optimal recovery of myocardial function. Although evidence of clinical superiority of any simple preservation solution is still lacking, some investigators theorize that the advantages of electrolyte modifications and additives will only be manifest in the setting of extended ischemic times or in marginal donors. Use of continuous perfusion storage systems will only become widespread after they have been technically simplified and after the issue of associated myocardial edema resolved. Continued research is necessary to address these ongoing debates over composition and delivery of cardioplegic-storage solutions.

The literature strongly suggests that oxygen-derived free radicals and leukocytes mediate reperfusion injury of the ischemic allograft. Promising experimental antioxidant therapy and leukocyte depletion techniques have demonstrated less dramatic results when applied clinically. Nevertheless, efforts to modify the untoward events of reperfusion should continue.

TABLE I.   Preservation Regimen for Cardiac Allografts at the Johns Hopkins Hospital

Donor management
  Optimize hemodynamic, ventilatory, and metabolic status
Procurement
  Single bolus of cold crystalloid cardioplegia through a 14-gauge catheter positioned proximal to the aortic
    crossclamp (at a pressure of 150 mmHg). All solutions are infused at a temperature of 2 to 4°C
  Topical cold saline concurrently poured into the pericardial well
Storage
  Allograft sequentially placed in two sterile bowel bags, each filled with cold saline, a saline filled air-tight
    container, and finally a standard cooler of ice
Implantation
  Donor heart remains in transport cooler until time of implantation
  Heart placed in bowl of cold saline where the anastomotic sites are prepared for implantation
  Cold sponge placed into pericardial well of recipient to provide insulation between donor heart and
    posterior mediastinum
  Vent positioned in the recipient left atrium through the right superior pulmonary vein or left atrial
    appendage for continuous aspiration of pulmonary venous return
  Continuous pericardial lavage with cold saline initiated after completion of posterior left atrial suture line
Reperfusion modification
  Mechanical neutrophil depletion with filter placed in cardiopulmonary bypass circuit (early clinical trials)

The critical components of successful preservation appear to involve meticulous donor management, hypothermia, and reperfusion modification. Improved outcome of heart transplantation in the future will rely on optimal donor selection and allograft preservation to attenuate myocardial insults incurred prior to implantation. The schema used currently at Johns Hopkins University developed upon the above-mentioned principles is summarized in Table 1.

REFERENCES

1. Breen TJ, Keck B, Daily OP, Hosenpud JD: The use of older donors results in a major increase in early mortality following orthotopic cardiac transplantation [abstract]. J Heart Lung Transplant 13(1):S51, 1994.
2. Bourge RC, Naftel DC, Costanzo-Nordin MR, et al: Pretransplantation risk factors for death after heart transplantation: A multi-institutional study. J Heart Lung Transplant 12:549–562, 1993.
3. The registry of the international society for heart and lung transplantation: Tenth official report—1993. J Heart Lung Transplant 12:541–548, 1993.
4. Stringham JC, Southard JH, Hegge J, et al: Limitations of heart preservation by cold storage. Transplantation 53:287–294, 1992.
5. McCord JM: Oxygen-derived free radicals in postischemic tissue injury. N Engl J Med 312(3):159–164, 1985.
6. Wheeldon DR, Potter CD, Oduro A, et al: Transplantation of marginal donors [abstract]. J Heart Lung Transplant 13(1):S51, 1994.
7. Jeevanadam V, Todd B, Eldridge C, et al: Reversal of donor myocardial dysfunction by triiodothyronine replacement therapy [abstract]. J Heart Lung Transplant 12(1):S70, 1993.
8. Wheeldon D, Sharples L, Wallwork J, et al: Donor heart preservation survey. J Heart Lung Transplant 11:986–993, 1992.
9. Ferrera R, Marcsek P, Larese A, et al: Comparison of continuous microperfusion and cold storage for pig heart preservation. J Heart Lung Transplant 12:463–469, 1993.
10. Bryne JG, Smith WJ, Murphy MP, et al: Complete prevention of myocardial stunning, contracture, low-reflow, and edema after heart transplantation by blocking neutrophil adhesion molecules during reperfusion. J Thorac Cardiovasc Surg 104:1589–1596, 1992.
11. Zehr KJ, Herskowitz A, Lee P, et al: Neutrophil adhesion inhibition prolongs survival of cardiac allografts with hyperacute rejection. J Heart Lung Transplant 12:837–845, 1993.
12. Pillai R, Bando K, Schueler S, et al: Leukocyte-depleted reperfusion of transplanted human hearts: A randomized, double-bind clinical trial. J Heart Lung Transplant 11:1082–1092, 1992.
13. Pearl JM, Drinkwater DC, Laks H, et al: Leukocyte-depleted reperfusion of transplanted human hearts: A randomized, doube-blind clinical trial. J Heart Lung Transplant 11:1082–1092, 1992.

Chapter 7

Techniques in Cardiac Transplantation

Robert W. Emery, MD
Kit V. Arom, MD, PhD

Surgical techniques of cardiac transplantation began when Carrel and Guthrie performed the first cardiac transplant into the neck of a dog. Although hemodynamically ineffectual, this procedure documented that the organ could be transplanted and would function. Later, Demikoff, with a series of elaborate experiments, was able to transplant thoracic organs in the dog without using cardiopulmonary bypass.[1] This work was performed during the 1930s, but did not come to light until much later. Thoracic transplantation techniques for orthotopic heart transplantation were at first cumbersome. They incorporated the anastomosis of four pulmonary veins, the great vessels, and the systemic venous system as separate anastomoses. Lower and Shumway created the first useful technique for orthotopic heart transplantation and reported this in 1960.[2] Many techniques for heterotopic heart transplantation in animals have been designed for experimental purposes; but discussion of these techniques are beyond the scope of this chapter, which instead focuses on the use of alterations of donor heart implantation in human situations.

THE DONOR HEART

Regardless of the technique of transplantation, appropriate donor cardiectomy is required. In all circumstances, a length of superior vena cava (SVC) extending at least to the azygos vein, and in certain situations longer, must be obtained. Length of the great vessels should be obtained to the aortic arch, occasionally beyond, and the pulmonary artery should include the bifurcation in all cases and longer lengths of individual pulmonary artery where indicated. Severance of the pulmonary veins should be undertaken at the level of the individual veins and the coalescence of these structures undertaken at a back table where visualization of the posterior portion of the heart is more easily obtained (Fig. 1). If necessary, a pedicled atrial flap for septal reconstruction may also be created. It is important that all structures be saved anatomically, and extra length obtained when variations in standard orthotopic transplantation procedures are anticipated. In this regard, the donor surgeon must know the recipient anatomy and the requirements of the donor organ to facilitate implantation. The atrial septum of the donor organ is inspected and a patent foramen ovale closed, if present. The great vessels are separated to obtain maximal length.

ORTHOTOPIC HEART TRANSPLANTATION

In 1960, Lower and Shumway reported a technique for orthotopic cardiac transplantation that has stood the test of time.[2] Although this technique is well known to surgeons performing transplantation, a brief reiteration is worthwhile. This technique was nicely illustrated by Copeland in 1988.[3] The recipient heart is excised at the level of the atrioventricular groove; and all excess donor atrium, particularly that of the left side including the left atrial (LA) appendage, is excised. The LA is inspected for any thrombus that may have occurred because of congestive heart failure or low output state. The right atrium (RA) is trimmed to the level of the cavae so that only excess tissue for anastomotic requirements is maintained.

The great vessels are divided at the level of the semilunar valves, preserving length of these vessels (Fig. 2). The implant procedure is undertaken beginning at the left lateral portion of the LA and taking a single 3-0 monofilament suture; the anastomosis is begun at the site of the atrial appendage on the donor heart, sewn to the level of the amputated atrial appendage of the recipient. The suture line is continued along the lateral and inferior portions of the atrium to the level of the interatrial septum. The

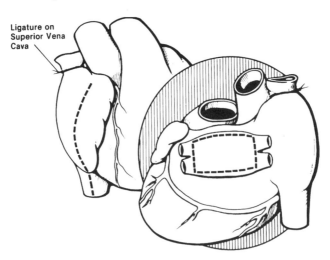

Ligature on
Superior Vena
Cava

FIGURE 1. The donor heart has been excised, maintaining as much length as possible on the great vessels, dividing the superior and inferior venae cavae at their entrance into the thoracic cavity and the pulmonary veins at their origin. An incision used for anastomosis of right atrium is shown in the upper left, extending toward the atrial appendage. An incision coalescing the entrances of the pulmonary vein is shown in the lower right. Variations of the latter incision may be necessary should additional left atrial wall be required. (From Copeland JG: Cardiac transplantation. In O'Rourke RA: Current Problems in Cardiology. Chicago, Year Book, 1988, with permission.)

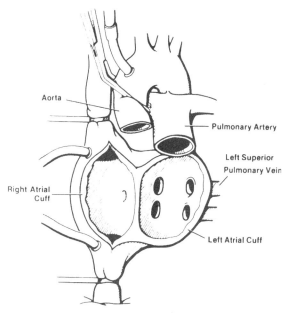

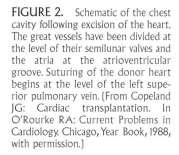

FIGURE 2. Schematic of the chest cavity following excision of the heart. The great vessels have been divided at the level of their semilunar valves and the atria at the atrioventricular groove. Suturing of the donor heart begins at the level of the left superior pulmonary vein. (From Copeland JG: Cardiac transplantation. In O'Rourke RA: Current Problems in Cardiology. Chicago, Year Book, 1988, with permission.)

remaining end of the double-ended suture is then taken and the dome of the atrium closed, followed by the interatrial septum. Before closure of the septum, the left atrium is filled with saline to eliminate as much air as possible. With completion of the suture line, an important part of the operative procedure, the insertion of a line for the infusion of cold saline into the LA appendage, is undertaken (Fig. 3). This cold saline serves two purposes: to continue to cool the endocardial surface of the heart during the implantation process and to evacuate residual air. The RA anastomosis is then undertaken using a similar suture, double-sewing the atrial septum, and continuing along the inferior portion of the RA. Traditionally, an incision is made through the pectinate muscles toward the atrial appendage (Fig. 3) to create the length necessary for atrial-to-atrial anastomosis. As one approaches the midportion of the right lateral wall of the atrium, the sutures are exchanged, sewing the dome of the atrium and the RA wall. The suture line is not completed, but a vent is placed in the right ventricle and the aortic anastomosis is completed in a single layer utilizing 4-0 monofilament suture (Fig. 4). The aorta is vented, the cold infusion line removed, the left atrial appendage ligated, and the cross-clamp removed. With a vent in the right ventricle, coronary sinus return is collected and the pulmonary anastomosis can be constructed in a blood-free environment. This anastomosis is also constructed with 4-0 monofilament suture. With the procedure completed, the heart is resuscitated, the air removed, and pacemaker wires applied. Cardiopulmonary bypass is discontinued when appropriate and the operation completed.

Although this traditional approach serves the purpose very well, problems with the operation exist. Redundant atrium with four separate atria in composite can lead to stasis and thrombus formation. Suture line complications have been reported.[4] Additionally, because of the double atrium, echocardiographically documented mitral and tricuspid insufficiency (which at times may be substantial) can occur. To ameliorate these problems, separate anastomosis of the superior and inferior vena cavae, as opposed to a RA to atrial anastomosis, as well as individual pulmonary venous implantation, has been proposed to eliminate atrial duplication and distortion.[5] This, however,

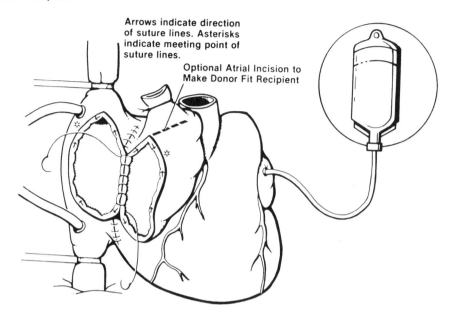

Arrows indicate direction of suture lines. Asterisks indicate meeting point of suture lines.

Optional Atrial Incision to Make Donor Fit Recipient

FIGURE 3. The left atrial anastomosis has been completed. A cold infusion line has been secured through the left atrial appendage for the infusion of saline (50 to 75 ml/min). The interatrial septum has been double-sewn, beginning the right atrial anastomosis. The dotted line indicates the site where an incision may be made to accommodate for excess recipient atrium. (From Copeland JG: Cardiac transplantation. In O'Rourke RA: Current Problems in Cardiology. Chicago, Year Book, 1988, with permission.)

has not become well accepted. More recently, Michler and his group have proposed a different RA incision to obviate the tricuspid insufficiency problem.[6] As opposed to curving the incision toward the atrial appendage through the pectinate muscles, the

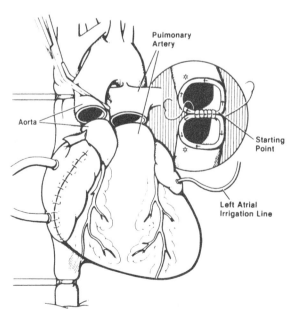

Pulmonary Artery

Aorta

Starting Point

Left Atrial Irrigation Line

FIGURE 4. The right atrial anastomosis has been completed and both great vessel anastomoses are undertaken. Rather than completing the right atrial anastomosis, the last several sutures are left incomplete and a vent is passed into the right atrium through the tricuspid valve. After completion of the aortic anastomosis, venting this structure, the cross-clamp may be released and the pulmonary arterial anastomosis completed in a blood-free environment. (From Copeland JG: Cardiac transplantation. In O'Rourke RA: Current Problems in Cardiology. Chicago, Year Book, 1988, with permission.)

incision is carried along the interatrial septum directly through the superior vena cava. There are two advantages to this incision that we we have come to use in our program routinely. First, RA anastomosis is completed using stronger musculature than the thin, fragile area of the pectinate portion of the RA. This allows for a more secure, hemostatic, and stable anastomosis. Second, no torsion on the heart distorts the tricuspid valve; and, as documented by Michler, tricuspid insufficiency is virtually absent, which is an advantage in patients with more elevated pulmonary vascular resistance.

When utilizing a *domino* donor, that is, an organ taken from a heart-lung transplant recipient, the LA, pulmonary artery and aortic anastomosis are performed in a similar fashion as already described. However, separate anastomoses to the inferior and superior vena cava are necessary.[7,8]

HETEROTOPIC HEART TRANSPLANTATION

Introduced by Barnard,[9] heterotopic heart transplantation has become a useful entity in four situations: (1) as a biologic *assist device*, (2) in cases where a donor heart is too small to occupy the anatomic location for which it is intended but immediate heart transplantation is warranted, (3) in patients with elevated pulmonary vascular resistance who have adapted right ventricles and the heterotopic heart acts as the functional left ventricular, and (4) as an adjunct assist to simultaneous procedures for the treatment of ischemic heart disease.[9a,10] The disadvantages of this procedure are its greater technical difficulty than orthotopic heart transplantation, that this extra heart takes up space in the right chest and can cause pulmonary compression, and, finally, that monitoring rejection may be difficult because of the abnormal lie of the organ.

The pericardium on the recipient's right side is freed and dropped into the right chest, exposing the atria on the right side. On cardiopulmonary bypass, an incision in the LA is made anterior to the pulmonary veins and this incision in the recipient is sewn to the site of the coalesced left pulmonary veins of the donor. The right pulmonary veins are previously securely ligated. The caval anastomosis is then undertaken by sewing the superior vena cava (SVC) of the donor to that of the recipient. The aorta-to-aortic anastomosis is undertaken in an end-to-side fashion; and, finally, the pulmonary artery to pulmonary artery anastomosis is conducted as an end-to-side process, often using prosthetic graft material to allow for length. The resultant anastomotic connections are shown in Figure 5.[11] The operation may be modified by sewing the pulmonary artery to the RA free wall in patients requiring only left ventricular assist where the patient's own right ventricle had adapted to elevated pulmonary artery pressures. In all hands, this technique has had fewer good results than that of orthotopic heart transplantation and is currently only uncommonly used.

Transplantation in Congenital Heart Disease

The techniques above sufficed for most transplant surgeons until the late 1980s, after cyclosporine was introduced and its use was well proved. Sporadic attempts at transplant therapy in congenital heart disease were undertaken in the early and middle 1980s; however, it was not until Bailey introduced the technique for cardiac transplantation in the hypoplastic left heart syndrome that an aggressive approach to pediatric and infant heart transplantation was undertaken.[12] Before this, transplantation in patients with congenital heart disease, or infants with cardiomyopathy, followed the lines of the Lower-Shumway procedure, or in procedures where the congenital anomaly (such as correct transposition of the great arteries) could be excised, leaving normal situs proximally and vessel distally, which would accept conduits in the anatomic position at the

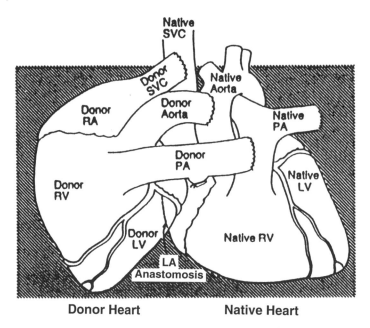

Donor Heart   **Native Heart**

FIGURE 5.   Schematic of heterotopic heart transplantation showing the completed anastomoses and position of the heterotopic heart relative to that of the native organ. (From Allen MD, Naasz CD, Popp RL, et al: Noninvasive assessment of donor and native heart function after heterotopic heart transplantation. J Thorac Cardiovasc Surg 95:75–81, 1988, with permission.)

level of the ligamentum arteriosus or with minor variations in donor harvest technique (Fig. 6). In these situations, lengthening the donor conduit or using prosthetic extension grafts sufficed to allow completion of the operation.[13] Since Bailey and his group performed the first orthotopic heart transplant for hypoplastic left heart syndrome using a nonhuman donor, surgeons at pediatric centers associated with heart transplant programs have devised ingenious techniques to correct for congenital problems that had heretofore obviated transplantation. These modifications relate to variations in situs and/or systemic venous return, corrections of atrial anomalies resulting from either congenital malformations or previous surgical interventions, dealing with pulmonary artery problems (most commonly those created at surgery or related to pulmonary atresia), and those dealing with the distal arterial circuit, such as hypoplastic left heart syndrome. In addition, palliative surgical procedures exist that have altered the venous and/or arterial anatomy for which techniques of transplantation require modification, such as the Stage I procedure for hypoplastic left heart syndrome. Transplant therapy may become necessary for complex corrected anatomy, as with atrial baffling procedures for physiologic correction of transposition of the great arteries, or modified Fontan procedures for complex single-ventricle anatomy where ventricular failure may intervene in subsequent years. Such surgically created anatomic abnormalities need to be addressed at the time of transplantation therapy. The need for transplantation in these latter groups will be increasing as the limits of aggressive surgical correction of congenital heart disease become better defined. Over the past 5 years the imaginative approaches taken to a variety of forms of congenital heart disease have required unique and ingenious modification of the transplant procedure or underlying recipient anatomy to allow implantation of the donor organ.

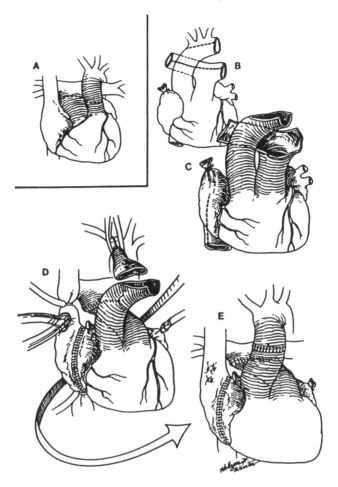

FIGURE 6.   The technique for completion of cardiac transplantation in patients with corrected transposition of the great vessels is demonstrated. Additional length of donor pulmonary artery and donor aorta are necessary. Utilizing this additional length, anatomic completion of the transplant procedure may be undertaken without the use of prosthetic conduits. (From Reitz BA, Jamieson SW, Gaudiani VA, et al: Method for cardiac transplantation in corrected transposition of the great arteries. J Cardiovasc Surg 23:293–296, 1982, with permission.)

VARIANCE IN SITUS

In situs inversus, situational correction of the atrial position becomes necessary before the ability to perform transplantation with a donor heart of normal situs. Several procedures are used in this unusual situation. The first is that described by Doty and coworkers (Figs. 7–9)[14] where, after excision of the ventricles is completed and a segment of SVC is transferred to the innominate vein, the atrial septum is divided. The RA segment is used to create a baffle from the left-lying inferior vena cava (IVC) along the diaphragmatic surface, so the entrance to this baffle lies on the recipient's right or anatomic side (Figure 8). The free LA is thus transposed to the patient's left and a standard donor-to-recipient LA anastomosis is created. The RA of the donor is modified and sewn to create a tunnel which the distal end being connected to the

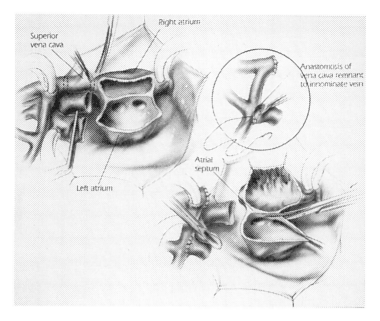

FIGURE 7. The technique of Doty and coworkers for transplantation with variance in situ is described. Following cannulation, the venous inflow through the left-lying superior vena cava is divided and over-sewn (see insert). A portion of the superior vena cava is then excised and sewn to the right side of the confluence of the innominate and jugular veins. The atrial septum is then split, dividing left and right atria. (From Doty DB, Renlund DG, Caputo GR, et al: Cardiac transplantation in situs inversus. J Thorac Cardiovasc Surg 99:493–499, 1990, with permission.)

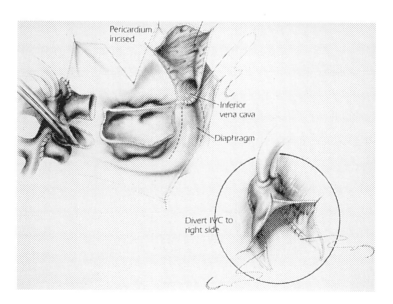

FIGURE 8. The right atrium of the recipient is then used to create a baffle along the diaphragmatic surface, returning inferior vena caval flow to the normal anatomic right-sided position. (From Doty DB, Renlund DG, Caputo GR, et al: Cardiac transplantation in situs inversus. J Thorac Cardiovasc Surg 99:493–499, 1990, with permission.)

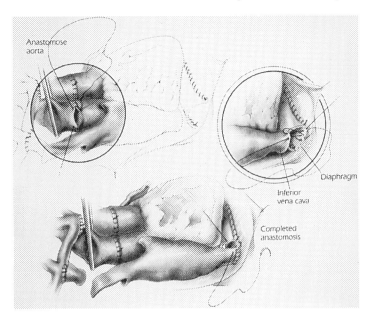

FIGURE 9. Transplantation is completed by modifying the right atrium of the donor to be sewn to the diaphragmatic baffle of the recipient. A composite superior vena cava is constructed for superior inflow. Great vessel anastomotic completion may then be undertaken with anatomic situs. (From Doty DB, Renlund DG, Caputo GR, et al: Cardiac transplantation in situs inversus. J Thorac Cardiovasc Surg 99:493–499, 1990, with permission.)

diaphragmatic IVC tunnel (Fig. 9). A superior portion is then extended as a composite superior vena cava and attached to the newly transposed superior systemic venous return. The great vessel anastomoses in this situation may be constructed in the standard fashion.

Vouche describes a true atrial neo-transposition with the right atrium being transposed anterior and to the right of the LA with septal reconstruction[15] (Fig. 10). In a third technique, a modified Senning operation may also be utilized (Fig. 11). The pulmonary venous atrium is opened anterior to the pulmonary veins, and the atrial septum is separated from its caudad and cephalad attachments to divert the pulmonary veins to the left-sided opening. This technique was described by Vouche et al.[15] In the case of situs inversus with azygos extension of the systemic venous return where atrial transposition is not feasible, atrial separation is carried out coupled with separation of the pulmonary veins and disconnection of the superior vena cava.[15] A baffle using the right atrium extending along the diaphragm is created (Fig. 12). Transplantation is then carried out as shown in Figure 13, connecting the left and right pulmonary venous return separately, the IVC to the baffled recipient return and extending the SVC to the donor atrial appendage. Great vessel connection is anatomic. These alterations in recipient anatomy allow the use of situs solitus organ donors for transplantation.

In the case of situs ambiguous, most commonly associated with heterotaxy syndrome, a single atrium is present that receives the systemic and pulmonary veins in a variety of locations. An interatrial baffle is constructed, partitioning the atrium into systemic and pulmonary sections, such that the pulmonary portion is referred to the patient's left and the systemic venous return to the patient's right (Fig. 14). If interruption of the hepatic segment of the inferior vena cava is present, superior vena caval anastomosis, baffling this structure into the systemic venous atrium, will be necessary.[16]

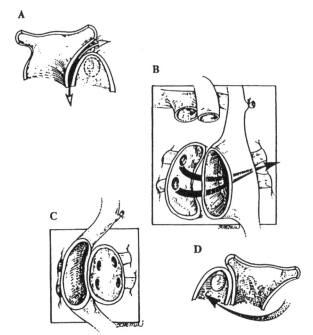

FIGURE 10. The technique of true atrial transposition is shown schematically. The left and right atria in situs inversus are separated and the left atrium is transposed behind the right atrium to create normal anatomic situs. (From Vouche PR, Tamisier D, Le Bidois J, et al: Pediatric cardiac transplantation for congenital heart defects: Surgical consideration and results. Ann Thorac Surg 56:1239–1247, 1993, with permission.)

FIGURE 11. Cardiac transplantation in situs inversus may also be carried out by creating a modified Senning procedure wherein an intraatrial baffle is created to divert the pulmonary venous return to the patient's left, and an incision is made in the remnant recipient right atrium. The left atrium of the donor is sewn to the incision to which the pulmonary venous return is directed, now lying on the recipient's left, and the right atrium of the donor is sewn to the residual portion of the atrium that receives the systemic venous blood flow, now lying on the patient's right. In this situation, transposition of the atria is not required. (From Vouche PR, Tamisier D, Le Bidois J, et al: Pediatric cardiac transplantation for congenital heart defects: Surgical consideration and results. Ann Thorac Surg 56:1239–1247, 1993, with permission.)

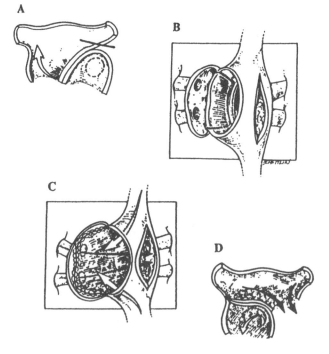

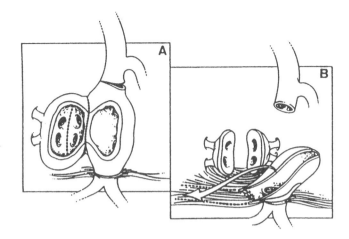

FIGURE 12.   Cardiac transplantation in patients with situs inversus and azygos continuation may also be carried out as shown in this schematic. The heart has been excised and the pulmonary venous inflow sites are separated. A baffle tunneling hepatic venous return to the recipient's right side is constructed. (From Vouche PR, Tamisier D, Le Bidois J, et al: Pediatric cardiac transplantation for congenital heart defects: Surgical consideration and results. Ann Thorac Surg 56:1239–1247, 1993, with permission.)

ANOMALIES OF SYSTEMIC VENOUS RETURN

Cardiac transplantation in the face of altered systemic venous return occurs in two major fashions. The first, and becoming more common, is that of surgically created cavopulmonary anastomosis, performed as a portion of a modified Fontan procedure, either unilateral or bilateral.[17] Most commonly, the SVC superiorly and inferiorly can

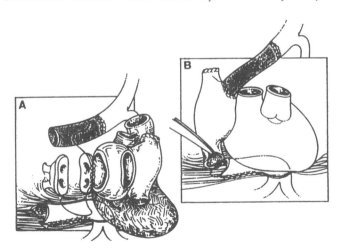

FIGURE 13.   Cardiac transplantation is carried out by separately sewing the right and left cuffs of the pulmonary vein. A pericardial baffle tunnels the hepatic venous return to the recipient's right, and an extension graft is placed from the superior vena cava with its inferior return toward the recipient's right. This extension of the superior vena cava is sewn to the atrial appendage of the donor heart, and the inferior vena cava of the donor heart is sewn to the inferior-lying diaphragmatic baffle (From Vouche PR, Tamisier D, Le Bidois J, et al: Pediatric cardiac transplantation for congenital heart defects: Surgical consideration and results. Ann Thorac Surg 56:1239–1247, 1993, with permission.)

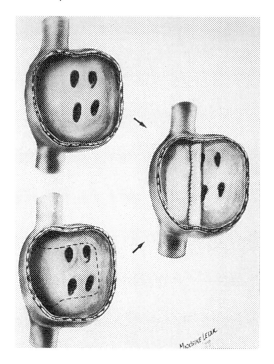

FIGURE 14. A common atrium, often present in heterotaxy syndrome with variable entry of the pulmonary veins, may be septated into the appropriate lying left and right atria so that an anatomically normal donor organ may be transplanted with usual techniques. (From Chartrand C: Pediatric cardiac transplantation despite atrial and venous return anomalies. Ann Thorac Surg 52:716–721, 1991, with permission.)

be removed from the pulmonary artery (Fig. 15), the pulmonary arteriotomy over-sewn, and a direct connection between the superior cava and the recipient atrium constructed (Figs. 16 and 17). The intraatrial baffle must be removed and the atria resepted. The use of a right-angle venous return cannula placed high in the superior vena cava facilitates this situation. Recipient IVC returns through the connected donor and recipient RAs.

In the case of persistent left superior vena cava (SVC), repair of the venous anatomy, either at the atrial or the systemic venous level, must be undertaken. With persistent LSVC in the presence of an innominate vein, the left cava may be safely ligated. It an innominate vein is absent and the left superior pulmonary vein drains to the coronary sinus, the heart is carefully excised such that the persistent superior vena cava and its connection to the recipient atrium are left intact. If this is not feasible, or there is double venous return with a persistent LSVC and right superior vena cava (RSVC), LSVC and RSVC repair described by Menkis et al,[19] using an extended length of donor SVC and the donor innominate vein to return both of these structures to the systemic venous atrium may be best applied (Fig. 18). When double venous return is persistent, or LSVC return to the left atrium is encountered, following excision of the recipient heart, baffling of the anomalous venous return to the superior or inferior atrial septum may be constructed (Fig. 19). In cases in which septal absence is also encountered (heterotaxy syndrome), unusual variants of atrial septation may also be applied[16] (Fig. 20).

Giant atrium, enlarged as a result of chronic congestive heart failure, may also be encountered. Variants in venous anatomy are of less concern in these situations; however, atrial reduction may be necessary to allow for size constraints of the donor organ. Allard and colleagues described the right atrial reduction by partial closure of the structure in continuity into the IVC.19 A wedge of LA may also be removed to reduce this structure to donor requirement (Fig. 21).

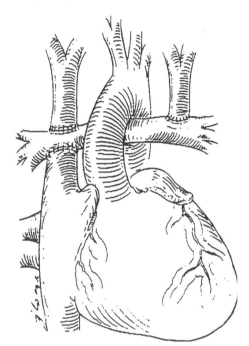

FIGURE 15. A completed modified Fontan procedure with bidirectional cavopulmonary anastomoses is shown in this schematic. Double venous return is present and situs solitus anatomy exists. (From Pearl JM, Laks H, Drinkwater DC: Cardiac transplantation following the modified fenton procedure. Transplant Sci 2:1–3, 1992, with permission.)

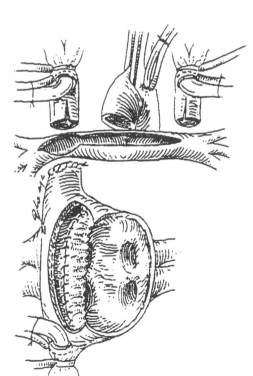

FIGURE 16. The heart has been excised; separate superior vena cava cannulas, as well as an inferior vena cava cannula, have been placed. Reconstruction of the intraatrial septum has been performed, separating the left from the right atrium. The proximal superior vena cava has been oversewn and the pulmonary artery widely opened. (From Pearl JM, Laks H, Drinkwater DC: Cardiac transplantation following the modified fenton procedure. Transplant Sci 2:1–3, 1992. with permission.)

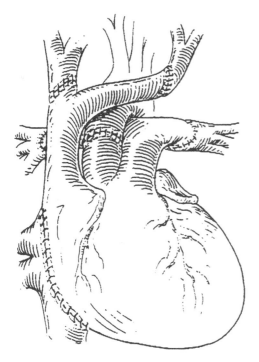

FIGURE 17. The heart transplantation procedure following modified Fontan method has been completed. The donor superior vena cava with an extension of the donor innominate vein is sewn to the double venous return. Right atrial to right atrial anastomosis, collecting inferior vena caval return, has been completed. Preservation of the pulmonary bifurcation has allowed repair of the pulmonary artery and the aortic anastomosis is constructed anatomically (From Pearl JM, Laks H, Drinkwater DC: Cardiac transplantation following the modified fenton procedure. Transplant Sci 2:1–3, 1992, with permission.)

Patients presenting with diminutive atria or cor triatriatum may require an enlargement procedure as shown in Figure 22 to allow unrestricted pulmonary venous outflow and completion of the transplant procedure.[16] Note that the wedge of tissue used to reconstruct the LA, as shown in the figure, may be created by incising three of four pulmonary veins in the donor heart, which results in a pedicled flap of homologous tissue that may be cut to the appropriate size and the enlargement constructed as part of the LA suture line.

HEART TRANSPLANTATION WITH SURGICALLY ALTERED ATRIA

The Senning, Mustard, and Shoemaker repairs of transposition of the great arteries require construction of intraatrial baffles to divert blood to the appropriate systemic ventricle. In each of these situations, the surgical repair must be taken down and a new septum must be placed using autologous pericardium, bovine pericardium, or polytetrafluoroethylene (PTFE) to separate the pulmonary and venous circuits. Situs solitus in routine transposition of the great arteries is most common. an example of such a reconstruction after Mustard's operation is shown in Figure 23.[16] Other atrioplastic techniques to correct malformation involving univentricular repairs may be constructed using a flap of donor LA constructed in the appropriate location by incising three of four donor veins.

HEART TRANSPLANTATION FOLLOWING OPERATIONS WITH ALTERATIONS OF THE PULMONARY ARTERIES

Pulmonary artery (PA) banding with resultant pulmonary artery stenosis is a common problem in congenital heart disease (Fig. 24).[20] If such stenoses are proximal, they can be excised and extension repair of the pulmonary arteries can be constructed.

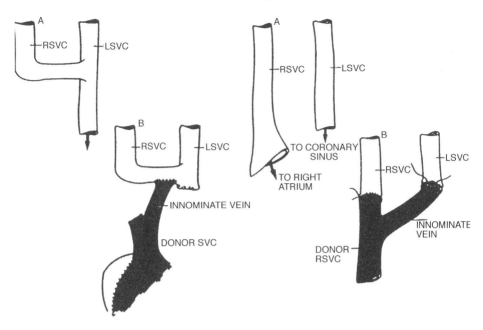

FIGURE 18. Construction of superior caval return in situations where anomalous venous return exists. With the presence of bilateral cavae, a single anastomosis using the donor innominate vein may be constructed to the recipient innominate vein. When this structure is absent, separate anastomoses to the right and left superior venae cavae must be constructed using the donor superior vena cava and the donor innominate vein as an extension graft. (From Menkis AH, McKenzie FN, Novick RJ, et al: Expanding applicability of transplantation after multiple prior palliative procedures. Ann Thorac Surg 52:722–726, 1991, with permission.)

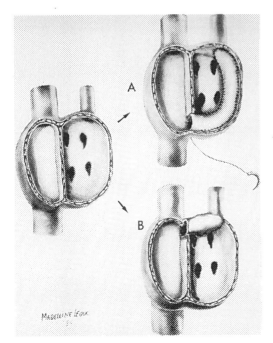

FIGURE 19. When double venous return is present with the left return to the left atrium, baffling of the left venous return to either the superior or inferior portion of the atrial septum must be constructed before transplantation, as shown in this figure. (From Chartrand C: Pediatric cardiac transplantation despite atrial and venous return anomalies. Ann Thorac Surg 52:716–721, 1991, with permission.)

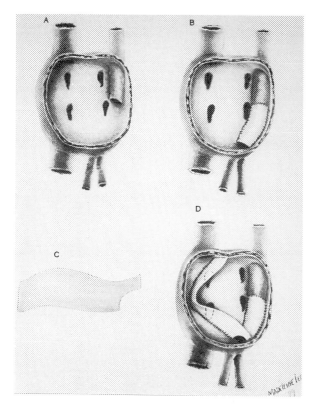

FIGURE 20. Variance of pulmonary venous return with double systemic venous return may also exist. In such cases, unusual baffling requirements may exist, such as that shown where baffling of the left superior vena cava is undertaken to the inferior left atrium and a creative septal baffle is constructed to separate the atria. (From Chartrand C: Pediatric cardiac transplantation despite atrial and venous return anomalies. Ann Thorac Surg 52: 716–721, 1991, with permission.)

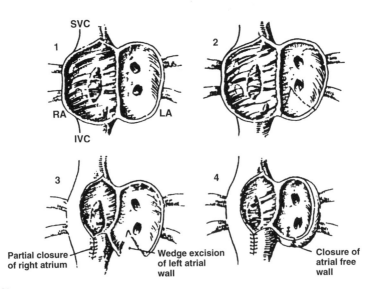

FIGURE 21.   In the case of giant left or right atrium, atrial reduction may be necessary. The right atrium may be reduced by creating a suture line from the inferior or superior cava to reduce the size of the anastomotic suture line. On the left side, a wedge of atrial tissue with excision of this tissue may be required. (From Allard M, Assaad A, Bailey L, et al: Surgical techniques in pediatric heart transplantation. J Heart Lung Transplant 10:808–827, 1991, with permission.)

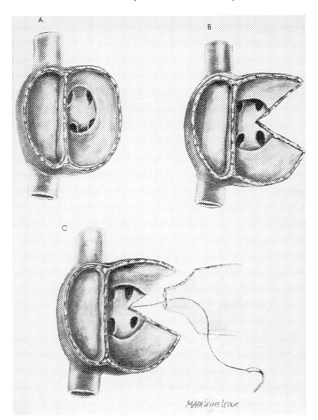

FIGURE 22. When a diminutive left atrium exists, or cor triatriatum is present, an incision on the left lateral aspect between the inferior and superior left pulmonary veins is made. A wedge of prosthetic material or a flap of donor atrial tissue reconstructs the defect and enlarges the left atrium and pulmonary venous outflow. (From Chartrand C: Pediatric cardiac transplantation despite atrial and venous return anomalies. Ann Thorac Surg 52: 716–721, 1991, with permission.)

If the stenosis is distal or continuous into the pulmonary bifurcation, a long reconstruction of the main pulmonary artery may be necessary (Fig. 25) using autologous donor tissue or patch angioplasty. If the left and right main PAs are hypoplastic or stenotic, an incision to the pericardial inlets, thus filleting this structure, will allow for an onlay patch of the opened donor pulmonary bifurcation (Fig. 26).[21]

In situations of hypoplastic left heart syndrome after stage I repair, the pulmonary bifurcation with the patch must be dissected completely and, by preserving length of donor vessel, direct anastomosis to the patch site may often be accomplished.

When modified Fontan repair of a univentricular heart has been accomplished using an atriocaval connection, simple primary repair of the pulmonary artery after takedown of this connection is most often sufficient, but patch or graft angioplasty may be necessary (Figs. 17 and 25).

Before transplantation, any peripheral pulmonary stenoses must be managed by any one or a combination of techniques, including, but not limited to, balloon dilatation, stenting and/or unifocalization to ensure pulmonary resistance is as low as possible to avoid any undue pressure load being placed on the newly transplanted right ventricle.

GREAT VESSEL RECONSTRUCTION

The most common great vessel variant, for which extensive reconstruction is necessary, is that first undertaken by Bailey and currently the most common indication for

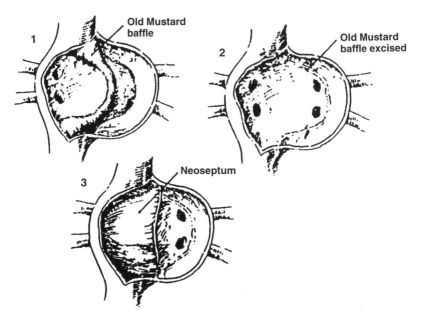

FIGURE 23. A Mustard operation for physiologic correction of transposition of the great arteries had been previously undertaken. Following excision of the heart, the Mustard baffle has been removed, creating a common atrium. A neoseptum has been constructed to separate the right and left atria anatomically. (From Allard M, Assaad A, Bailey L, et al: Surgical techniques in pediatric heart transplantation. J Heart Lung Transplant 10:808–827, 1991, with permission.)

neonatal and infant heart transplantation: hypoplastic left heart syndrome.[12] In this anomaly a hypoplastic or absent left ventricle with a diminutive aorta is present. Most commonly, a coarctation is present and requires intervention at the time of

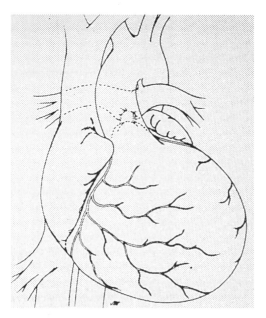

FIGURE 24.   Placement of a pulmonary band, used to prevent pulmonary volume overload, is demonstrated. (From Cooper MM, Fuzesi L, Addonizio LJ, et al: Pediatric heart transplantation after operations involving the pulmonary arteries. J Thorac Cardiovasc Surg 102:386–395, 1991, with permission.)

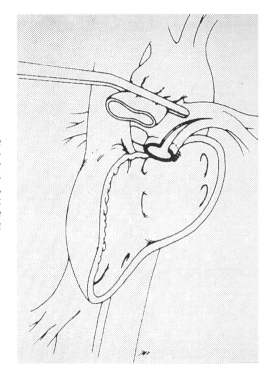

FIGURE 25. The heart is excised; the common atrium requires septation, and extension of the incision in the pulmonary artery to enlarge the site of band-induced fibrosis may be necessary. (From Cooper MM, Fuzesi L, Addonizio LJ, et al: Pediatric heart transplantation after operations involving the pulmonary arteries. J Thorac Cardiovasc Surg 102:386–395, 1991, with permission.)

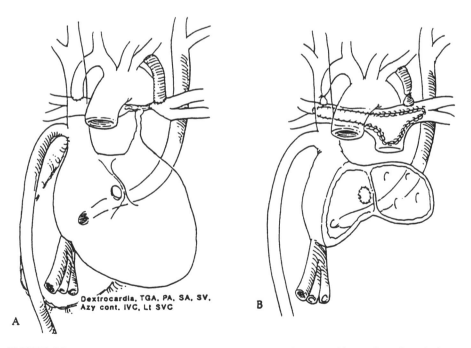

Dextrocardia, TGA, PA, SA, SV, Azy cont. IVC, Lt SVC

A

B

FIGURE 26. Stenotic or hypoplastic pulmonary arteries may be repaired by patch graft angioplasty following excision of the heart (see also Figs. 16 and 27). (From Turrentine MW, Kesler KA, Cadwell R, et al: Cardiac transplantation in infants and children. Ann Thorac Surg 57:546–554, 1994, with permission.)

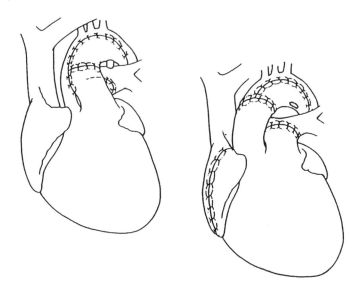

FIGURE 27. Transplantation of the heart following Stage I repair of hypoplastic left heart syndrome is shown in this schematic. Note the repair of the great vessels includes the preserved neopulmonary artery. The pulmonary bifurcation with its patch is dissected completely, the patch is removed and direct pulmonary artery anastomosis is accomplished. Note the shunt has been completely divided to free the pulmonary bifurcation. (From Cooper MM, Fuzesi L, Addonizio LJ, et al: Pediatric heart transplantation after operations involving the pulmonary arteries. J Thorac Cardiovasc Surg 102:386–395, 1991, with permission.)

transplantation. To perform transplantation, a period of deep hypothermic circulatory arrest is necessary. A schematic of this lesion from Bove is shown in Figure 27.[22] Cannulation is undertaken through the pulmonary artery with the cannula extended into the descending thoracic aorta. Double venous cannulation is used. The patient is cooled to deep hypothermic levels. Once appropriate temperatures have been reached, the heart is excised in standard fashion and the diminutive aorta is ligated at the arch. Remnant structures after excision of the heart are clearly shown in Figure 28. The diminutive aorta, with connecting ductal structure, is evident. The donor organs brought onto the field and the left atrial anastomosis is first completed under low flow perfusion with the cannula remaining in place through the clamped pulmonary artery (Fig. 29). With completion of the left atrial anastomosis, hypothermic arrest is achieved, the great vessels snared, and the ductal structure divided. The aorta is opened beyond the aortic arch, as shown in Figure 30. An island of the great vessels on the donor aorta is excised (Fig. 29), allowing a wide orifice to patch the incision of the recipient's vessels. Anastomosis between the donor and recipient aorta is undertaken during this shortened period of deep hypothermic circulatory arrest. The donor aorta acts as an onlay patch on the recipient aorta (Fig. 30). With aortic anastomosis completed, the cannula is replaced into the donor ascending aorta, as shown in Figure 31, and the pulmonary artery and right atrial anastomosis may be completed in standard fashion with reperfusion of both systemic circulation and the donor organ. The completed procedure is shown in Figure 32. This operation was first described by Bailey and later modified to its current form by Mavroudis and associates, to minimize the period of deep hypothermic circulatory arrest.[23,24] Other modifications in the procedure may be required if anomalies of venous inflow also exist.[25]

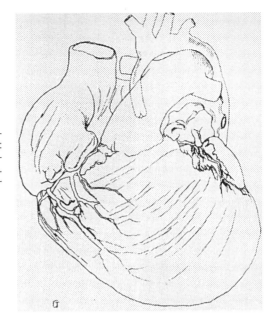

FIGURE 28. Schematic of the hypoplastic left heart syndrome. (From Bove EL: Transplantation after first-stage reconstruction for hypoplastic left heart syndrome. Ann Thorac Surg 52:701–707, 1991, with permission.)

Other malformations of the great vessels that need to be dealt with include transplantation carried out after the arterial switch for treatment of d-transposition of the great arteries, with or without ventricular septal defect. To accomplish arterial switch, the LeCompte maneuver, in which the pulmonary arteries are passed anterior to the

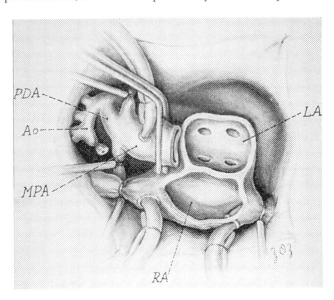

FIGURE 29. The systemic perfusion cannula has been inserted through the pulmonary artery; two venous cannulas are in place. The diminutive aorta has been ligated at the level of the arch and the heart excised at the level of the atria. (From Backer CL, Idriss FS, Zales VR, Mavroudis C: Cardiac transplantation for hypoplastic left heart syndrome: A modified technique. Ann Thorac Surg 50:894–898, 1990, with permission.)

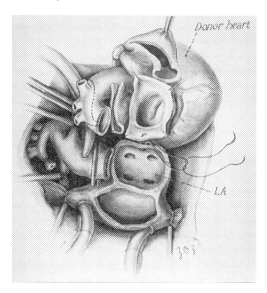

FIGURE 30. The donor left atrial anastomosis is constructed. An island of great vessels is excised from the donor aorta, leaving a patulous opening for reconstruction of the recipient diminutive aortic structures. (From Backer CL, Idriss FS, Zales VR, Mavroudis C: Cardiac transplantation for hypoplastic left heart syndrome: A modified technique. Ann Thorac Surg 50:894–898, 1990, with permission.)

aorta, is completed. To perform cardiac transplantation, this maneuver needs to be *undone*. The cardiopulmonary bypass is initiated with the cannula near the arch of the aorta. Extensive dissection of the anterior pulmonary arteries to their entrance into the pericardium at the hilar structures is carried out, as well as of the ascending aorta. As shown in Figure 33, from Vouche, the great vessels may then be unwound to their

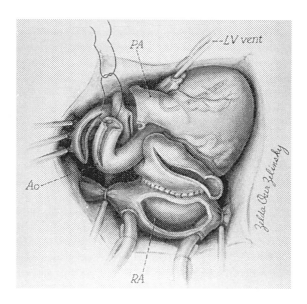

FIGURE 31. The aortic anastomosis is constructed following completion of the left atrial anastomosis. With completion of aortic reconstruction, systemic and cardiac reperfusion may be reinitiated, minimizing the time of hypothermic arrest. Note the perfusion cannula has been removed and the pulmonary artery trimmed to the appropriate length. (From Backer CL, Idriss FS, Zales VR, Mavroudis C: Cardiac transplantation for hypoplastic left heart syndrome: A modified technique. Ann Thorac Surg 50:894–898, 1990, with permission.)

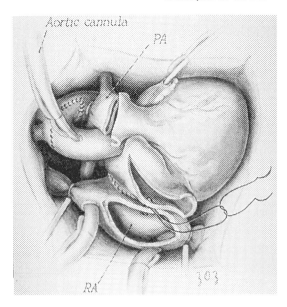

FIGURE 32. The aortic reconstruction has been completed and the perfusion cannula replaced in the donor ascending aorta. The operation may then be completed in standard fashion. (From Backer CL, Idriss FS, Zales VR, Mavroudis C: Cardiac transplantation for hypoplastic left heart syndrome: A modified technique. Ann Thorac Surg 50:894–898, 1990, with permission.)

anatomic position and standard transplantation with primary anastomosis to the great vessels accomplished.[15]

In simple, uncorrected transposition or malposition of the great vessels, the situs is normal at the level of the ligamentum arteriosum. After excision of the heart at the level of the great vessels, as shown in Figure 34, extensive dissection to the level of the ductus with ligation and division of this structure allows mobilization of the aorta and

FIGURE 33. The completed transplantation procedure for treatment of hypoplastic left heart syndrome. (From Backer CL, Idriss FS, Zales VR, Mavroudis C: Cardiac transplantation for hypoplastic left heart syndrome: A modified technique. Ann Thorac Surg 50:894–898, 1990, with permission.)

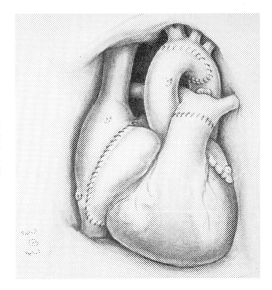

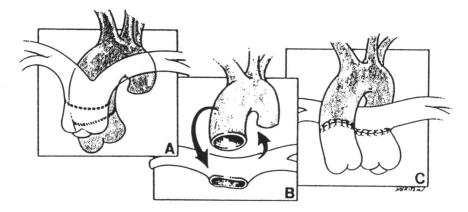

FIGURE 34.   Great vessel reconstruction following the LeCompte maneuver. The great vessels are extensively dissected following excision of the heart, when the great vessels are unwound to perform transplantation in the anatomic position. (From Vouche PR, Tamisier D, Le Bidois J, et al: Pediatric cardiac transplantation for congenital heart defects: Surgical consideration and results. Ann Thorac Surg 56: 1239–1247, 1993, with permission.)

the pulmonary artery to allow enough flexibility, in most instances, for anatomic reconstruction.[15] An extension graft to the pulmonary artery is occasionally necessary and easily achieved.

In surgically altered malposition of the great arteries, such as that seen in tetralogy of Fallot with pulmonary atresia, where a conduit from the right ventricle is extended to the pulmonary artery on either the patient's left or right side (Fig. 35), division of the conduit with construction of the pulmonary anastomosis to the area of conduit insertion, or to a retained portion of the conduit itself, may be completed.

Much has occurred to improve the probability of transplantation in patients with congenital heart disease over the decade of the 90s. Currently, even the most difficult

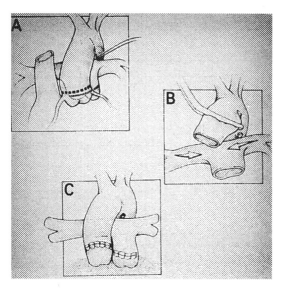

FIGURE 35.   When transposition or malposition of the great vessels is present, situs solitus lie of the structures recurs at the level of the ligamentum arteriosum. The heart is excised at the level of the atrioventricular groove and the similunar valve (A). Extensive dissection of the aorta and pulmonary arteries is carried out to mobilize these structures to the level of the ligamentum, which is divided (B). Enough flexibility of the great vessels is then present to allow standard orthotopic transplantation (C), often without use of a prosthetic extension graft. (From Vouche PR, Tamisier D, Le Bidois J, et al: Pediatric cardiac transplantation for congenital heart defects: Surgical consideration and results. Ann Thorac Surg 56:1239–1247, 1993, with permission.)

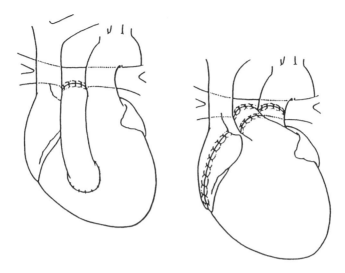

FIGURE 36. When conduit replacement of the main pulmonary artery has been accomplished to either an anatomic or nonanatomic location, excision of the heart and aorta is carried out as usual. A portion of the implanted conduit may be retained, however, in order to add length to the pulmonary artery to create a connection with the donor pulmonary artery. (From Cooper MM, Fuzesi L, Addonizio LJ, et al: Pediatric heart transplantation after operations involving the pulmonary arteries. J Thorac Cardiovasc Surg 102:386–395, 1991, with permission.)

complex congenital anomalies may be approached with transplantation of an anatomically normal cardiac donor using one, or a combination, of the aforementioned techniques. The thrust of transplantation for congenital heart disease begun in the late 1980s is peaking in the mid-90s and maturation of these processes over the next five to 10 years will certainly occur.

REFERENCES

1. Copeland JG, Emery RW: The history of cardiothoracic transplantation. In Emery RW, Pritzker MR (eds): State of the Art Reviews: Cardiothoracic Transplantation. Philadelphia, Hanley & Belfus, 1989, pp 535–540.
2. Lower RR, Shumway NE: Studies on orthotopic homotransplantation of the canine heart. Surg Forum 11:18–20, 1960.
3. Copeland JG: Cardiac transplantation. In O'Rourke RA (ed): Current Problems in Cardiology. chicago, Year Book Medical Publishers, 1988, pp 179–183.
4. Wolfsohn AL, Walley VM, Masters RG, et al: The surgical anastomoses after orthotopic heart transplantation: Clinical complications and morphologic observations. J Heart Lung Transplant 13:455–465, 1994.
5. Dreyfus G, Jebara V, Mihaileanu S, Carpentier AF: Total orthotopic heart transplantation: An alternative to the standard technique. Ann Thorac Surg 52:1181–1184, 1991.
6. Michler RE, Smith CR, Quaegebur JM, et al: Surgical lessons learned in heart transplantation for complex congenital heart disease. J Thorac Cardiovasc Surg (in press).
7. Baumgartner WA, Traill TA, Cameron DE, et al: Unique aspects of heart and lung transplantation exhibited in the "domino-donor" operation. JAMA 261:3121–3125, 1989.
8. Yacoub M, Khagani A, Aravot D, et al: Cardiac transplantation from live donors [abstract]. J Am Coll Cardiol 11:102A, 1988.
9. Barnard CN, Losman JG: Left ventricular bypass. S Afr Med J 49:303–312, 1975.
9a. Losman JG: Review of the Capetown experience with heterotopic heart transplantation. Bull Texas Heart Inst 4:243–255, 1977.
10. Ridley PD, Khaghani A, Musumeci F, et al: Heterotopic heart transplantation and recipient heart operation in ischemic heart disease. Ann Thorac Surg 54:333–337, 1992.

11. Allen MD, Naasz CA, Popp RL, et al: Noninvasive assessment of donor and native heart function after heterotopic heart transplantation. J Thorac Cardiovasc Surg 95:75–81, 1988.
12. Bailey LL, Concepcion W, Shattuck H, Huang L: Method of heart transplantation for treatment of hypoplastic left heart syndrome. J thorac Cardiovasc Surg 92:1–5, 1986.
13. Reitz BA, Jamieson SW, Gaudiani VA, et al: Method for cardiac transplantation in corrected transposition of the great arteries. J Cardiovasc Surg 23:293–296, 1982.
14. Doty DB, Renlund DG, Caputo GR, et al: Cardiac transplantation in situs inversus. J thorac Cardiovasc Surg 99:493–499, 1990.
15. Vouche PR, Tamisier D, Le Bidois J, et al: Pediatric cardiac transplantation for congenital heart defects: Surgical consideration and results. Ann thorac Surg 56:1239–1247, 1993.
16. Chartrand C: Pediatric cardiac transplantation despite atrial and venous return anomalies. Ann Thorac Surg 52:716–721, 1991.
17. Pearl JM, Laks H, Drinkwater DC: Cardiac transplantation following the modified Fontan procedure. Transplant Sci 2:1–3, 1992.
18. Menkis AH, McKenzie FN, Novick RJ, et al: Expanding applicability of transplantation after multiple prior palliative procedure. Ann Thorac Surg 52:722–726, 1991.
19. Allard M, Asaad A, Bailey L, et al: Surgical techniques in pediatric heart transplantation. J Heart Lung Transplant 10:808–827, 1991.
20. Cooper MM, Fuzesi L, Addonizio LJ, et al: Pediatric heart transplantation after operations involving the pulmonary arteries. J Thorac Cardiovasc Surg 102:386–395, 1991.
21. Turrentine MW, Kesler KA, Caldwell R, et al: Cardiac transplantation in infants and children. Ann Thorac Surg 57:546–554, 1994.
22. Bove EL: Transplantation after first-stage reconstruction for hypoplastic left heart syndrome. Ann thorac Surg 52:701–707, 1991.
23. Backer CL, Idriss FS, Zales VR, Mavroudis C: Cardiac transplantation for hypoplastic left heart syndrome: A modified technique. Ann Thorac Surg 50:894–898, 1990.
24. Mavroudis C: Commentary: Orthotopic cardiac transplantation in neonates. Ann Thorac Surg 52:705–706, 1991.
25. Spray TL, Huddleston CB, Canter CE: Technique of transplantation for hypoplastic left heart syndrome with left superior vena cava. Ann Thorac Surg 55:779–781, 1993.

Immunosuppression in Heart Transplantation: History and Current and Future Regimens

Chapter 8

Michel Carrier, MD
Pasquale Ferraro, MD

Immunosuppression is an essential part of transplant management. This aspect of patient care has been the focus of much attention, clinical experience, research, and publications. In a survey of transplant program directors in the United States, Evans et al.[1] reported wide variations in the use of immunosuppressive agents and combination protocols within the heart transplant community. As the number of centers performing heart transplantation increases and with the current leveling off in organ donation, most centers have seen their volume of transplants grow smaller. Future development of immunosuppressive agents and protocols thus depends on results of multicenter clinical trials, whereas individual physicians will base their selection of agents and protocols on conference consensus[2] and practical guidelines.[3]

The current practice of immunosuppression in heart transplantation is based on the clinical experience with cyclosporine over the last 15 years. The purpose of this review is to summarize the variety of immunosuppressive agents as they apply to clinical transplantation of the heart and to explain our bias, choice of agents, dosages, and protocols.

CYCLOSPORINE MAINTENANCE THERAPY

Cyclosporine was introduced into clinical practice 15 years ago.[4] Trials in recipients of kidney allografts demonstrated the superiority of cyclosporine over a conventional

88   Chapter 8

TABLE I.   Immunosuppressive Regimens: The Maintenance of Immunosuppression

Conventional immunosuppression protocol or the pre-cyclosporine era
  Azathioprine and prednisone
Cyclosporine maintenance therapy
  Double drug treatment: Cyclosporine and prednisone
  Triple drug treatment: Cyclosporine, prednisone, azathioprine
  Steroid-sparing treatment: Cyclosporine, azathioprine

combination of azathioprine and prednisone in improving patient and graft survival.[5,6] Historically, three combinations of immunosuppressive agents have been developed and used following heart transplantation: the *double drug treatment* of cyclosporine and prednisone[7]; the *triple drug treatment* of cyclosporine, azathioprine, and prednisone; and the *steroid-sparing treatment* including cyclosporine, azathioprine, and prednisone, tapered and discontinued (Table 1).

The *double therapy* initially used by the Stanford group[7] was rapidly replaced by *triple therapy*. Adding azathioprine to cyclosporine and prednisone allowed clinicians to reduce cyclosporine dosage and to improve the short- and mid-term renal function of transplant recipients.[9] Later, attempts to wean patients from oral prednisone led to the current approach of steroid-sparing treatment with the hope that a steroid-free protocol will decrease the incidence of several clinical side effects following transplantation.[10,11]

Results of these various protocols of cyclosporine maintenance have not been validated in clinical trials and remain based mostly on a single-center clinical cohort of patients, who were at best compared with an historical group. In this regard, collaborative studies and registry data may help improve the power of these observations. Between 1985 and 1992, Opelz and the collaborative Transplant Study[12] have collected data on 12,857 heart patients who had transplants in 104 centers in 24 countries. In this study, cyclosporine maintenance protocols were clearly superior to the conventional treatment of azathioprine and prednisone (Fig. 1). Graft survival with the three cyclosporine-based maintenance treatments appears similar despite a trend favoring the triple drug and the steroid-sparing approaches over cyclosporine and prednisone alone.

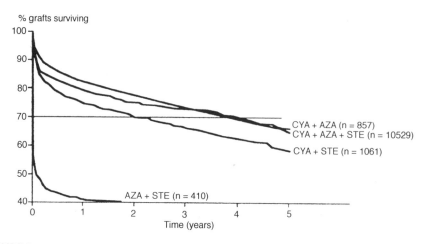

FIGURE I.   Graft survival from the Collaborative Transplant Study. CYA = cyclosporine; AZA = azathioprine; STE = steroid. (Dr. Opelz, personal communication.)

TABLE 2.   Immunosuppressive Regimens: Induction of Immunosuppression with Antibodies

Antilymphocyte/antithymocyte antibodies	Monoclonal antibody
1.1 Minnesota ALG	2.1 OKT3
1.2 ATGAM (Upjohn)	
1.3 RATG (Stanford, Pittsburgh)	

INDUCTION OF IMMUNOSUPPRESSION: ANTILYMPHOCYTE ANTIBODIES

To induce immunosuppression immediately after transplantation, antilymphocyte antibodies have been in use since the first few heart transplantations were performed in the late sixties.[13] Antithymocyte and antilymphocyte antibodies from the horse and then from the rabbit were both used (Table 2). One of the most popular polyclonal antibody preparations was the rabbit antithymocyte globulin (RATG).[13–15] The latter was shown to reduce early acute rejection after transplantation, to allow the late initiation of maintenance cyclosporine treatment after transplantation, and thus to help prevent early renal insufficiency resulting from cyclosporine toxicity.[15,16]

The monoclonal antibody OKT3 is an anti-CD3 antibody that has recently been recommended as part of an early prophylactic regimen after transplantation. Conflicting results, however, have been reported. Renlund et al. suggested that OKT3 prophylactic treatment was superior to the equine antithymocyte globulin,[17] whereas Kormos et al. reported similar results when comparing OKT3 and RATG perioperative immunosuppression.[18] A meta-analysis including 1881 patients from 38 studies published between 1985 and 1991 on the prophylactic effect of OKT3 treatment against acute rejection after cardiac, renal, and liver transplantation concluded that OKT3 treatment did not improve patient survival. Whereas rabbit ATG proved superior to OKT3 in preventing acute rejection, the latter was better than all other regimens studied.[19] Moreover, OKT3 treatment effectively delayed the occurrence of the first episode of acute rejection after heart transplantation (Figs. 2 and 3).

The Collaborative Transplant Study showed that the prophylactic use of cytolytic agents (OKT3 or ATG) did not affect graft survival in the 12,604 patients studied after heart transplantation (Fig. 4). Furthermore, Opelz et al.[20] reported that the incidence of non-Hodgkin lymphoma was higher among heart transplant recipients than among kidney recipients (relative risk of 3.00), and suggested that prophylactic OKT3 might increase the incidence of lymphoproliferative disorders after heart transplantation (Table 3). Swinnen and colleagues[21] reported a higher incidence of lymphoma in heart transplant patients who received OKT3 as a prophylactic agent, and as treatment of acute rejection episodes.

A NEW GENERATION OF CYCLOSPORINE: NEORAL CYCLOSPORINE

Cyclosporine is a lipophilic polypeptide with a marked variability in pharmacokinetic profiles within and among patients administered the soft capsules.[22] The absorption of cyclosporine is influenced by bile flow, coadministration of food, and gastrointestinal motility.[23] Studies of the pharmacokinetic properties of Neoral, a new microemulsion formulation of cyclosporine, resulted in an increased "area under the concentration curve," a decreased "time to maximal blood concentration," and increased "maximal blood concentration," and much less variability in intestinal absorption.[24,25] The new microemulsion formulation of cyclosporine depends less on bile for intestinal absorption after liver transplantation, a characteristic that can be of great benefit to patients immediately after transplantation.[26]

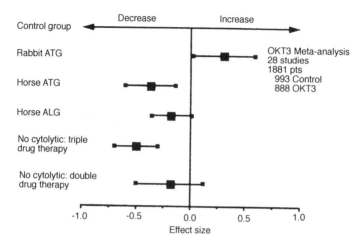

FIGURE 2.   Effect of prophylactic OKT3 in induction of immunosuppression on the incidence of acute rejection after transplantation. OKT3 patients had a higher incidence of acute rejection than RATG-treated patients and a lower rejection rate than the other group of patients. (Adapted from Carrier M, Jenicek M, Pelletier LC: Value of monoclonal antibody OKT3 in solid organ transplantation: A meta-analysis. Transplant Proc 24:2586–2591, 1992.)

Clinical trials are currently testing the new formulation of cyclosporine. Preliminary data in kidney allograft recipients suggest the Neoral cyclosporine results in more predictable absorption, pharmacokinetic profiles, and blood levels, without potentiating its toxicity.[27,28] Larger and completed experimental trials are needed to evaluate the clinical impact of this new generation of oral cyclosporine.

CLINICAL EXPERIENCE WITH VARIOUS IMMUNOSUPPRESSION REGIMENS AT THE MONTREAL HEART INSTITUTE

Between 1983 and 1987, the double drug treatment of cyclosporine and prednisone was used as recommended by the Stanford group.[7] In 1987, the triple drug treatment with the addition of azathioprine was introduced to decrease cyclosporine dosage and to try to improve long-term renal function (Table 4). A year after transplantation,

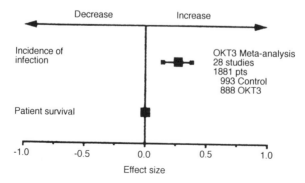

FIGURE 3.   Infection and survival rates after prophylactic OKT3. Patients given OKT3 had a higher incidence of infection and a similar survival rate when compared with patients in the control group. (Adapted from Carrier M, Jenicek M, Pelletier LC: Value of monoclonal antibody OKT3 in solid organ transplantation: A meta-analysis. Transplant Proc 24:2586–2591, 1992.)

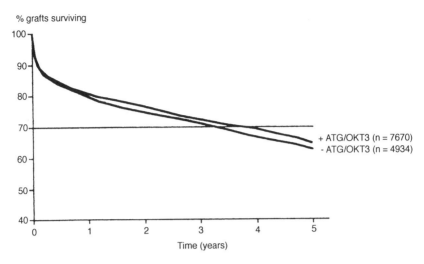

% grafts surviving

+ ATG/OKT3 (n = 7670)
- ATG/OKT3 (n = 4934)

Time (years)

FIGURE 4.   Graft survival from the Collaborative Transplant Study comparing patients treated with ATG or OKT3 and patients without a cytolytic agent. (Dr. Opelz, personal communication.)

creatinine levels were higher and clearance of creatinine lower in patients treated with the double drug treatment as compared with patients on the triple drug regimen. Nevertheless, the early renal failure related to cyclosporine remained a significant concern with these immunosuppression regimens.

To postpone administration of cyclosporine to the third day after transplantation, at the time when hemodynamic stability is reached in most patients, RATG is used for induction of immunosuppression immediately after transplantation (Table 4). This quadruple drug treatment of RATG, azathioprine, prednisone, and cyclosporine resulted in similar clinical results in terms of survival, rejection, and infection, whereas renal function remained normal in the immediate postoperative period. The quadruple drug treatment, which includes azathioprine in the maintenance protocol and rabbit ATG in the induction regimen, resulted in excellent overall clinical results and was effective in protecting early and late renal function from cyclosporine toxicity.

At present, we continue to use the quadruple drug regimen but attempt to decrease prednisone dosage at 5 mg/day 1 year after transplantation. Diabetics and patients who never demonstrated histologic rejection are then weaned off prednisone, whereas others are maintained at the lowest possible oral dosage of maintenance prednisone, that is

TABLE 3.   Incidence of Non-Hodgkin's Lymphoma—The Collaborative Transplant Study

Drug Regimens	Heart Transplant Recipients (no.)	Lymphoma Cases (no)	Relative Risk
Triple drug/steroid-sparing treatment	6,585	80	0.98
(CYA, AZA ± STE)	5,255	66	1.11
ATG/ALG/OKT3	4,072	42	0.91
ATG/ALG	1,183	24	3.12*
OKT3			

Relative risk: Calculated from data of Opelz[20] comparing the specified drug regimen against all others.

TABLE 4. Immunosuppressive Regimens: The Experience at the Montreal Heart Institute

	Double Drug Treatment	Triple Drug Treatment	Triple Drug and RATG Induction
No. patients	24	13	77
Years	1983–1987	1987	1988–1992
Preoperative			
Cyclosporine	10 mg/kg PO	6 mg/kg PO	None
Azathioprine	None	4 mg/kg PO	4 mg/kg PO
Intraoperative			
Methylprednisolone	500 mg IV	500 mg IV	500 mg IV
Postoperative			
RATG	None	None	125 mg IV infusion/day for 3 days
Methylprednisolone	125 mg IV for 3 days	125 mg IV for 3 days	125 mg IV for 3 days
Azathioprine	None	150 mg/day, taper to keep WBC > 5000	150 mg/day, taper to keep WBC > 5000
		4 mg/kg/day PO serum level	100 mg every 12 h, day 3
Cyclosporine	4 mg/kg/day PO serum level	200–300 mmol/L	200 mg/every 12 h, day 4 serum level 200–300 mmol/L
Prednisone	100 mg taper to 20 mg/day at 1 month	100 mg taper to 14 mg/day at 1 month	100 mg/day at 1 month 5 mg/day at 12 months
Rejection (no./patient)	1.3 ± 1	0.8 ± 1	0.6 ± 0.1
Infection (no./patient)	1.7 ± 4	0.3 ± 1	0.9 ± 0.1
Creatinine peak value at 1 week (mmol/L)	215 ± 21*	215 ± 21*	148 ± 9
Creatinine at 1 year (mmol/L)	157 ± 7*	116 ± 7	123 ± 4

* Mean of double and triple drug treatment patients.
(Adapted from Carrier M, Pelletier GB, Leclerc Y, et al: Effet de la cyclosporine sur la fonction rénale après transplantation cardiaque: Peut-on diminuer la toxicité? Can J Surg 33:243–247, 1990; and from Carrier M, Pelletier GB, Cartier R, et al: Induction of immunosuppression with rabbit antithymocyte globulin: Five-year experience in cardiac transplantation. Can J Cardiol 9:171–176, 1993.)

5 mg/day or 5 mg every other day (or 2.5 mg/day). More than 47 (of 160) transplant patients are currently receiving less than 5 mg/day or no maintenance dosage of oral prednisone. This late and selective approach to steroid weaning was suggested by Miller and coworkers[11] because weaning of prednisone in the immediate postoperative period was not tolerated in 50% of patients.[10] Moreover, it has yet to be shown that patients without prednisone have a better clinical outcome than patients maintained on low doses of maintenance prednisone.

We have used the new microemulsion of cyclosporine (Neoral) in two patients. In the first case, Neoral was initiated with a dosage of 100 mg twice a day starting on the second day after transplantation, and the trough levels were immediately stable averaging 200 mmol/L (Fig. 5). This patient was maintained on Neoral for 1 month and all results from endomyocardial biopsies were normal. The second patient was maintained on Neoral for a few days when the patient was in hepatic and renal failure following cardiogenic shock. Unfortunately, this latter patient died of related complications. Thus, our initial experience with the use of this new generation of cyclosporine, although limited, supports the results that were presented with liver transplant patients[26]

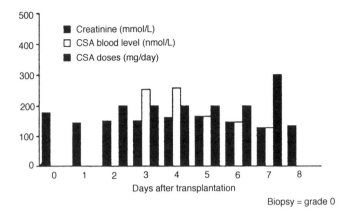

FIGURE 5.   Clinical case treated with Neoral cyclosporine. Blood levels stabilized immediately after the first doses of Neoral.

and suggests that improvement in intestinal absorption and stable trough levels can be achieved in the immediate postoperative period after heart transplantation, whereas renal function appears to remain normal. Clinical trials to confirm these hypotheses are needed, but we can already suggest that the new microemulsion of cyclosporine may be easier to use in the immediate postoperative period, challenging the need for antibody induction treatment. Moreover, the pharmacokinetic profile of Neoral differs greatly from that of the soft capsule of cyclosporine. Thus, current clinical outcomes, patient and graft survival, acute and chronic rejection, as well as infection, and drug side effects may be significantly improved with Neoral microemulsion of cyclosporine.

ALTERNATIVE AND ADJUNCT APPROACHES TO IMMUNOSUPPRESSION

Several other approaches to immunosuppression have been studied and used. Bromocriptine, an inhibitor of pituitary release of prolactin, was shown to have a synergistic effect with cyclosporine in decreasing incidence of early acute rejection after heart transplantation.[29] Moran and associates[30] suggested that prostaglandin E improves renal function and reduces incidence of acute rejection in renal transplant recipients treated concurrently with cyclosporine and prednisone. Cyclophosphamide was successfully substituted for azathioprine in triple drug regimen when patients showed signs of azathioprine-induced hepatotoxicity[31] or in patients with histologic evidence of vascular rejection.

Major histocompatibility antigens play a critical role in acute rejection of allografts. Opelz and the Collaborative Transplant Study[32] found that patients who received a perfectly human leukocyte antigen (HLA)-matched donor had a better long-term survival rate than mismatched patients (Fig. 6). Patients with two HLA-A, B, or DR mismatches had a 25% greater likelihood of failed grafts within 3 years of transplantation when compared with transplants with either no mismatches or only one. Whereas donor-recipient matching for HLA antigen is not yet practical, development of better methods of preservation of donor hearts and of DNA typing techniques for HLA determination, as well as the use of mechanical assist devices for mid- and long-term support of the failing heart, will likely make the donor-recipient matching for major histocompatibility loci more accessible to the clinical practice of heart transplantation in the near future.

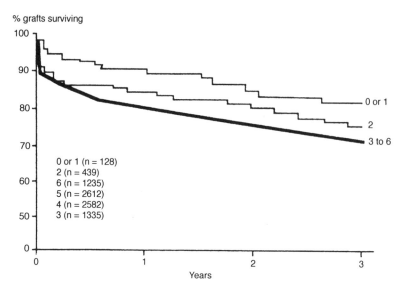

FIGURE 6.   Graft survival from the Collaborative Transplant Study according to the number of HLA-A, B, or DR mismatches. (Adapted from Opelz G, Wujciak T: The influence of HLA compatibility on graft survival after transplantation. N Engl J Med 330:816–819, 1994.)

CONCLUSION

Cyclosporine has been the key to all clinical immunosuppression regimens for the last 15 years. An understanding of the clinical use of cyclosporine and pharmacokinetic studies resulting in wide application of blood-level measurements of the molecule have led to the current development of heart transplantation. Although as yet undocumented, the new microemulsion formulation of cyclosporine will likely improve control of the pharmacokinetic and blood levels of the drug, and as such clinical results will likely improve. Meanwhile, newer compounds and drug combinations need to be tested in controlled clinical trials to determine their potential use and benefit in clinical transplantation of the heart.

REFERENCES

1. Evans R, Manninen DL, Dong FB, et al: Immunosuppressive therapy as a determinant of transplantation outcomes. Transplantation 55:1297–1305, 1993.
2. Hunt SA: 24th Bethesda Conference. J Am Coll Cardiol 22:1–64, 1993.
3. O'Connell JB, Bourge RC, Costanzo-Nordin MR, et al: Cardiac transplantation: Recipient selection, donor procurement, and medical follow-up. Circulation 86:1061–1079, 1992.
4. Calne RY, White DJG, Evans DB, et al: Cyclosporin A initially as the only immunosuppressant in 34 recipients of cadaveric organs: 32 kidneys, 2 pancreases, and 2 livers. Lancet 17:1033–1036, 1979.
5. European Multicenter Trial: Cyclosporin A as sole immunosuppressive agent in recipients of kidney allografts from cadaver donors. Lancet 2:57–60, 1982.
6. The Canadian Multicenter Transplant Study Group: A randomized clinical trial of cyclosporine in cadaveric renal transplantation. N Engl J Med 309:809–815, 1983.
7. Oyer PE, Stinson EB, Jamieson SW, et al: Cyclosporin A in cardiac allograft: A preliminary experience. Transplant Proc 15:1247–1252, 1983.
8. Bolman RM, Cance C, Spray T, et al: The changing face of cardiac transplantation: The Washington University Program, 1985–1987. Ann Thorac Surg 45:192–197, 1988.
9. Carrier M, Pelleter GB, leclerc Y, et al: Effet de la cyclosporine sur la fonction rénale après transplantation cardiaque: Peut-on diminuer la toxicité? Can J Surg 33:243–247, 1990.

10. Price GD, Olsen SL, Taylor DO, et al: Corticosteroid-free maintenance immunosuppression after heart transplantation: Feasibility and beneficial effects. J Heart Lung Transplant 11:403–413, 1992.
11. Miller LW, Wolford T, McBride LR, et al: Successful withdrawal of corticosteroids in heart transplantation. J Heart Lung Transplant 11:431–434, 1992.
12. Opelz G, Wujciak T: The influence of HLA compatibility on graft survival after heart transplantation. N Engl J Med 330:816–819, 1994.
13. Bieber CP, Griepp RB, Oyer PE, et al: Use of rabbit antithymocyte globulin in cardiac transplantation: Relationship of serum clearance rates to clinical outcome. Transplantation 22:478–488, 1976.
14. Carey JA, Frist WH: Use of polyclonal antilymphocytic preparations for prophylaxis in heart transplantation. J Heart Transplant 9:297–300, 1990.
15. Copeland JG, Icenogle TB, Williams RJ, et al: Rabbit antithymocyte globulin. A 10-year experience in cardiac transplantation. J Thorac Cardiovasc Surg 99:852–860, 1990.
16. Carrier M, Pelletier GB, Cartier R, et al: Induction of immunosuppression with rabbit antithymocyte globulin: Five-year experience in cardiac transplantation. Can J Cardiol 9:171–176, 1993.
17. Renlund DG, O'Connell JB, Gilbert EM, et al: A prospective comparison of murine monoclonal CD-3 (OKT3) antibody-based and equine antithymocyte globulin-based rejection prophylaxis in cardiac transplantation . Transplantation 47:599–605, 1989.
18. Kormos RL, Armitage JM, Dummer S, et al: Optimal perioperative immunosuppression in cardiac transplantation using rabbit antithymocyte globulin. Transplantation 49:306–311, 1990.
19. Carrier M, Jenicek M, Pelletier LC: Value of monoclonal antibody OKT3 in solid organ transplantation: A meta-analysis. Transplant Proc 24:2586–2591, 1992.
20. Opelz G, Henderson R: Incidence of non-Hodgkin lymphoma in kidney and heart transplant recipients. Lancet 342:1514–1516, 1993.
21. Swinnen LJ, Constanzo-Nordin MR, Fisher S, et al: Increased incidence of lymphoproliferative disorder after immunosuppression with the monoclonal antibody OKT3 in cardiac transplant recipients. N Engl J Med 323:1723–1728, 1990.
22. Kahan BD: Cyclosporine. N Engl J Med 9:587–593, 1989.
23. Lemaire M, Fahr A, Maurer G: Pharmacokinetics of cyclosporin: Inter- and intra-individual variations and metabolic pathways. Transplant Proc 22:1110–1112, 1990.
24. Browne BJ, Jordan S, Welsh MS, et al: Diet and cyclosporin A—pharmacokinetic comparison between Neoral and Sandimmune gelatin capsules. The Third International Congress on Cyclosporine, Seville, Spain, 1994, p 84.
25. Kahan BD, Dunn J, Fitts C, et al: American study in renal transplantation. The Third International Congress on Cyclosporine, Seville, Spain, 1994, p 130.
26. Trull AK, Tan KKC, Tan EF, et al: Improved absorption of cyclosporine from new microemulsion formulation in 9 liver transplant recipients. The Third International Congress on Cyclosporine, Seville, Spain, 1994, p 87.
27. Holt DW: The pharmacokinetics of Sandimmune Neoral—A new oral formulation of cyclosporine. The Third International Congress on Cyclosporine, Seville, Spain, 1994, p 128.
28. Neumayer HH, Faber L, Haller P, et al: Conversion from Sandimmune to Sandimmune Neoral— Experience in 300 patients after renal transplantation. The Third International Congress on Cyclosporine, Seville, Spain, 1994, p 131.
29. Carrier M, Wild J, Pelletier LC, Copeland JG: Bromocriptine as an adjuvant to cyclosporine immunosuppression after heart transplantation. Ann Thorac Surg 49:129–132, 1990.
30. Moran M, Mozes MF, Maddux MS, et al: Prevention of acute graft rejection by the prostaglandin E_1 analogue misoprostol in renal-transplant recipients treated with cyclosporin and prednisone. N Engl J Med 322:1183–1188, 1990.
31. Wagoner LE, Olsen SL, Bristow MR, et al: Cyclophosphamide as an alternative to azathioprine in cardiac transplant recipients with suspected azathioprine-induced hepatotoxicity. Transplantation 56:1415–1418, 1993.
32. Opelz G, Wujciak T: the influence of HLA compatibility on graft survival after heart transplantation. N Engl J Med 330;816–819, 1994.

Tacrolimus (FK506)—How We Do It in Pittsburgh

Chapter 9

Bartley P. Griffith, MD

In a systematic screening program initiated by the Fujisawa Pharmaceutical Company in 1982, Goto and Kino described the immunosuppressive qualities of a fermentation product of *Streptomyces tsukubarnis* in 1984.[1,2] The drug named at that time FR-900506 was further evaluated by Calne and Ochiai, and their in vitro and in vivo work was presented at the 1986 Transplant Society meeting in Helsinki. By 1987 the drug's name was shortened to FK506, and animal studies presented at a satellite symposium of the European Society of Transplantation in Sweden interested Dr. Thomas Starzl.[3] Starzl, not willing to discard this potentially powerful immunosuppressant because of described associated vasculitis, encouraged his colleague Saturo Todo and the Fujisawa Corporation to permit further preclinical studies to be performed in Pittsburgh. Zeevi and others at our center confirmed the one hundred times greater potency of FK506 versus cyclosporine (CsA) and importantly demonstrated this in donor-specific mixed lymphocyte cultures with host cells obtained from endomyocardial biopsies in rejecting human recipients.[4] Dr. Todo and his colleagues had success in primate renal models. The first clinical trial began at the University of Pittsburgh in 1988 as a rescue for recipients with chronic liver rejection and was followed in that same year as a primary immunosuppressant in liver, kidney, heart, and lung.[5-14] Additional organs, including intestines and bone marrow, have been added, and recently national and international trials have helped to define the role for this important immunosuppressant. In 1994 FK506 was approved by the FDA and accepted by Medicare for approved transplant procedures. The generic name of FK506 is now tacrolimus, and it is marketed under the trade name Prograf. This paper reviews its pharmacology and immunology, and our experience with its use in recipients of heart and/or lung allografts.

PHARMACOLOGY

Tacrolimus is a lipophilic macrolide lactone (Fig. 1) supplied in 1- and 5-mg capsules. It is prepared at 5 mg/ml in the expedient cremophor for intravenous administration and is diluted in D_5W to .002 to .004 mg/ml. Unlike cyclosporine, its absorption does not depend on intact enterohepatic circulation and thereby represents a significant advantage for use in liver transplantation. The same drugs that alter cyclosporine metabolism can be expected to accelerate or inhibit tacrolimus. It is metabolized by microsomal P_{450} enzymes in the liver and intestine, and less than 5% of the drug is excreted unmetabolized in the stool. Of clinical interest and compatible with observed augmented toxicities when cyclosporine and tacrolimus are combined has been the recognition that tacrolimus inhibits the cyclosporine $P_{450}III^A$ enzyme oxidase, resulting in sustained cyclosporine levels. Individual variation in absorption and metabolism has resulted in a poor correlation between the dose of tacrolimus and blood levels, necessitating blood-level monitoring. Fortunately, unlike cyclosporine, overall drug exposure, as described by cumulative area under the blood-level concentration curve, correlated with trough drug level ($R \geq 0.93$) (Fig. 2).[15] The new Neoral microemulsion preparation of cyclosporine was formulated to improve availability of cyclosporine. Most of our original work used a monoclonal enzyme immunoase (EIA) to measure plasma levels. Currently, a whole-blood antibody technique (IMX) is used because it is faster (1 to 3 hours) and, as a whole blood measurement, avoids possible inaccurate measurement caused by the shift of drug into red blood cells as the specimen cools to room temperature. Based on dose optimization studies in kidney recipients (FDA Advisory Committee, 11/22/93), we target the tacrolimus dose to reach 15 to 20 ng/ml whole blood (IMX) during the first 3 postoperative months and reduce it to 10 ng/ml relative to the clinical balance between rejection and drug toxicity. Higher doses with levels greater than 20 ng/ml, although associated with a lower rate of rejection, have required downward adjustments in up to 65% because of toxicities. Lower doses are associated with less toxicity but have been less effective. Because thoracic organ recipients are often hemodynamically unstable perioperatively, we have adopted a low dose (0.075 mg/kg twice daily) for oral initiation of the drug on the first postoperative day. The dose is progressively increased (0.15 mg/kg per day) toward the 15 to 20 ng/ml target, usually within 5 days. When oral or gavage dosing is not possible because of gastrointestinal

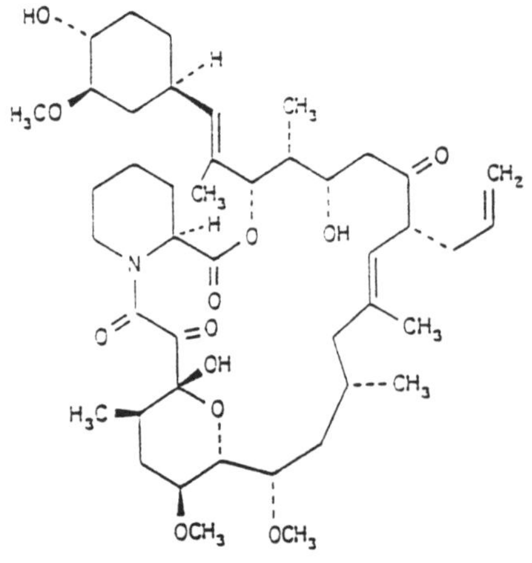

FIGURE I.   Chemical structure of tacrolimus.

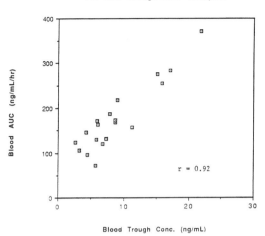

FIGURE 2. Tacrolimus drug exposure as described by cumulative area under the blood level concentration curve.

impairment, tacrolimus may be given intravenously with a 24-hour dose of 0.036 mg/kg that is progressively increased to target levels. Like cyclosporine, intravenous use of tacrolimus has a higher incidence of acute renal failure.

IMMUNOSUPPRESSIVE EFFECTS

To the extent that it is reasonable to generalize, it is probable that, like cyclosporine, the chief effect of tacrolimus is based upon its ability to restrict T-cell proliferation by limiting the calcium-dependent transcription of factors that initiate genes for the production of cytokines (IL-2) for other soluble mediators, including IL-3 and interferon gamma.[16] The events subsequent to the presentation of antigen embedded in MHC protein to the TcR-CD3 complex on T-cells cause recruitment of intracellular and extracellular calcium required for activation of the serine/threonine phosphatase calcineurin. A substrate of calcineurin includes the cytoplasmic component of nuclear factor of activated T-cells (NF-AT). With dephosphorylization of NF-AT and simultaneous activation by ras of c-fos and c-jun, lymphokine genes are transcribed. The critical calcineurin step is blocked when tacrolimus combines with an intracellular binding protein (immunophilin family) called FKBP. Cyclosporine also combines with an immunophilin called cyclophylin, and both inhibit the subsequent serine/threonine phosphatase, calcineurin. Because the block of calcineurin occurs in all cells, not just the dividing lymphocytes, it is not surprising that both of these medications have similar toxicities.

CLINICAL EXPERIENCE

Cardiac Transplantation

We first reported our experience with tacrolimus in adult cardiac recipients in 1991.[13] This and subsequent use after cardiac transplantation in our institution was not controlled prospectively against cyclosporine-based immunotherapy.[14] Adult patients received moderate doses of tacrolimus (0.15 mg/kg/bid), 0.15 mg/kg prednisone, and azathioprine. Steroids were weaned relative to rejection whenever possible. A 93% 1-year survival rate was achieved in this initial group despite inclusion of a significant number of high-risk recipients. Freedom at 3 months from grade ≥ 3a was 41%, and the linearized rate was 0.95 per patient. At 1 year, 30% were not receiving steroids, and those who did averaged 8.5 mg/kg per day. Compared with our most contemporary cyclosporine-based protocols, which included induction of therapy with the cytolytic monoclonal antibody OKT3 plus maintenance with prednisone and azathioprine, survival and freedom from rejection were similar, but only 28% of the patients given tacrolimus versus 48% of those given cyclosporine had repeat episodes of rejection. Left ventricular ejection fraction in this group of 70 patients averaged 66% and ranged between 48 and 75% at 1 year, and of the 35 who had annual coronary arteriography, 4 (11%) had evidence of mild coronary arteriopathy. The importance of this finding moderates initial concerns about the possibility of drug-associated vasculitis, previously seen in some animal species. Based on our continued experience with tacrolimus, incidence of graft vascular disease is similar with both therapies. Side effects were not major problems and included hypertension in 54%, new onset diabetes in 18%, hyperkalemia in 10%, and neuromuscular abnormalities including seizure, tremors or hallucinations in 10%. Currently we are following 81 consecutive patients treated with tacrolimus (unpublished). This group has achieved an actual survival of 79% at 2.9 ± 1.3 years of follow-up. Compared with cyclosporine plus cytolytic induction therapy, the tacrolimus group has had a higher incidence of grade >2 rejection (57 vs. 40%, p = 0.07). In contract there appears to be less endocardial fibrosis and fewer Quilty lesions (55 vs. 89%, p < 0.01) in 12-month biopsies, suggesting a better long-term outlook for patients treated with tacrolimus.

Rescue Therapy after Heart Transplant

We have been fortunate to evaluate the usefulness of tacrolimus as a rescue from persistent cardiac rejection (≥3a) in an additional 26 recipients who have averaged 435 days of cyclosporine-based and augmented steroid plus cytolytic therapy.[14] All have been successfully treated. In 20, tacrolimus alone was successful within 2 weeks. Two patients required additional methylprednisolone, and one additional OKT3 and methylprednisolone. The average dose of prednisone was reduced in this group from 20 mg/day to 12.5 mg. Over the period of treatment, creatinine rose insignificantly from 1.5 to 2.0 mg/dl. Because of additive toxicities, cyclosporine was discontinued for 2 to 3 days before tacrolimus, which was slowly increased to 0.15 mg/kg twice daily with a serum trough of 1.0 to 2.0 mg/ml (TDX). Serum creatinine levels were carefully followed during the conversion and thereafter. In view of the heavy immunosuppressants received by these patients, it is not surprising that four had major infections (one each with disseminated tuberculosis, nocardiosis, mucormycosis, and aspergillosis). Additionally, four (15%) developed posttransplant lymphoproliferative disease (PTLD). Six of the 26 died between 4 months and 4 years of the switch to tacrolimus (PTLD, 3; suicide, 1; osteosarcoma, 1; glioblastoma multiforme, 1). Because all patients demonstrated stabilized biopsies and none died with acute or chronic failure, we concluded that tacrolimus is an effective agent for refractory rejection and likely should be used earlier before heavy doses of adjunct immunosuppressive therapy.

Lung Transplantation

Between October 1991 and March 1993, 74 lung transplants (35 single lung transplants, 39 bilateral lung transplants) were performed on 74 recipients who were randomly assigned to receive either tacrolimus or cyclosporine.[17] Thirty-eight recipients (19 single lung transplants, 19 bilateral lung transplants) received tacrolimus, and 36 recipients (16 single lung transplant, 20 bilateral lung transplant) received cyclosporine. Recipients receiving tacrolimus or cyclosporine were similar in age, gender, preoperative New York

Heart Association functional class, and underlying disease. Acute rejection was assessed by clinical, radiographic, and histologic criteria. Acute rejection was treated with methylprednisolone, 1g IV/day, for 3 days or rabbit antithymocyte globulin if steroid-resistant.

During the first 30 days after transplant, one patient in the tacrolimus group died of cerebral edema, whereas two recipients treated with cyclosporine died, one of bacterial pneumonia and one of cardiac arrest. Although 1-year survival was similar between groups, the number of recipients free from acute rejection in the tacrolimus group was significantly higher when compared with the cyclosporine group. The mean number of episodes of acute rejection/100 patient days was significantly fewer in the tacrolimus group (1.2) as compared with the cyclosporine group (2.0). Although only one recipient (1/36, i.e., 3%) in the group treated with cyclosporine remained free from acute rejection within 120 days of transplantation, 13% (5/38) of the group treated with tacrolimus remained free from acute rejection during this interval. Prevalence of bacterial infection in the cyclosporine group was 1.5 episodes/100 patient days and 0.6 episodes/100 patient days in the tacrolimus group. The prevalence of cytomegaloviral and fungal infection was similar in both groups. Acute rejection occurred less frequently in the tacrolimus-treated group compared with the cyclosporine-treated group in the early postoperative period (< 90 days). Early graft survival at 30 days was similar in the two groups, but intermediate graft survival at 6 months was better in the tacrolimus group compared with the cyclosporine group. Although transient renal dysfunction immediately after transplantation was frequently observed with intravenous administration of tacrolimus or cyclosporine, the majority of cases were well controlled with concomitant administration of low-dose prostaglandin E_1. Notably absent in the tacrolimus group were complaints of gingival hyperplasia or hirsutism, frequently diagnosed in recipients treated with cyclosporine. Systolic and diastolic arterial pressures were similar in the two groups during this observational period. Twelve recipients in the tacrolimus group (12 of 38) and 15 recipients in the cyclosporine group (15 of 36) required antihypertensive therapy, consisting of enalapril maleate or diltiazem hydrochloride.

This randomized trial of tacrolimus versus cyclosporine after isolated pulmonary transplantation suggests that tacrolimus-based immunosuppression resulted in less frequent moderate and severe acute rejection. Follow-up studies in continuation of this trial continue to suggest this difference. Overall, 11% of the tacrolimus patients were free from rejection at 6 months after transplantation whereas virtually none of the cyclosporine recipients were free of at least one episode. We hope this improved freedom in numbers of rejection and those with recurrent rejection will translate into a reduced incidence of obliterative bronchiolitis, although it is unclear at present whether tacrolimus will be associated with reduced incidence of chronic rejection.

Toxicity

Because inhibition of calcineurin phosphatase activity is the common mode of biologic action of both tacrolimus and cyclosporine, it is not surprising that most of the toxicities overlap. Although little is known about the toxic effects of the drugs or their metabolites, it is known that calcineurin is critical to all nerve cells and that it is involved in the regulation of nitric oxide synthetase activity. We have found this might explain the high evidence of neurologic toxicity and that most of these toxicities have been minor and certainly not a significant impediment to the use of the drug.[18] We have noted that tacrolimus is not associated with lanugo, hair growth, facial brutalization, or gingival hyperplasia. These benefits significantly improve the quality of our recipients' lives. Tacrolimus does seem to have a very similar nephrotoxicity diabetogenic potential and perhaps similar or a bit less associated hypertension.[19] The mean creatinine value at

1 year in our heart transplant survivors treated with tacrolimus has been 2.2 ± 1.2 mg/dl compared with our cyclosporine A group (2.1 ± 0.09, p = 0.05).

SUMMARY

It has been stimulating to be part of the clinical introduction of the much heralded tacrolimus for heart and lung transplant recipients. Although we initially had hoped it would provide a more uniform ability to treat patients with a low-risk monoimmuno-suppressant therapy, we have learned, as in most clinical situations, that over time, our expectations have been reduced. Without question we favor tacrolimus in our compo-nent therapy following transplantation, which now includes azathioprine and steroids. For those interested in switching to tacrolimus, it is important to remember that cy-closporine must be withheld for a number of days. When using this medication as a primary immunosuppressant instead of cyclosporine, it is suggested that it be used liter-ally as a substitute for cyclosporine, in a protocol with which a center is comfortable— for example, one associated with induction, triple drug therapy, or another means.

REFERENCES

1. Kino T, Hatanaka H, Miyata S, et al: FK-506, a novel immunosuppressant isolated from a Streptomyces. I. Fermentation, isolatin and physicochemical and biological characteristics. J Antibiot (Tokyo) 40:1249–1255, 1987.
2. Kino T, Hatanaka H, Miyata S, et al: FK-506, a novel immunosuppressant isolated from a Streptomyces. II. Immunosuppressive effect of FK-506 in vitro. J Antibiot (Tokyo) 40:1256–1265, 1987.
3. Ochiai T, Nagata M, Nakajima K, et al: Studies of the effects of FK506 on renal allografting in the beagle dog. Transplantation 44:729–733, 1987.
4. Zeevi A, Duquesnoy RJ, Eiras G, et al: Immunosuppressive effect of FR-900506 on in-vitro lymphocyte alloactivation: Syndergism with cyclosporin A. Transplant Japonica 19(6):40, 1988.
5. Fung JJ, Todo S, Jain A, et al: Conversion from cyclosporine to FK 506 in liver allograft recipients with cyclosporine-related complications. Transplant Proc 22:6-12, 1990.
6. Fung J, Abu-Elmagd K, Jain A, et al: A randomized trial of primary liver transplantation under im-munosuppression with FK 506 vs cyclosporine. Transplant Proc 23:2977–2983, 1991.
7. Takaya S, Bronsther O, Todo S, et al: Retransplantation of liver: A comparison of FK 506 and cy-closporine-treated patients. Transplant Proc 23:3026–3028, 1991.
8. Tzakis AG, Reyes J, Todo S, et al: FK 506 versus cyclosporine in pediatric liver transplantation. Transplant Proc 23:3010–3015, 1991.
9. Uemoto S, Ozawa K, Tanaka K, et al: Experience with FK 506 in living related donor liver transplanta-tion. Transplant Proc 23:3007–3009, 1991.
10. Shapiro R, Jordan M, Scantlebury V, et al: FK 506 in clinical kidney transplantation. Transplant Proc 23:3065–3067, 1991.
11. Japanese FK 506 Study Group: Clinicopathological evaluation of kidney transplants in patients given a fixed dose of FK 506. Transplant Proc 23:3111–3115, 1991.
12. Jensen CWB, Jordan ML, Schneck FX, et al: Pediatric renal transplantation under FK 506 immunosup-pression. Transplant Proc 23:3075–3077, 1991.
13. Armitage JM, Fricker FJ, del Nido P, et al: The clinical trial of FK 506 as primary and rescue immuno-suppressive in pediatric cardiac transplantation. Transplant Proc 23:3058–3060, 1991.
14. Armitage JM, Kormos RL, Fung J, Starzl TE: The clinical trial of FK 506 as primary and rescue im-munosuppression in adult cardiac transplantation. Transplant Proc 23:3054–3057, 1991.
15. Regazzi MB, Rondanelli R, Biol D, et al: Optimization of sampling time for cyclosporine monitoring in transplant patients. J Clin Pharmacol 32:978–981, 1992.
16. Steinmuller DR: Medical Intelligence Unit FK506 and Organ Transplantation. Georgetown, TX, RG Landes Company, 1994.
17. Griffith BP, Bando K, Hardesty RL, et al: A prospective randomized trial of FK506 versus cyclosporine after human pulmonary transplantation. Transplantation 57:848–851, 1994.
18. Fung JJ, Alessiani M, Abu-Elmagd K, et al: Adverse effects associated with the use of FK 506. Transplant Proc 23:3105–3108, 1991.
19. Tauxe WN, Mochizuki T, McCauley J, et al: A comparison of the renal effects (ERPF, GFR, and FF) of FK 506 and cyclosporine in patients with liver transplantation. Transplant Proc 23:3146–3147, 1991.

Chapter 10

Steroid Withdrawal in Cardiac Transplantation

Leslie W. Miller, MD
Thomas L. Wolford, MD
Thomas Donohue, MD

Corticosteroids have been a component of every immunosuppressive regimen to prevent allograft rejection since the beginning of clinical solid organ transplantation.[1] The daily maintenance dose has been reduced over time, especially since the advent of triple drug immunosuppression[2] (i.e., the addition of azathioprine to cyclosporine and prednisone), which allowed a reduction in the dosage of each of the three components of that regimen. Chronic corticosteroid use is associated, however, with very substantial dose-related morbidity, including osteoporosis, glucose intolerance, growth suppression, salt and water retention, and hyperlipidemia. As a result, there has been increasing interest in investigating the possibility of totally withdrawing corticosteroids from the maintenance immunosuppressive regimen and using only cyclosporine and azathioprine long-term.[3-6] Although this concept seems attractive and potentially obviates most, if not all, of the morbid complications of corticosteroids, total withdrawal of steroids may also be associated with several potential problems, including whether cyclosporine and azathioprine alone would provide adequate immunosuppression and whether the dosage of cyclosporine would have to be increased (to provide adequate immunosuppression) to a level associated with increased side-effects such as nephrotoxicity and hypertension. In addition, debate is ongoing whether corticosteroids are atherogenic and potentiate the accelerated coronary disease seen in cardiac transplant recipients, or whether they are protective by their role in inhibiting T-cell activation through a blockade of interleukin (IL)-1 production and thereby provide a critical component of inhibition to the immune-mediated component of accelerated coronary artery disease.

Yacoub[3] is credited with the initial report of successful withdrawal of corticosteroids in heart transplant recipients in the early 1980s. Since his original study, which was performed by stopping steroids by day 3 posttransplant, two approaches have evolved to timing of withdrawal of steroids posttransplant, namely *early*—within 3 to 4 weeks of transplantation, and almost always in conjunction with the use of a 10 to 14 day course of cytolytic (induction) therapy,[4–9] or *late*—which delays the initiation of withdrawal to a minimum of 3 months after transplant and may not employ the routine use of induction therapy.[10–12] The Utah transplant program has published the largest experience with early steroid withdrawal, again in conjunction with the use of a course of induction therapy utilizing OKT-3[6–8] They found withdrawal of steroid during or immediately after the 14-day course of OKT-3 was associated with a significant increase in rejection in the ensuing 1 to 2 weeks,[13] and therefore most patients were given a substantial dose of methylprednisolone beginning at 1.0 mg/kg/day for 7 days on the last day of prophylactic OKT-3, then tapered off over 2 weeks to prevent a rebound in the immune response after OKT-3 was completely discontinued. Steroids were therefore usually totally withdrawn within 4 weeks after transplant. The success with this approach (i.e., percentage of patients able to remain free of chronic maintenance steroids) is reported 50-60% at 1 year and 40 to 50% at 2 years.[8]

The ability to withdraw patients from steroids was reported to be one of the benefits of induction therapy, but the contribution of induction therapy to the success of steroid withdrawal was unclear. Because incidence of rejection was confined nearly totally to the first 6 months after transplant in our program, we elected to initiate our experience with steroid withdrawal in patients who were at least 6 months posttransplant. Initially, we withdrew steroids only from male patients who had experienced no rejection in the first 6 months. However, when the very high success rate in that specific population of patients without induction therapy was evident, we extended our inclusion criteria to all patients, and gradually shortened the time posttransplant to initiate withdrawal to an average of 4 months to further evaluate the importance of time. This also resulted from a desire to eliminate additional biopsies in these patients by taking advantage of their normal protocol biopsy schedule earlier posttransplant.

The immunosuppressive regimen used in our program with steroid withdrawal is outlined in Table 1. The dosage of corticosteroids is tapered progressively to none by an average of 5 months after transplant. None of the patients receive induction therapy perioperatively. the dose of cyclosporine was not empirically increased and in fact was reduced gradually over time in an attempt to minimize hypertension and nephrotoxicity. The dose or azathioprine was not changed, but often dose reduction was required when steroids were totally discontinued because of the loss of the demarginating effect on white blood cell count of corticosteroids. The biopsy schedule is outline in Table 2. Steroids were tapered by 2.5 mg/day every other week. Patients were biopsied at the onset of steroid withdrawal (at a time when they were usually receiving 5 mg/day of methylprednisolone), after 4 weeks (or when a dose of 2.5 mg/day was reached), at the

TABLE 1.   Immunosuppression Protocol for Steroid Withdrawal

		Months Posttransplant				
	Pretransplant	1	2	3	4	5
Steroid*	10	0.3	0.2	0.1	.05	off
Cyclosporine A*	1–3 IV	4.4	3.9	3.7	3.6	3.7
Azathioprine*	2	1.9	1.8	1.8	1.7	1.7

* mg/kg

TABLE 2.   Biopsy Schedule

Routine	SW (Late)
Weekly × 4	5 mg
Bi-weekly × 3	2.5 mg
Monthly × 6	0
Bi-monthly × 2	Monthly × 3
Every 3 mo × 4	Every 3 mo × 6
Yearly	Every 4 mo

time they became totally free of corticosteroids, then monthly for 3 months, every 3 months for the following 6 months, and then every 4 months thereafter. Only ISHLT biopsy grade 3A rejection or greater or any biopsy associated with hemodynamic compromise was treated. A treatment course consisted of 10 mg/kg of intravenous methylprednisolone daily for 3 days. initially patients were returned to the level of corticosteroids they had been taking before biopsy evidence of rejection (typically, no steroid). More recently, we have returned the patients to 10 mg of oral prednisone for 1 week, then tapered the dose by 2.5 mg per week until off and then resumed the original biopsy schedule.

Overall success of steroid withdrawal with "late" steroid withdrawal in our program is approximately 70% at a mean follow-up of 27 months. The criteria for failure of steroid withdrawal included (1) two rejections that occurred at any time during follow-up off steroids; (2) any episode associated with hemodynamic compromise; (3) cyclosporine-related toxicity (primarily neurotoxicity); (4) white blood cell count below 4,000; or (5) intolerable symptoms of arthralgias or arthritis. Half of the protocol failures, or approximately 15% of the patients in whom steroid withdrawal was attempted, returned to steroids because of rejection, 20% because of neutropenia (white blood cell count below 4,000) or unwillingness to use monotherapy in this population of patients; 20% because of increased cyclosporine toxicity; and 10% as a result of intolerable arthritic complaints.

Although steroid withdrawal has been successful in over 70% of our patients, several obvious nonrejection parameters such as blood lipids, hypertension, and body weight did not change significantly. Unlike the Utah experience, where total cholesterol was very significantly lower in the patients successfully withdrawn from steroids,[7] compared with patients returned to steroids at 1 year (270 mg/dl vs. 215 mg/dl), the mean cholesterol level at the time of initiating steroid withdrawal in our program was only 215 mg/dl, which is nearly identical to the cholesterol level at 1 year in patients taken off steroids at Utah.

This was felt to be due to the relatively low total dose of steroids in our patients in the first 6 months posttransplant. No difference existed in the incidence of coronary artery disease by angiography in patients on or off steroids at a mean of 47 months posttransplant, nearly 2 1/2 years of follow-up off steroids. The lack of an adverse impact of steroid withdrawal on the incidence of allograft coronary artery disease was similarly noted in the Utah program with early withdrawal[13] and UCLA with late withdrawal.[10]

Several factors have been found to be associated with successful steroid withdrawal, including male gender, patients over 50 years of age, and patients with no rejection prior to steroid withdrawal. The UCLA program has noted that patients (n = 70) with at least one match at the DR locus have had nearly 95% successful withdrawal of corticosteroids.[10] Only 40% of our (n = 24) with one DR match, however, were successfully withdrawn. However, only three (12%) of these patients were returned to steroids because of rejection vs. 29% in patients with no DR match.. The success rate of steroid withdrawal in women has been as low as 15%[8-10] and as high as 40%, but it is significantly lower than in male counterparts in whom steroid withdrawal is initiated at a similar time posttransplant. This is discouraging in that the increased risk of osteoporosis in women patients[14,15] makes them one of the major target groups for this approach to immunosuppression.

The success of steroid withdrawal seems to vary with time of initiation (early vs. late). The long-term success of patients who are withdrawn early would seem to be inferior to patients in whom steroid withdrawal was accomplished later (> 4 months) without the use of induction therapy. The only exception is the one prospective trial, but there was a 40% crossover from steroid-free to chronic steroid group.[16] However, criteria for defining rejection, the ISHLT biopsy grade to initiate rejection therapy, doses of maintenance immunosuppression used, and the number of rejections required to meet protocol failure are very different between the 2 approaches of early or late withdrawal, thereby severely limiting the ability to compare the results directly. One major question regarding steroid withdrawal is the effect it might have on allograft coronary disease (ACD). Data from Utah[17] suggest no difference in the incidence of ACD. UCLA[18] has recently shown a significantly lower incidence of ACD in patients successfully withdrawn from steroids compared to patients continued on maintenance steroids.

It seems clear, however, that the patients successfully withdrawn from corticosteroids represent an immunologically privileged group. The greatest success includes men patients over 50 years of age who have had limited or no rejection in the 3 months before initiating steroid withdrawal. Although success in female patients is uniformly inferior to age-matched male cardiac transplant recipients, the addition of methotrexate to cyclosporine and azathioprine or substitution for azathioprine has been associated with increased success of steroid withdrawal in female patients in our program. A majority of patients can be successfully managed without corticosteroids for long-term immunosuppression and nearly all patients can be maintained on a relatively low dose of approximately 5 mg of methylprednisolone a day. Steroid withdrawal may offer substantial benefit to transplant candidates with diabetes, obesity, preexisting mild osteoporosis, and children in whom growth-retarding effects are substantial and with whom early experience with steroid withdrawal has been encouraging.[19,20] Longer-term follow-up is required to assess accurately the impact of steroid withdrawal on allograft CAD. Prospective randomized trials in a nonselected consecutive group of patients will be required to measure the benefit of steroid withdrawal, but results thus far are very encouraging.

REFERENCES

1. Bolman RM, Elick B, Olivari MT, et al: Improved immunosuppression for heart transplantation. Heart Transplant 4:315–318, 1985.
2. Miller LW: Steroid withdrawal in heart transplantation [editorial]. J Heart Lung Transplant 11(2):401–402, 1992.
3. Yacoub M, Alivizatos P, Radley-Smith R, et al: Cardiac transplantation: Are steroids really necessary? [abstract]. J Am Coll Cardiol 5:533, 1985.
4. Katz MR, Barnhart GR, Szentpetery S, et al: Are steroids essential for successful maintenance of immunosuppression in heart transplantation? J Heart Transplant 6:293–297, 1987.
5. Esmore DS, Spratt PM, Keogh AM, et al: Cyclosporine and azathioprine immunosuppression without maintenance steroids: A prospective randomized trial. J Heart Transplant 8:194–199, 1989.
6. Renlund DG, O'Connell JB, Gilbert EM, et al: Feasibility of discontinuation of corticosteroid maintenance therapy. J Heart Transplant 6:71–78, 1987.

7. Renlund DG, Bristow M, Crandall BG, et al: Hypercholesterolemia after heart transplantation: Amelioration by corticosteroid-free maintenance immunosuppression. J Heart Transplant 7:214–220, 1988.

8. Price GD, Olsen SL, Taylor DO, et al: Corticosteroid-free maintenance immunosuppression after heart transplantation: Feasibility and beneficial effects. J Heart Lung Transplant 11(2):403–414, 1992.

9. Keogh A, Macdonald P, Harvson A, et al: Initial steroid-free versus steroid-based maintenance therapy and steroid withdrawal after heart transplantation: Two views of the steroid question. J Heart Lung Transplant 11(2):421427, 1992.

10. Kobashigawa J, Stevenson LW, Brownfield ED, et al: Initial success of steroid weaning late after heart transplantation. J Heart Lung Transplant 11(2):428–430, 1992.

11. Miller LW, Wolford T, McBride LR, et al: Successful withdrawal of corticosteroids in heart transplantation. J Heart Lung Transplant 11(2):431–434, 1992.

12. Pritzker MR, Lake KD, Reutzel TJ, et al: Steroid-free maintenance immunotherapy: Minneapolis Heart Institute experience. J Heart Lung Transplant 11(2):415–420, 1992.

13. O'Connell JB, Renlund DG, DeWitt CW, et al: Sensitization to OKT3: Correlation with early allograft loss [abstract]. J Heart Transplant 8:95, 1989.

14. Sambrook P, Birmingham J, Kelly P, et al: Prevention of corticosteroid osteoporosis. A comparison of calcium, calcitriol, and calcitonin. N Engl J Med 328:1747–1752, 1993.

15. Meunier PJ: Is steroid-induced osteoporosis preventable? N Engl J Med 328:1781–1782, 1993.

16. Keogh A, Macdonald P, Mundy J, et al: Five year follow-up of a randomized double-drug versus triple-drug therapy immunosuppressive trial after heart transplantation. J Thorac Cardiovasc Surg 100:6–12, 1990.

18. Kobashigawa JA, Gleeson MP, Stevenson LW, et al: Late steroid weaning in cardiac transplant patients is not associated with an increase in transplant coronary artery disease. J Heart Lung Transplant 13(1)(part 2):S48, 1994.

19. Au J, Gregory JW, Colquhoun IW, et al: Pediatric cardiac transplantation with steroid-sparing maintenance immunosuppression. Arch Dis Child 67:1262–1666, 1992.

20. Canter CE, Moorhead S, Saffitz JE, et al: Steroid withdrawal in the pediatric heart transplant recipient initially treated with triple immunosuppression. J Heart Lung Transplant 13(1):74–80, 1994.

Chapter 11

New Immunosuppressive Drugs for Transplantation

Randall E. Morris, MD

We are at the beginning of a revolution in the discovery, development, and application of drugs for the control of graft rejection. This revolution is being driven by the success of the so-called xenobiotic immunosuppressants; these are low-molecular-weight drugs produced by microorganisms or by organic synthesis. The number of these new drugs that have advanced to clinical use in only the last 4 years is more than double the number of xenobiotic immunosuppressants approved for use in the last 35 years. In addition, many of these new drugs suppress the immune system by novel mechanisms of action. These new compounds have generated a momentum that will sustain new developments in immunosuppression for many years to come.

Even if not all of the current new xenobiotic immuno-suppressants are approved and widely adopted for clinical use, information gained from the study of these compounds will be the foundation for further immunosuppressive drug development. For example, when specific benefits and limitations of the xenobiotics now in clinical trials become more clearly defined, strategies for improving these drugs and for developing different agents will come into clearer focus. In addition to the value of the study of these drugs in patients, these compounds have proven to be essential to the understanding of fundamental immunologic processes. Because these drugs block different steps leading to immune cell activation, these agents have been wielded creatively as molecular tools to discover and dissect new biochemical pathways critical to the immune cell response. Information from these studies is being used to draw blueprints of the immune system's circuitry that will be harnessed to design even more effective, specific, and safer means of controlling the immune response.

The immune system is so complex and redundant, we cannot even begin to contemplate all the possible ways to suppress its actions. Many other approaches to immunosuppression have been, and continue to be, explored that differ from the actions of the known xenobiotic immuno-suppressants. Although many of these other means of suppressing the immune system are highly promising, their promise remains unfulfilled. All too often a particular way of suppressing the immune response is seductively elegant in concept and may even prove to be effective in vitro or in certain animal models, only to fail in clinical trials. Unlike xenobiotics, which often fail because of unexpected toxicity, nonxenobiotic immunosuppressants are often so specific in their actions that the overall immune response remains minimally suppressed. A case in point is the use of certain monoclonal antibody immunosuppressants. Although short-term immunosuppression is clearly produced by antibodies that deplete all T cells, other monoclonal antibodies directed to T-cell subsets or to cell-surface antigens present on activated immune cells have yet to demonstrate substantial immunosuppressive efficacy in human graft recipients. Because the nonxenobiotic immunosuppressants appear to be drugs of the future, this review of new immunosuppressants for transplantation limits its scope to xenobiotic drugs.

Regardless of what roles xenobiotic or nonxenobiotic drugs play in the future of immunosuppression for transplantation, effective, specific, and safe control of the response to graft antigens will continue to be the most significant barrier to continued progress in clinical transplantation. Ultimately, a chapter on heart and lung transplantation will need to discuss only the following areas: surgical technique, surgical complications, and suppression of rejection. Other topics such as management of infections, malignancy, drug toxicity, and issues concerning diagnosis and treatment of rejection, rehabilitation, cost-effectiveness, and the use of human donors would become obsolete if the immune response could be controlled optimally. Although heart and lung transplantation have evolved into life-saving procedures that are now acceptable treatments for end-stage cardiopulmonary diseases, these options are available to only a very small proportion of the patients who could benefit from them. For those fortunate enough to be recipients, transplantation is palliative, not curative. Complications that are a direct cause of imperfect immunosuppression adversely affect the recipients' quality of life and rehabilitation and make the care of these patients labor-intensive and extremely costly. The ultimate goal of transplantation is to have all recipients of nonhuman donor tissues or cells accept these transplants indefinitely without rejection and without nonspecific suppression of the immune system or systemic toxicity. This goal can be attained only by research designed to explore new ways of controlling the immune system.

Although the new xenobiotic immunosuppressants are far from ideal, they represent important advances that are the result of intense research in immune suppression over the last 6 years. The field of immunosuppression is changing so rapidly that this chapter should be viewed as a snap-shot of this discipline in mid-flight in 1995. No other chapter in this book is as likely to become obsolete as rapidly as this one. For this reason, the goal of this chapter is to introduce the reader to new drugs now in clinical trials with the potential to be used in recipients of heart and lung grafts. This introduction endeavors to provide a logical framework that can be referred to as new information about these agents becomes available. Concepts of each drug's mechanism of action, rather than precise details, are provided, because this area is being actively investigated and a specific account of our current beliefs implies a level of confidence that does not truly exist. Similarly, the results of clinical trials are not discussed in detail because most clinical data are from uncontrolled studies. Because the field of immunosuppression is so dynamic, this chapter should be read in conjunction with the most up-to-date articles and reviews devoted to these drugs' mechanisms of action and clinical trial results. A brief annotated bibliography is provided at the end of the text.

CATEGORIES OF NEW XENOBIOTIC IMMUNOSUPPRESSANTS

In the past, new immunosuppressants were introduced infrequently enough for those in the field to become familiar with each agent before the next new drug appeared. For example, from approximately 1960 to the mid-1980s, only three new xenobiotic drugs were widely adopted for use in transplantation: steroids, azathioprine, and cyclosporine (CsA). Poly- and monoclonal anti-T-cell antibodies were also introduced during that time. In the last 12 years, nine new xenobiotics have entered clinical trials, and eight of these began testing in the last 4 years alone. This explosion of new agents is a considerable challenge to those who realize that to understand the future of transplantation, one must understand the differences and similarities among these new drugs. The rate of progress is now so rapid that instead of learning about one new drug every few years, several drugs must be understood simultaneously. To minimize confusion, these drugs can be categorized by structure, origin, and mechanism of action. These categories provide an outline that enables the drugs to be grouped in ways that compare their similarities and contrast their differences.

The structures of CsA and several of the new xenobiotic immunosuppressants are shown in Figure 1. Two of the new agents, cyclosporine G (CsG) and IMM 125 are structurally related analogues of CsA and are not shown. The structures of the other seven new drugs are shown. Only two of these seven drugs bear some structural resemblance to each other: FK506 (tacrolimus) and rapamycin (RPM, sirolimus). The remaining five drugs are leflunomide (LFM), mizoribine (MZR), mycophenolate mofetil (MMF), Brequinar sodium (BQR) and deoxyspergualin (DSG). None of these five compounds is structurally related to each other or to the other four new agents. The structures shown in Figure 1 are the structures of the drugs in the forms in which they

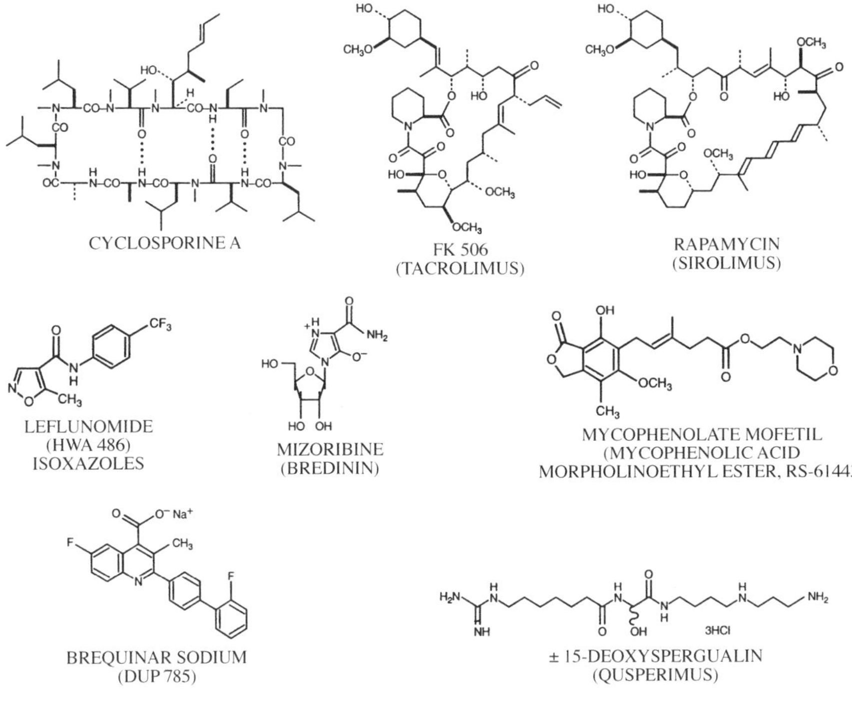

FIGURE 1.   Structures of new immunosuppressive drugs.

are administered. LFM, MZR, and MMF are pro-drugs and undergo a change in structure to become the active form of the drug. Before MMF was produced, the active form of the drug, mycophenolic acid (MPA), was administered. Therefore, MMF and MPA will be referred to interchangeably.

Categorizing the nine new xenobiotics by origin is relatively simple. For example, the CsA analogue, CsG, as well as FK506, RPM, and MZR are metabolic products of bacteria or fungi. BQR and LFM are produced by total organic synthesis. The other CsA analogue, IMM 125, as well as MMF and DSG are fermentation products that have been modified chemically after their isolation. Therefore, the origins of these new agents fall into the following categories: natural product, synthetic, or semi-synthetic.

The most important categorization of these new drugs is by their mechanisms of immunosuppressive action. These are shown in Figure 2. Despite similarities and differences among these drugs' structures and origins, no clear relationship exists between these categories and the drugs' mechanisms of action (Table 1). CsA and its analogues are structurally distinct from FK506 but all these compounds suppress immune cell function by inhibiting cytokine synthesis. RPM is structurally similar to FK506, yet RPM does not block cytokine synthesis. RPM is a natural product that is structurally dissimilar to the synthetically-produced LFM, yet both block the action of growth factors. MZR and MMF are structurally dissimilar, but both block purine synthesis. BQR and LFM are the only drugs that block pyrimidine synthesis. DSG does not inhibit the synthesis or action of cytokines and does not block DNA synthesis, but does suppress the maturation of immune cells.

As the mechanisms of action of these drugs have begun to be more clearly understood, it has become possible to reconcile the apparent incongruity between a drug's structure and its effect on the immune system. Structure-function relationships are discussed in more detail later in this chapter. Regardless of how well we now understand the relationship between structure and function, it is important to appreciate that the proposed mechanisms of immunosuppressive action for all of these new drugs are derived from studies done completely in vitro. Therefore, it remains to be proved

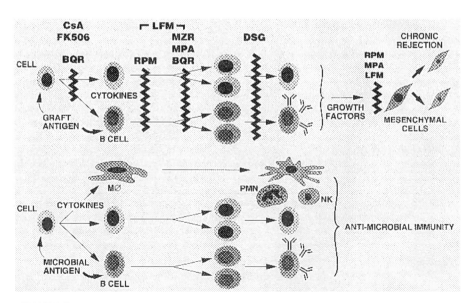

FIGURE 2.   Effects of new xenobiotic immunosuppressants on antigraft and antimicrobial immunity.

TABLE I. Mechanisms of Action of New Immunosuppression Drugs for Transpantation

Immunosuppressant	Origin	Mechanism				
		Block Cytokine Synthesis	Inhibit Growth Factors	Inhibit Purine Synthesis	Inhibit Pyrimidine Synthesis	Inhibit Immune Cell Maturation
Cyclosporine (CSA, CSG)	N	+				
FK506 (Tacrolimus)	N	+				
Rapamycin (Sirolimus)	N		+			
Leflunomide (LFM)	OS		+		+	
Mizoribine (MZR)	N		+	+		
Mycophenolate Mofetil (MMF)	SS		+	+		
Brequinar sodium (BQR)	OS		+		+	
Deoxysperqualin (DSG)	SS		+			+

N = Natural; OS = Organic synthesis; SS = Semisynthetic.

that the proposed mechanisms outlined in Figure 2 faithfully represent the actions of these drugs in vivo. Furthermore, as more is learned about these drugs, other mechanisms of immunosuppressive action are likely to be discovered.

The remainder of this chapter discusses each drug as part of the category that best describes its mechanism of action. Recently, detailed information on each of these new agents has been summarized in reviews or proceedings of conferences. These references and these articles should be referred to for additional information.

CYTOKINE SYNTHESIS INHIBITORS

Three of the newest immunosuppressants have mechanisms of action that mimic CsA. It is now known that CsA binds to proteins in the cytoplasm known as cyclophilins. The drug-cyclophilin complex then inhibits the enzymatic activity of another protein, calcineurin. Calcineurin is believed to play an important role in the cascade of events that leads to the transcription of certain cytokine genes (such as the gene for interleukin (IL)-2). By inhibiting transcription of lymphocyte-specific growth factors, the proliferation and activation of T cells is halted. Although CsA cannot directly inhibit B cell activation, T-cell-dependent B cell responses are inhibited.

CsA is close to the ideal immunosuppressant because it does not depend on T-cell depletion for its actions and because its immunosuppressive effects are restricted T cells undergoing activation. The primary drawbacks to the use of CsA are the nephrotoxicity and hypertension associated with its administration. It now appears that the toxic effects of CsA are mediated by complexes among CsA, cyclophilin, and calcineurin. As a result, it has been difficult to create analogues of CsA that retain immunosuppressive efficacy and are also less toxic. Recently, two new analogues, CsG and IMM 125, have begun to be evaluated in the clinic. CsG appeared to have a greater therapeutic index than its parent. IMM 125 was found to be hepatotoxic. Clinical trials for both drugs have ceased. So much effort has been expended in the search for analogues with greater therapeutic indexes that this research effort is reaching the point of diminishing returns. Because the initial steps in the pathways leading to suppression of T-cell proliferation and to toxicity appear to be identical and because CsA and its analogues block these steps, there is little opportunity to design molecules that are at once immunosuppressive and not at all toxic; rational drug design may be the only answer.

The third drug that mediates its immunosuppressive effects by interfering with the transcription of cytokine genes is FK506. FK506 also inhibits the activity of calcineurin after the drug has complexed with its cytoplasmic binding protein, FKBP. Because FK506 binds to FKBP much more avidly than CsA binds to cyclophilin, FK506 is a more potent immunosuppressant. In certain instances, FK506 has been able to reverse rejection that has been resistant to conventional immunosuppression. Although the greatest experience with FK506 has been in liver-allograft recipients, this drug has also been evaluated in renal and heart transplant patients. FK506 has been used to prevent and to treat liver and heart graft rejection with good results. It is less clear whether this drug offers a significant improvement over CsA in kidney graft recipients. The use of FK506 appears to have several advantages. First, the need for conventional immunosuppressants has been reduced. Second, FK506 can be used to treat rejection simply by increasing the dose.

As expected from its mechanism of action, the toxicity profile of FK506 is similar to that of CsA. FK506 is nephrotoxic and blood levels must be kept within narrow limits to ensure that nephrotoxicity is minimized. It is unlikely that analogues of FK506 will offer vastly superior therapeutic indexes, because the mechanisms of immunosuppressive action of FK506 appear to be inseparable from the biochemical pathways that cause toxicity.

INHIBITORS OF CYTOKINE ACTION

Two drugs define this new class of immunosuppressants: RPM and LFM. Neither inhibits the synthesis of cytokines, but both block the actions of immune, as well as nonimmune, cytokines and growth factors. Although both RPM and LFM appear to affect cells in the same way, the precise mechanisms by which they mediate their effects are probably quite different. Unlike CsA and its analogues and FK506, RPM and LFM also act directly on B cells to inhibit their functions.

RPM is structurally similar to FK506 and must bind to FKBPs to be immunosuppressive. Because the RPM-FKBP complex does not interact with calcineurin, the toxicity profile of RPM differs from those of CsA and FK506. Preclinical animal toxicology indicates that RPM is not as nephrotoxic as FK506. The exact biochemical events responsible for the inhibition of cytokine and growth factor action by the RPM-FKBP complex are far from clear, but the pharmacologic target of the complex now appears to be a lipid kinase. T cells can be stimulated to proliferate by pathways (calcium-independent signalling) (Fig. 2) that bypass the T-cell receptor, and these pathways are not blocked by CsA or FK506. Stimulation of T-cell proliferation through the CD28 pathway or by the interaction of IL-2 with its receptor are blocked by RPM.

RPM is clearly an unusually potent drug for prevention and treatment of allograft rejection in experimental animals. Its ability to prevent graft vascular disease in rat heart allografts may result from a combination of its suppressive effects on T and B cells and its ability to block the effects of growth factors that stimulate proliferation of intimal smooth muscle cells. The ultimate importance of this drug will have to await the outcome of clinical trials that are now underway. Phase I studies are being conducted to determine the maximum tolerated dose of this drug and its dose-limiting side effects. These data plus information from Phase II efficacy studies in transplant patients will determine the therapeutic index of this agent.

LFM is a prodrug that is converted almost immediately after administration to the active form of the drug. Current speculation regarding the mechanism of action of LFM is that it blocks the activity of selected tyrosine kinases associated with cell surface growth factor receptors. As a result, the normal transduction of signals after the interaction of a growth factor with its receptor is blocked. LFM has been studied most thoroughly in patients with rheumatoid arthritis and has been quite effective for treatment of advanced forms of this conditions. Analysis of the safety data from this study is incomplete, but so far it does not appear that LFM has any substantial toxic effects on specific organ systems. Information on the immunosuppressive efficacy of LFM in animal transplant recipients is limited, but the data show that it very effectively prolongs the survival of kidney, skin, and heart grafts in rodents. Recent studies have shown it to be an effective agent for suppression of acute rejection in nonhuman and dog organ allograft recipients when combined with CsA.

In preclinical transplant animal models, both RPM and LFM have been shown to be highly effective when combined with CsA. It is likely that this type of combination therapy could be useful in the clinic, because it may allow doses of CsA to be reduced to nonnephrotoxic levels. The use of drugs that block distinct steps in the immune response and that have nonoverlapping toxicity is a rational means of improving immunosuppressive while at the same time reducing systemic toxicity.

INHIBITORS OF DNA SYNTHESIS

There are three drugs in this category: MZR, MPA (or its prodrug form MM), and BQR. Each of these is a potential alternative to azathioprine. Both MZR and MPA have an important theoretic advantage over azathioprine. T cells and B cells rely, more than other cells, on a de novo pathway for synthesis of purine nucleotides. Unlike other cells, T cells and B cells cannot use the alternative salvage pathway for purine biosynthesis. MZR and MMF are relatively selective inhibitors of T-cell and B-cell DNA synthesis because both these drugs block the activity of a single critical enzyme responsible for the synthesis of purines in the de novo pathway. In contrast, azathioprine blocks many enzymes required for DNA synthesis and is a less specific inhibitor or immune cell proliferation than either MZR or MMF.

MZR has been used as an alternative for azathioprine for about a dozen years in transplant recipients in Japan. In those studies, less myelotoxicity was noted in patients on MZR compared with azathioprine. More extensive studies in transplantation have been done with MMF. Preclinical work has shown that this compound prolongs the survival of organ allografts in rodents and large animals. It has also been found to be effective for the reversal of ongoing rejection in these models. Most of the clinical studies have concentrated on the effects of MMF in renal transplant patients. These Phase II trials have shown that there is a relationship between the dosage level and the incidence of graft rejection. Other studies showed that MMF is able to reverse rejection in patients that were refractory to treatment with conventional immunosuppressants. MMF has been used in rodent transplant models to prevent graft vascular disease, and this application may also be relevant to its use in patients.

BQR does not directly inhibit purine synthesis, but does block the action of a key enzyme in the pathway leading to pyrimidine synthesis. BQR also differs from MZR and MPA because it inhibits both DNA and RNA synthesis. Although BQR failed as an anticancer agent, its use in patients with malignant diseases provided information on its safety and pharmacokinetics. Because high doses of BQR and its continued use have been shown to be myelotoxic, the rationale for its use as an immunosuppressant depends on the assumption that immune cells are more sensitive to its antimetabolic effects than nonimmune cells. This assumption has been borne out in studies of the immunosuppressive efficacy of BQR in rodent graft recipients. These experiments have shown that BQR is able to prevent rejection and very effectively halts ongoing rejection. It has also been used effectively for the prolongation of hamster to rat xenografts.

Experiments that are currently ongoing will determine the efficacy of this drug in large animal recipients of organ allografts. Because BQR has been shown to produce immunosuppression in rodent allograft recipients that is at least additive when combined with CsA, it is likely that BQR will be used as adjunctive therapy in patients. This drug is in Phase II trials in renal transplant recipients. Current clinical development is on hold. LFM has also recently been found to inhibit pyrimidine synthesis in vitro.

INHIBITOR OF CELL MATURATION

DSG not only has a structure that differs from all the other new xenobiotic immunosuppressants, it also suppresses the immune system by means distinct from those of other agents. For example, in vitro studies have shown that DSG is not an effective inhibitor of cytokine synthesis, the actions of cytokines, or DNA synthesis. Despite its apparent inability to suppress these steps in immune activation that are the target of other drugs. DSG is an effective immunosuppressant. Its true mechanism of immunosuppressive action is unknown, but by a process of elimination, it appears that DSG blocks the immune response by halting the maturation of T and B cells into fully functional effector cells. This drug, like RPM, LFM, and the antimetabolites directly suppresses T cells and B cells in vitro.

In vivo, DSG has been used to prevent rejection of rodent allografts and xenografts. In nonhuman primates treated with a short course of DSG plus long-term therapy with CsA, prolonged graft survival was seen. DSG has also been found to halt advanced rejection in rodent and large animal graft recipients. These results prompted the first clinical trials in Japan in renal allograft recipients. These patients had continued to reject despite a variety of conventional immunosuppressive treatments. Although the trials were not controlled, the results appeared to support the belief that this drug was effective for this application. Clinical trials are now being conducted in the United States in high-risk renal allograft recipients who have previously rejected one or more grafts within a year of transplantation. DSG can now only be administered intravenously, so these patients are receiving a short induction course in conjunction with conventional immunosuppressants. If the results of this trial indicate that DSG is effective, a more extensive and controlled Phase III trial will be undertaken.

SUMMARY

The proliferation of new xenobiotic drugs offers the potential to benefit transplantation in many ways. In theory, the use of drugs with different mechanisms of action and nonoverlapping toxicities should increase the overall immunosuppressive efficacy without increasing systemic toxicity. The variety of new drugs will enable this assumption to be tested in the clinic. Already these new molecules have been used to uncover new knowledge of how immune cells respond to activation. This understanding, in turn, will be the foundation for the discovery and development of a new generation of immunosuppressants. In the meantime, currently available drugs need to be studied much more thoroughly in vitro, in animal transplant models, and in clinical trials so that they can be used intelligently and to their maximum advantage. We now have more drugs than ever before that directly suppress B-cell function, and these drugs may be especially valuable for xenograft recipients.

Compared with the last 30 years, the number and variety of new immunosuppressants are very great. It is important to remember, however, that the immune system is exceedingly complex. Therefore, in the future the number of new drugs of all types will continue to increase. As the complexity of immunosuppression increases, a greater premium will be placed on drugs that are clearly safer and more effective than the drugs that now exist. This competitive environment will ensure that continued progress is made.

SELECTED BIBLIOGRAPHY

1. Morris RE: Overview of immunosuppressive drugs for transplantation: Where are we? How did we get here? and Where are we going? Clin Transplant 7:138–146, 1993.
2. Morris RE: Immunopharmacology of new xenobiotic immunosuppressive molecules. Semin Nephrol 12:304–314, 1992.
3. Thomson AW (ed): The Molecular Biology of Immunosuppression. New York, John Wiley and Sones, 1992.
4. Ten Years of cyclosporine in clinical practice. Past, present and future in transplantation immunology. Transplant Proc 25:1–99, 1992.
5. Morris RE: Rapamycins: Antifungal, antitumor and immunosuppressive macrolides. Transplant Rev 6;39–87, 1992.
6. Sigal NH, Dumont FJ: Cyclosporin A, FK-506 and rapamycin: Pharmacological probes of lymphocyte signal transduction. Annu Rev Immunol 10:519–560, 1992.
7. Dayton JS, Turka LA, Thompson CB, Mitchell BS: Comparison of the effects of mizoribine with those of azathioprine, 6-mercaptopurine and mycophenolic acid and T lymphocyte proliferation and purine ribonucleotide metabolism. Molecular Pharmacol 41;671–676, 1992.
8. Cramer DV, Chapman FA, Jaffee BD, et al: The effect of new immunosuppressive drug, brequinar sodium, on heart, liver and kidney allograft rejection in the rat. Transplantation 53:303–308, 1992.
9. Annual American Society of Transplant Surgeons postgraduate course: advances in immunosuppression. Clin Transplant 5(part 2):475–599, 1991.

Acute Cardiac Allograft Rejection: Diagnosis and Treatment

Chapter 12

Pasquale Ferraro, MD
Michel Carrier, MD

Diagnosis of acute allograft rejection by the endo-myocardial biopsy (EMB) technique initially developed by Caves,[1] and later characterized by Billingham,[2] has had a significant impact on the clinical success of heart transplantation. Although invasive, biopsy of the allograft heart remains the gold standard for diagnosis of acute rejection. In treatment of acute episodes of rejection, the great majority of American transplant program directors, in a recent survey, favored the use of intravenous steroids as the most effective approach.[3]

Whereas EMB and intravenous steroids form the basis of the diagnosis and treatment of acute rejection after heart transplantation, many ancillary techniques to the diagnosis of rejection and several alternatives to the treatment of resistant rejection have been proposed. This review summarizes the current clinical approach to diagnosis and treatment of acute allograft rejection and describes our choice of agents, dosages, and protocols.

DIAGNOSIS OF ACUTE REJECTION: ENDOMYOCARDIAL BIOPSY AND ANCILLARY TECHNIQUES

Histologic nomenclature for diagnosis of heart rejection was recently standardized by a study group of pathologists headed by Billingham.[4] The grading of cellular rejection ranges from grade 0 (no signs of acute rejection) to grade 4 (severe rejection) (Table 1). This grading system has been useful in following patients after transplantation, in selecting

TABLE 1.   Standardized Cardiac Biopsy Grading

Grade	Formulation	Description
0	—	No rejection
1A	Focal, mild	Focal infiltrate without necrosis
1B	Diffuse, mild	Diffuse infiltrate without necrosis
2	Focal. moderate	One focus of aggressive infiltration and/or focal myocyte damage
3A	Multifocal, moderate	Multifocal aggressive infiltrates and/or myocyte damage
3B	Diffuse, borderline severe	Diffuse inflammatory process with borderline severe necrosis
4	Severe	Diffuse aggressive infiltrate, edema, hemorrhage, vasculitis, with necrosis

(Adapted from Billingham ME, Cary NRB, Hammond ME, et al: A working formulation for the standardization of nomenclature in the diagnosis of heart and lung rejection: Heart rejection study group. J Heart Transplant 9:587–593, 1990.)

which patients need to be actively treated for acute rejection, in monitoring the resolution of rejection episodes and, in treating the occasional patient with an infectious myocarditis.

Clinical evaluation is an important aspect of patient management and may help detect an early episode of rejection. Specifically, one must look for cardiac arrhythmias, signs of congestive heart failure, decrease in exercise tolerance, and changes in heart size on chest roentgenogram. With the advent of cyclosporine and better immunosuppression, however, most episodes of acute rejection appear insidiously without any specific symptoms. Routine EMB has therefore been recommended in the follow-up of patients after heart transplantation. Transplant centers employ a schedule of routine cardiac biopsies that reflects the higher incidence of rejection episodes during the first 6 to 12 months following transplantation (Table 2). In a survey of 104 American heart transplant programs, Evans and coworkers[5] found that 97% of centers consider heart biopsy monitoring an important and essential approach to successful clinical outcome.

Myocardial biopsy remains the only reliable and definitive way to diagnose and assess severity of acute allograft rejection. Monitoring transplanted hearts with routine EMB is nonetheless associated with several disadvantages. Although overall complication rates are low (1% to 2%) and procedure-related deaths are exceedingly rare (0.05%),[6] the technique is both invasive and expensive. Furthermore, histologic changes in acute rejection may present asymmetric patterns[7] contributing to the sampling error inherent to the biopsy technique. Misinterpretation of the biopsy specimen and inter-observer variability have been reported,[8] and diagnosis may be difficult in cases of vascular (humoral) rejection as shown by Hammond.[9] The latter type of rejection, defined by immunofluorescent findings of immunoglobulins (IgG or IgM) and complement (C3) in a vascular pattern, is related to a positive donor-specific crossmatch, to a higher incidence of resistant rejection with hemodynamic compromise, and to graft loss with poorer patient survival.[9] Immunofluorescence analysis of cardiac biopsy, in addition to routine histologic evaluation, is therefore essential in selected cases of refractory rejection.

TABLE 2.   Schedule of Routine Endomyocardial Biopsy at the Montreal Heart Institute

Time after Transplantation	Routine Cardiac Biopsy
First month	Every week
Second and third months	Every 2 weeks
Fourth to twelfth months	Every 1 to 2 months
After first year	Yearly/according to clinical indication/if there is a change in medication

ANCILLARY DIAGNOSTIC METHODS

To find a reliable noninvasive method for screening acute rejection and evaluating therapy, a variety of ancillary techniques have been developed and reported. To date, however, few have had a significant impact on clinical practice.[10] These methods are either directed at evaluating the systemic immune process of rejection or detecting with greater specificity changes in allograft function.

Allograft rejection is characterized by a systemic process of cellular immunity and by a local immune effect leading to destruction of the allograft tissue.[11] The techniques used to evaluate induction and expression of systemic immunity include cytoimmuno-logic monitoring and T-cell analysis.[12-14] These methods, however, have proved unreliable, and in a review of several clinical studies (Table 3), sensitivity and specificity of these tests averaged 75% and 67%, respectively. Furthermore, if these techniques had been used in our patient population characterized by a 14% prevalence of acute rejection at biopsy, 43% of all episodes of rejection would have been missed, an unacceptable rate of failure.[10] Recent studies have shown greater density of donor-specific cytotoxic lymphocytes within the transplanted heart when compared with the peripheral blood.[15,16] These findings suggest that differentiation and proliferation of lymphoblasts during the initial phase of acute rejection takes place within the graft itself, thus explaining the lack of sensitivity and specificity of methods monitoring changes in the peripheral blood.

A number of noninvasive techniques directed at allograft function, including surface ECG, intramyocardial ECG, radionuclide scanning, and magnetic resonance imaging (MRI), have been tested. Once again, results have been disappointing with wide variations in sensitivities and specificities (6 to 97%) in detecting acute rejection.[10] Echocardiography seemed promising at first, because several specific morphologic and functional changes associated with rejection were identified.[17] Recent studies, however, one of which included 1400 serial echocardiograms in 130 patients within 24 hours of EMB, have confirmed the poor sensitivity of echocardiography to diagnose both mild and some cases of moderate rejection.[18,19]

Some authors have advocated intramyocardial electrograms as a reliable means of detecting rejection.[20] This technique, however, requires a dual-chamber pacemaker and has only a 50% sensitivity in the presence of mild rejection. Two imaging techniques,

TABLE 3.   Noninvasive Diagnostic Methods—Comparison of Two Groups of Methods

	Monitoring of Immunologic Events (CIM)	Monitoring of Allograft Events (Echo, Scintigraphy)
No. clinical studies	13	9
% Sensitivity (mean ± SEM)	75 ± 7	93 ± 3
% Specificity (mean ± SEM)	67 ± 8	87 ± 3
Prevalence of rejection 14% of 568 biopsies or 80 episodes (our series)		
Posttest probability of acute rejection, % (mean ± SEM)		
Positive	34 ± 6	57 ± 6
Negative	7 ± 1	3 ± 1
Nondiagnosed episodes of acute rejection	34 (34/80, 43%)	15 (15/80, 19%)

CIM = cytoimmunologic monitoring
(Adapted from Carrier M: Noninvasive assessment of cardiac transplant rejection: A critical look at the approach to acute rejection. Can J Surg 34:569–572, 1991.)

MRI scanning[21] and positron emission tomography (PET) with N-ammonia uptake[22] are presently under study. Although initial results seem encouraging, the cost and practicality of this sophisticated technology have yet to be evaluated.

Despite the great amount of clinical and experimental effort that has gone into the development of a noninvasive method to diagnose acute allograft rejection, 80 to 90% of transplant directors in Evans' survey[5] believe that cytoimmunologic monitoring, electrocardiograms, and echocardiography are unnecessary and of little value. Thus, our present noninvasive techniques have not yet acquired the necessary diagnostic accuracy and reliability to replace EMB as the clinical method of choice in monitoring cardiac rejection after transplantation. Ultimately, techniques aimed at detecting changes in cellular metabolism and function during acute rejection will be developed.

TREATMENT OF ACUTE ALLOGRAFT REJECTION

With the great number of regimens currently in use for maintenance and induction immunosuppression, an equally important number of protocols exists for the treatment of acute rejection following heart transplantation. Selection of treatment protocols varies according to several factors including timing of episode with respect to the transplantation, severity of rejection (Billingham's Classification), the patient's clinical status, previous history of rejection, inpatient or outpatient therapy, and local institutional bias. Thus, therapeutic decision-making remains difficult. Studies have shown that anti-rejection therapy greatly influences the rate of infectious complications and allograft rejection is still an important cause of early and late deaths after transplantation.[23-25] Appropriate therapy of graft rejection is thus an essential component of patient management following transplantation.

Intravenous and Oral Prednisone

In Evans' survey of transplant program directors, intravenous steroids were recommended for acute or resistant rejection by 92% of respondents.[3] The use of steroids has represented the mainstay of therapy since its initial recommendation by the Stanford group in 1971.[26] The regimen consists of intravenous methylprednisolone (Solu-Medrol) 1000 mg/day or 15 mg/kg/day, if weight < 50 kg) for 3 consecutive days, while the usual maintenance therapy is administered. Results with this protocol have been excellent with response rates varying from 90% to 96%.[27-29]

Two issues concerning intravenous steroids, ideal route and dosage, are still unresolved. In one report, reduced doses of methylprednisolone (200 mg/day vs. 500 mg/day vs. 1000 mg/day) were studied in histologically proven rejection.[28] The effectiveness of the three regimens was similar. The authors, however, were unable to document reduced steroid side effects with smaller doses.

The possible role of oral prednisone (bolus and tapered) in the treatment of acute rejection without hemodynamic compromise has also been studied. Generally, prednisone is increased to 100 mg daily for 3 days and then tapered by 5 to 10 mg/day until the previous maintenance dose has been reached. Early reports showed success rates in the range of 80 to 90% for moderate acute rejection (Billingham's grades 2 and 3A) treated with oral prednisone.[30,31] In a recent randomized trial with asymptomatic patients presenting grade 3A rejection, similar resolution rates were obtained with intravenous and oral steroids.[29] An advantage of oral prednisone is the reduce rate of infectious complications.[30,32] Also, there is no need for hospitalization during treatment.

TABLE 4.   Choice of Immunosuppression Regimen in the Treatment of Rejection

Medication	Indication	Success Rate
Solu-Medrol IV	Grades 3 and 4 Early rejection (< 2–3 months)	95%
Oral prednisone	Grade 3A Late rejection (> 2–3 months) Outpatient treatment	90%
ATG/ALG/OKT3	Grades 3 and 4 Hemodynamic compromise Persistent/recurrent	60–90%*
Methotrexate	Grade 2 or 3 persistent or recurrent	60–90%*

* High rate of recurrence despite immediate success, high rate of infection after treatment, and rate of malignancy?

Choice of Immunosuppression Regimen

An area of controversy lies in deciding what episodes of rejection should be treated based on EMB results. Our current policy with acute allograft rejection at the Montreal Heart Institute is summarized in Table 4. The need for aggressive treatment of patients with severe rejection, grades 3B and 4 (diffuse inflammatory infiltrates with necrosis, edema, and hemorrhage) is not a matter for debate. Intravenous methylprednisolone is recommended as first-line therapy (1000 mg daily for 3 days) in these cases. Polyclonal antilymphocyte globulins (ATG, ALG) or OKT3 may be administered as rescue therapy therapy for refractory episodes or simultaneously in selected patients.[3,27,33,34]

Routine EMB in asymptomatic patients may reveal mild rejection (grades 1A, 1B, and 2) defined as focal or diffuse lymphocytic infiltrates with possible myocyte damage. Additional immunosuppressive treatment in these cases is generally unnecessary.[33–35] Several studies have shown that without any change in maintenance immunosuppression, mild rejection will progress to moderate or more severe forms in only 18% to 41% of patients (i.e., 60 to 80% spontaneous resolution).[35–37] Once an episode of mild rejection has been documented, however, repeat biopsy is recommended 7 to 14 days later or earlier if symptoms develop. If the rejection process has progressed, therapy is indicated in most patients. We favor oral prednisone (bolus and tapered) if the patients remain asymptomatic and if the episode occurs more than 3 months after transplant. Other acceptable alternatives include the standard intravenous steroid regimen or increased oral cyclosporine.[37] Management of asymptomatic patients showing persistent mild rejection without any signs of progression ("dirty biopsy") remains controversial. What effect this form of rejection has on late graft function or on coronary artery disease is unknown. Hosenpud[31] recommends treatment of mild rejection if it persists on three successive biopsies.

Moderate acute rejection (grade 3A) is characterized on biopsy by a multifocal inflammatory infiltrate (large aggressive lymphocytes) with myocyte damage. Treatment of these episodes depends on several factors. In one study, the authors recommended intravenous steroids for moderate rejection occurring within 1 month of transplantation, whereas asymptomatic patients who presented more than 1 months after surgery were observed and rebiopsied 5 to 7 days later.[38] Interestingly, they found spontaneous resolution of the rejection process in 50% of cases. Patients with persistent moderate rejection were treated with increased oral prednisone, whereas patients who progressed were subjected to an intravenous steroid regimen. Regardless of the latter experience and in accordance with most authors, we advocate intravenous methylprednisolone for episodes of moderate rejection (grade 3A) occurring within 3 months of transplantation.[27,28,33,34] Oral prednisone (bolus and tapered) is probably a valid alternative in selected asymptomatic patients presenting early episodes and in patients without hemodynamic compromise more than 3 months postoperatively. This approach has been used in the great majority of patients at the Montreal Heart Institute with an overall resolution rate of more than 90%. Close follow-up and repeat biopsies are essential when treating these episodes.

Although timing of allograft rejection may influence therapy, both the severity of the rejection process as determined by biopsy and the patient's clinical status are more important. Patients presenting with clinical or echocardiographic signs of heart failure or graft dysfunction require hospitalization, intravenous steroids, and possibly OKT3 or ALG/ATG. It is imperative to begin anti-rejection therapy at once even if confirmation of diagnosis by EMB has not been obtained. In a recent study based on data from the Transplant Cardiologists Research Group, 143 episodes of rejection with hemodynamic compromise were reviewed.[29] Very little correlation was found between histologic findings and allograft dysfunction because 61% of these patients only had signs of mild or moderate rejection on biopsy.

Refractory or Recurring Rejection

Refractory or recurring episodes of moderate rejection are of concern because in some patients they may lead to loss of graft function, to severe coronary atherosclerosis, and to occurrence of significant side effects of cumulative immunosuppression such as infection and malignancy. Refractory or recurring rejection may require other forms of therapy including ALG, ATG, OKT3, and methotrexate.[3,34,39,40] Newer agents such as FK506[41] and mycophenolate mofetil[42] may also be of benefit; clinical trials are forthcoming.

Antilymphocyte antibodies (ALG, ATG) and the monoclonal antibody OKT3 have been used successfully to control persistent, recurrent, or severe episodes of acute rejection with hemodynamic compromise.[39,43–45] OKT3's mechanism of action includes opsonization of circulating T cells, which causes a rapid decrease in their number, and interference with the T-cell antigen recognition apparatus rendering the lymphocytes incapable of interacting with foreign antigen (antigenic modulation). Its mechanism of action is different from that of cyclosporine, antimetabolites, or steroids, and thus OKT3 possesses a specific toxicity profile. Although most of the adverse effects of OKT3 are easily dealt with, a substantial increase in the incidence of lymphoproliferative disorders has been reported[46] and remains a concern for patients requiring multiple courses of OKT3. Nonetheless, a meta-analysis including 384 patients from eight studies published between 1985 and 1991 on the treatment of acute rejection with OKT3 concluded that patients treated with this agent had better chances of resolution of rejection than control patients with an odds ratio of 3.0.[47]

At the Montreal Heart Institute, we have used RATG to treat 13 episodes of early grade 4 or recurrent moderate acute rejection in 10 patients (Table 5). Although initial results were excellent with a resolution rate of 90%, 60% of patients had a recurrent episode of rejection within the following 3 months.

Methotrexate, a folic acid analogue, interferes with DNA and purine synthesis and possesses cytotoxic inhibitory effects on both cellular and humoral immunity.[48] The use of methotrexate in the treatment of cardiac allograft rejection was first reported by Costanzo-Nordin.[49] A number of studies have since confirmed the effectiveness of methotrexate therapy in selected patients with recurrent or refractory rejection.[40,50–52]

TABLE 5.   Treatment of Refractory or Recurrent Acute Rejection: Experience at the Montreal Heart Institute with RATG and Methotrexate

	RATG	Methotrexate
No. of patients	10	8
Dosage	125 mg IV	2.5–5 mg/week
Duration of treatment	3 ± 6 days	4 ± 1 months
Time after transplantation	59 ± 20 days	9 ± 3 months
No. of previous rejections	2 ± 1	2 ± 1
Resolution of rejection	9/10	5/8
Recurrence after treatment	6/10	1/8
Infection after treatment	1/10	0/8
Malignancy after treatment	0/10	0/8
Survival	8/10	8/8
Total follow-up (months)	45 ± 13	11 ± 1

This therapy, however, may be associated with severe leukopenia, significant infectious complications, and recurrent episodes of acute rejection.

In our experience, methotrexate has been administered to eight patients with persistent late acute rejection grade 2 or 3A (Table 5). These patients have had multiple episodes of acute rejection treated, but overall remained in stable clinical condition. Low doses of methotrexate added to the maintenance regimen while carefully following the white cell count were well tolerated and effective in resolving rejection episodes in five patients. Following this therapy, incidence of rejection episodes was reduced to 0.1 ± 0.1 episode/patient. We believe that methotrexate could play a significant role in the management of recurrent and persistent rejection processes.

Experimental Approaches to Acute Rejection

Other agents and treatment modalities for acute rejection are currently under investigation. One such immunosuppressive agent is FK506, a macrolide antibiotic. Introduced in 1989, FK506 was first used for liver transplant recipients with refractory rejection. In a recent clinical trial, FK506 was employed as baseline immunosuppression in cardiac transplantation and as rescue therapy for episodes of acute allograft rejection.[41] Preliminary results showed a small number of rejection episodes and a low rate of recurrence. FK506 was also effective in treating cardiac rejection refractory to conventional immunotherapy. A number of significant adverse effects, however, have been reported. These include renal dysfunction, hypertension, neurotoxicity (central and peripheral), diabetes, and lymphoproliferative disorders. The exact role of FK506 has yet to be established, whereas long-term effects on graft function and coronary artery disease are unknown. The potential complications associated with this agent may limit its use in clinical transplantation.

Mycophenolate mofetil, formerly known as RS-61443, is a lymphocyte-specific inhibitor of purine synthesis with antiproliferative effects on T and B lymphocytes. This agent possesses many of the properties of azathioprine. It has been tested in a preliminary trial as maintenance immunosuppression and was effective and well tolerated.[42] Whether or not it will pay a significant role in the treatment of acute rejection remains to be seen. Two other modalities, total lymphoid irradiation and photochemotherapy (photopheresis), discussed in chapter 20, are also currently being developed and tested in clinical trials.[53–55]

CONCLUSION

In the transplant program at the Montreal Heart Institute, we have individualized our approach to patients presenting with acute allograft rejection after heart transplantation. Therapeutic decision-making is based on several clinical variables and includes the use of intravenous and oral steroids in most patients. RATG, OKT3, and methotrexate are employed selectively in severe, refractory, or persistent episodes of rejection. The ultimate goal of immunotherapy remains the induction of a level of graft tolerance to minimize treatable rejection episodes. Newer immunosuppressive agents and modalities, better combinations of existing drugs, or possibly improved donor-recipient HLA matching may help achieve this goal in the not so distant future.

REFERENCES

1. Caves PK, Stinson EB, Billingham ME, Shumway NE: Percutaneous transvenous endomyocardial biopsy in human heart recipients. Ann Thorac Surg 16:325–326, 1973.
2. Billingham ME: Diagnosis of cardiac rejection by endomyocardial biopsy. Heart Transplant 1:25–30, 1980.
3. Evans RW, Manninen DL, Dong FB, et al: Immunosuppressive therapy as a determinant of transplantation outcomes. Transplantation 55:1297–1305, 1993.
4. Billingham ME, Cary NRB, Hammond ME, et al: A working formulation for the standardization of nomenclature in the diagnosis of heart and lung rejection: Heart rejection study group. J Heart Transplant 9:587–593, 1990.
5. Evans RW, Manninen DL, Dong FB, et al: The medical and surgical determinants of heart transplantation outcomes: The results of a consensus survey in the United States. J Heart Transplant 12:42–45, 1993.
6. Wilansky S, Radonancevic B: Endomyocardial biopsy in cardiac transplantation. ACC Curr J R, March/April 22–24, 1994.
7. Haverich A, Scott WC, Dawkins KD, et al: Asymmetric pattern of rejection following orthotopic cardiac transplantation. J Heart Transplant 4:280–285, 1984.
8. Billingham ME: Dilemma of variety of histopathologic grading systems for acute cardiac allograft rejection by endomyocardial biopsy. J Heart Transplant 9:272–276, 1990.
9. Hammond EH, Yowell RL, Nunada S, et al: Vascular (humoral) rejection in heart transplantation: Pathologic observations and clinical implications. J Heart Transplant 8:430–443, 1989.
10. Carrier M: Noninvasive assessment of cardiac transplant rejection: A critical look at the approach to acute rejection. Can J Surg 34:569–572, 1991.
11. Barry WH: Mechanisms of immune mediated myocyte injury. Circulation 89:2421–2432, 1994.
12. Hoshinaga K, Mohanakumar T, Pascoe EA, et al: Expression of transferrin receptors on lymphocytes: Its correlation in the T-helper T-suppressor cytotoxic ratio and rejection in heart transplant recipients. J Heart Transplant 9:198–204, 1990.
13. Fieguth MG, Haverich A, Schafers MG, et al: Cytoimmunologic monitoring in early and late acute cardiac rejection. J Heart Transplant 7:95–101, 1988.
14. May RM, Cooper DKC, Dutoit ED, et al: Cytoimmunologic monitoring after heart and heart lung transplantation. J Heart Transplant 9:133–135, 1990.
15. Suitters AJ, Rose ML, Dominguez MJ, et al: Selection for donor specific cytotoxic T lymphocytes within the allografted human heart. Transplantation 49:1105–1109, 1990.
16. Breuer M, Schutz A, Engelhardt M, et al: Intragraft events after heart transplantation: An experimental study comparing cytology in coronary sinus blood, peripheral blood, and daily histology. Transpl Int 7:22–26, 1994.
17. Hsu DT, Spotnitz HM: Echocardiographic diagnosis of cardiac allograft rejection. Prog Cardiovasc Dis 33:149–160, 1990.
18. Dodd DA, Brady LD, Carden KA, et al: Pattern of echocardiographic abnormalities with acute cardiac allograft rejection in adults: Correlation with endomyocardial biopsy. J Heart Lung Transplant 12:1009–1018, 1993.
19. Ciliberto GR, Mascarello M, Gronda E, et al: Acute rejection after heart transplantation: Noninvasive echocardiographic evaluation. J Am Coll Cardiol 23:1156–1161, 1994.
20. Grauhan O, Warveuke H, Muller J, et al: Intramyocardial electrogram recordings for diagnosis and therapy monitoring of cardiac allograft rejection. Eur J Cardiothorac Surg 7:49–494, 1993.
21. Mousseaux E, Farge D, Guilleurain R, et al: Assessing human cardiac allograft rejection using MRI with Gd-DOTA. J Comput Assist Tomogr 17;237–244, 1993.

22. Hoff SJ, Stewart JR, Frist WH, et al: Noninvasive detection of heart transplant rejection with positron emission scintigraphy. Ann Thorac Surg 53:572–577, 1992.
23. Mason JW, Stinson EB, Hunt SA, et al: Infections after cardiac transplantation: Reaction to rejection therapy. Ann intern Med 85:69–72, 1976.
24. Kirklin JK, Naftel DC, McGriffin DC, et al: Analysis of morbid events and risk factors for death after cardiac transplantation. J Am Coll Cardiol 11:917–924, 1988.
25. Sweeney MS, Macris MP, Frazier OH, et al: The treatment of advanced cardiac allograft rejection. Ann Thorac Surg 46:378–381, 1988.
26. Griepp RG, Stinson EB, Dong E, et al: Determinants of operative risk in human heart transplantation. Am J Surg 122:192–197, 1971.
27. Miller LW: Treatment of cardiac allograft rejection with intravenous corticosteroids. J Heart Transplant 9:283–287, 1990.
28. Wahlers T, Heublein B, Cremer J, et al: Treatment of rejection after heart transplantation: What dosage of pulsed steroids is necessary? J Heart Transplant 9:568–574, 1990.
29. Kobashigawa JA, Kirklin JK, Naftel DC, et al: Pretransplantation risk factors for acute rejection after heart transplantation: A multi-institutional study. J Heart Lung Transplant 12:355–366, 1993.
30. Michler RE, Smith CR, Drusin RE, et al: Reversal of cardiac transplant rejection without massive immunosuppression. Circulation 74(Suppl III):III-68, 1986.
31. Hosenpud JD, Norman DJ, Pantely GA: Low dose oral prednisone in the treatment of acute cardiac allograft rejection not associated with hemodynamic compromise. J Heart Transplant 9:292–296, 1990.
32. Dresdale AR, Drusin RE, Lamb J, et al: Reduced infection in cardiac transplant recipients. Circulation 72(Suppl I):II-237, 1985.
33. McGoon MD, Fronty RP: Techniques of immunosuppression after cardiac transplantation. Mayo Clin Proc 67:56–595, 1992.
34. O'Connell JB, Bourge RC, Costanzo-Nordin MR, et al: Cardiac transplantation: Recipient selection, donor procurement, and medical follow-up. Circulation 86:1061–1079, 1992.
35. Lloveras JJ, Escourrou G, Delisle MB, et al: Evolution of untreated mild rejection in heart transplant recipients. J Heart Lung Transplant 11:751–756, 1992.
36. Imakita M, Tazelaar D, Billingham ME: Heart allograft rejection under varying immunosuppressive endomyocardial biopsy. J Heart Transplant 5:279–25, 1986.
37. Kobashigawa J, Stevenson LW, Moriguchi J, et al: Randomized study of high dose oral cyclosporine therapy for mild acute cardiac rejection. J Heart Transplant 8:53–58, 1989.
38. Hutter JA, Wallwork J, English TAH: Management of rejection in heart transplant recipients: Does moderate rejection always require treatment? J Heart Transplant 9:87–91, 1990.
39. Deeb GM, Bolling SF, Steimle CW, et al: A randomized prospective comparison of MALG with OK3 for rescue therapy of acute myocardial rejection. Transplantation 51:180–183, 1991.
40. Hosepud JD, Hershberger RE, Ratkovec RR, et al: Methotrexate for treatment of patients with multiple episodes of acute cardiac allograft rejection. J Heart Lung Transplant 11:739–745, 1992.
41. Armitage JM, Korures RL, Morita S, et al: Clinical trial of FK 506 immunosuppression in adult cardiac transplantation. Ann Thorac Surg 54:205–211, 1992.
42. Taylor DO, Ensley D, Olsen SL, et al: Mycophenolate mofetil (RS-61443): Preclinical, clinical and three year experience in heart transplantation. J Heart Lung Transplant 13:571–52, 1994.
43. Sweeney MS, Macris MP, Frazier OH, et al: The treatment of advanced cardiac allograft rejection. Ann Thorac Surg 46:378–31, 1988.
44. Klein JB, McLeish KR, Bunke CM, et al: Use of OKT3 monoclonal antibody in the treatment of acute cardiac allograft rejection. Transplantation 45:727–729, 1988.
45. Bristow MR, Gilbert EM, Renlund DG, et al: Use of OKT3 monoclonal antibody in heart transplantation: Review of the initial experience. J Heart Transplant 7:1–11, 1988.
46. Swinnen LJ, Constanzo-Nordin MR, Fisher SG, et al: Increased incidence of lymphoproliferative disorder after immunosuppression with the monoclonal antibody OKT3 in cardiac transplant recipients. N Engl J Med 323:1723–1728, 1990.
47. Carrier M, Jenicek M, Pelletier LC: Value of monoclonal antibody OKT3 in solid organ transplantation: A meta-analysis. Transplant Proc 24:2586–2591, 1992.
48. Rosenthal GJ, Weigand GW, Germolec DR: Suppression of B cell function by methotrexate and trimetrexate. Evidence of inhibition of purine biosynthesis as well as a major mechanism of action. J Immunol 141:410–146, 1988.
49. Constanzo-Nordin MR, Grusk BB, Silver MA, et al: Reversal of recalcitrant cardiac allograft rejection with methotrexate. Circulation 78(Suppl III):III47–III57, 1988.
50. Olsen SL, O'Connell JB, Bristow MR, Renlund DG: Methotrexate as an adjunct in the treatment of persistent mild cardiac allograft rejection. Transplantation 50:773–775, 1990.
51. Bourge RC, Kirklin JK, Williams CW, et al: Methotrexate pulse therapy in the treatment of recurrent acute heart rejection. J Heart Lung Transplant 11:1116–1124, 1992.

52. Bouchart F, Gundry SR, Gonzalez JVS, et al: Methotrexate as rescue/adjunctive immunotherapy in infant and adult heart transplantation. J Heart Lung Transplant 12:427–433, 1993.
53. Salter M, Kirklin JK, Bourge RC, et al: Total lymphoid irradiation in the treatment of early or recurrent heart rejection. J Heart Lung Transplant 11:902–912, 1992.
54. Rose EA, Ban ML, Xn H, et al: Photochemotherapy in human heart transplant recipients at high risk for fatal rejection. J Heart Lung Transplant 11:746–750, 1992.
55. Meiser BM, Km F, Reichen-Spurner H, et al: Reduction of the incidence of rejection by adjunct immunosuppression with photochemotherapy after heart transplantation. Transplantation 57:563–568, 1994.

Chapter 13

Nonspecific Graft Dysfunction in Cardiac Transplantation

Leslie W. Miller, MD
Thomas L. Wolford, MD
Thomas Donohue, MD

Impairment of contractile function of the transplanted heart may occur at any time following implantation, but is usually divided into "early" allograft dysfunction, which is the most common time, and later, or so-called *nonspecific* graft dysfunction. Data from the Cardiac Transplant Research Database[1] and the Registry of the International Society for Heart and Lung Transplantation[2] show the highest risk of graft failure as well as overall mortality occurs during the first 30 days following transplantation. Etiology of early allograft dysfunction is outlined in Table 1 and includes (1) primary graft dysfunction, which may result from traumatic, metabolic, or hemodynamic injury to the heart before explantation as well as prolonged warm ischemia, poor preservation, or prolonged cold ischemia; (2) hyperacute rejection; (3) technical problems; (4) unresponsive pulmonary hypertension, or finally, (5) acute cellular or antibody-mediated rejection.

The clinical features of primary graft failure are often evident with minutes of reperfusion and may be manifest as global and/or focal wall hypokinesis, low cardiac output and hypotension, high pacing threshold, high intracardiac filling pressures especially in patients with prolonged ischemia times, and dependence requirement for multiple inotropes and pressor agents to maintain blood pressure. Risk factors for primary graft failure include requirement for high doses of vasopressor agents in the donor before explantation, older donors where occult coronary disease may cause impaired delivery of cardioplegia solutions, donors with an electrocardiogram

TABLE 1.   Causes of Early Allograft Dysfunction

Primary graft failure	Hyperacute rejection
Trauma	Technical problems
Metabolic (thyroid)	Fixed pulmonary hypertension
Catecholamine excess	Acute cellular and/or antibody-mediated rejection
Warm ischemia	
Poor preservation	
Prolonged cold ischemia	

demonstrating left ventricular hypertrophy, or patients with focal or global wall motion abnormalities before explantation.

Treatment of primary graft failure includes use of inotropic and pressor drugs and for extreme cases, use of intraaortic balloon pump or even more sophisticated forms of mechanical support. Recently, the beneficial effects of supplementing the donor with active thyroid hormone have been shown to improve cardiac performance in otherwise marginal donors.[3] Donors who require high doses of pressor agents may sustain catecholamine-induced subendocardial or focal myocardial injury that may be evident as contraction band necrosis of myocytes on pathologic examination on early biopsy.[5] Early allograft dysfunction related to prolonged cold ischemia time may improve within hours of reperfusion, particularly the component of diastolic dysfunction, which may also be evident as high cardiac filling pressures resulting from passive accumulation of fluid in the myocardium during preservation.

Technical problems remain another source of early allograft dysfunction, and they usually manifest while still in the operating room. The most common problem is torsion of the pulmonary artery anastomosis, particularly in patients who have had multiple previous sternotomies where adhesions may fix the posterior wall of the heart and great vessels. This torsion will create a gradient across the anastomosis and impair right ventricular emptying with secondary distension of the right ventricle, elevated right atrial pressure, and low cardiac output. This diagnosis can be confined by direct needle puncture measurement of the pressure on either side of the pulmonary artery anastomosis. Demonstration of a gradient above 5 mm warrants revision. Another technical problem encountered in the operating room is air embolism, often preferentially into the right coronary artery because of sequestration of air into the pulmonary veins or ventricular apex during implantation. This air can often be clinically visible in the coronaries and may cause dysfunction for 1 to 5 days. Perhaps the most common technical problem is bleeding, particularly because many patients undergoing transplant have had multiple previous sternotomies and are being maintained on anticoagulant agents pretransplant.

The final cause of early allograft dysfunction manifesting in the operating room is hyperacute rejection. This should largely be anticipated by routine panel reactive antibody screen in the recipient at the time of listing for transplantation. The specificity of a circulating antibody should be able to be defined and therefore anticipated.[5,6] However, because the donor-specific crossmatch is almost never available until after the heart has been implanted, demonstration of a positive crossmatch may never be confirmed later. Treatment of hyperacute rejection is based on attempts to remove circulating antibody and to suppress its subsequent development with therapies such as plasmapheresis,[7] exchanging 1 to 2 plasma volumes and replacing them with type-specific plasma and albumin. In addition, cytolytic therapy with agents such as OKT-3 and more B-cell specific therapy such as cyclophosphamide are optimal strategies.[8] Many hearts undergoing hyperacute rejection will develop a blue, mottled appearance related to direct cellular damage as well as probable myocardial ischemia and vasospasm. Prognosis is extremely poor, and early consideration for mechanical assistance is indicated, with the total artificial heart being the optimal device by totally removing the source of foreign antigen. Retransplantation in this setting may be the only definitive solution but only with a donor whose human leukocyte antigen profile is devoid of the offending antigens, and success is seen as very poor.

The leading cause of early allograft dysfunction outside of the operating room is right ventricular failure resulting from relatively fixed pulmonary hypertension in the recipient. This entity should also be anticipated before transplantation from preoperative hemodynamic screening of the recipient during candidate evaluation.[1,9] Although complete hemodynamic monitoring may seem optimal immediately posttransplant, direct measurement of pulmonary artery (PA) pressure may be deceiving because the unconditioned donor right ventricle may fail in attempting to eject against a new and extreme afterload, resulting in decreased PA flow and therefore lowered PA pressure, thus erroneously implying improvement. Direct measurement of RA pressure is actually the most important hemodynamic parameter in patients with pulmonary hypertension. The finding of mean RA pressure greater than 20 mmHg more than 12 hours postimplantation represents a very high risk for subsequent irreversible right ventricular failure. Treatment should include early initiation of vasodilator drugs such as nitroprusside, or if this proves inadequate, use of prostaglandins, and minimal use, if not total avoidance, of vasopressor agents. Inotropic support should include use of isoproterenol, a good beta-agonist, which is devoid of any alpha-vasoconstrictive properties. Use of combinations of beta-agonists such as isoproterenol and dobutamine should be avoided because they have identical mechanisms of action and may accelerate development of receptor down regulation and unresponsiveness to these agents. Recently, the phosphodiesterase inhibitor agent, milrinone,[10] which is an extremely potent vasodilator drug as well as an inotrope, has been shown to be an effective inotrope in this setting and a good agent to lower pulmonary resistance. Sustained use of high doses of beta-agonists may result in early down regulation of beta-receptors; thus serious consideration should be given to use of a combination conversion to the phosphodiesterase type drugs if impaired right ventricular function and pulmonary hypertension persist. This topic is covered in detail elsewhere in the text.

The final cause of early allograft dysfunction includes acute rejection. This may occur as early as 3 to 4 days posttransplant. Patients at highest risk for early rejection include patients under 40 years of age, women, positive panel reactive antibody pretransplant, use of a female donor, underlying inflammatory or immune mediated heart disease in the recipient, or patients in whom suboptimal immunosuppressive drug doses are used because of underlying renal insufficiency or preexisting infection.[11] Diagnosis of acute cellular rejection should be confirmed by endocardial biopsy. Patients with acute rejection associated with hemodynamic compromise and graft dysfunction warrant cytolytic therapy, most commonly with the drug OKT-3. Hemodynamic monitoring of these patients often shows a restrictive physiology with elevated chamber pressures throughout, decreased cardiac output, as well as relative bradycardia and/or evidence of heart block, supraventricular or ventricular arrhythmias, pericardial effusion, and uncommonly, but on occasion, a patient may have fever, confusing the diagnosis of infection versus acute rejection.

Biopsies from patients with hemodynamic compromise and graft dysfunction should also be carefully screened for histologic evidence of vasculitis. Failure to find any evidence of cellular-mediated rejection may warrant fluorescent staining of the biopsy specimen with fluorescent antibodies against immunoglobulins and complements.[12] It is uncommon for humoral rejection to occur in the absence of cellular rejection except in multiparous women and patients previously transfused. Demonstration of any evidence of antibody-mediated rejection warrants use of plasmapheresis and cytolytic therapy such as OKT-3. One helpful test to confirm potential antibody-mediated rejection is to obtain a repeat routine panel reactive antibody screen to demonstrate the presence of circulating antibodies.

Graft dysfunction may also occur several weeks to months posttransplant. The first step in evaluating such a patient is to perform an endomyocardial biopsy. Occasionally, these patients may exhibit no clear evidence of cellular or antibody-mediated rejection. They may, however, respond to a course of rejection therapy with methylprednisolone and/or cytolytic therapy.[13] There have been several anecdotal reports of reversal of nonspecific graft dysfunction with the use of plasmapheresis. This therapy has limited morbidity and, again, may be specifically indicated in patients who demonstrate circulating antibodies. The other consideration in patients in whom allograft dysfunction occurs or persists in the absence of demonstrable evidence of rejection or failure to respond to a course of rejection therapy is the possibility of coronary disease in the allograft. This usually results from unsuspected significant preexisting coronary stenosis in the donor, especially if > 50 years old but even in younger donors, or in patients who have had clinical cytomegalovirus infection. Failure to respond to rejection therapy warrants coronary angiography. Although significant focal epicardial stenoses may occur, perhaps the more common finding is diffuse small vessel obliteration and global ischemia.

Persisting and/or progressive graft dysfunction that does not respond to rejection therapy, particularly that which appears to result from diffuse small vessel disease, carries a very poor prognosis, and retransplantation may be the only definitive option.

The increase in the number of patients on the waiting list for transplantation has caused most centers to liberalize their criteria for selection for cardiac donors.[14] With increasing evidence of significant underlying coronary disease in older donors, however, this expansion of the donor pool may be limited. Undoubtedly many hearts are not used because of concerns of possible early allograft dysfunction posttransplant, but most donor hearts can be supported and will function promptly and adequately postimplantation. Future use of agents such as active thyroid hormone and improved preservation solutions with the addition of critical substrate deficiencies may help improve impaired donor function preexplantation. The majority of other causes of graft dysfunction, particularly early posttransplant, should be anticipated and treatment strategies implemented as early as possible.

REFERENCES

1. Bourge R, Naftel D, Costanzo-Nordin M, et al: Pretransplantation risk factors for death after heart transplantation: A multiinstitutional study. J Heart Lung Transplant 12:549–562, 1993.
2. Kaye MP: The Registry of the International Society for Heart and Lung Transplantation: Tenth official report—1993. J Heart Lung Transplant 12:541–548, 1993.
3. Jeevanandam V, Todd B, Regillo T, et al: Reversal of donor myocardial dysfunction in predicting survival after orthotopic heart transplantation. J Heart Lung Transplant 13:194–201, 1994.
5. Jarcho J, Naftel D, Shroyer TW, et al: Influence of HLA mismatch on rejection after heart transplantation: A multiinstitutional study. J Heart Lung Transplant 13:583–596, 1994.
6. Lavee J, Kormos RL, Duquesnoy RJ, et al: Influence of panel-reactive antibody and lymphcytotoxic crossmatch on survival after heart transplantation. J Heart Lung Transplant 10:921–930, 1991.
7. Partanen J, Nieminen M, Krogerus L, et al: Heart transplant rejection treated with plasmapheresis. J Heart Lung Transplant 11:301–305, 1992.
8. Miller LW, Wesp A, Jennison SH, et al: Vascular rejection in cardiac transplant recipients. J Heart Lung Transplant 12(2):S147–S152, 1993.
9. Warner-Stevenson L, Miller LW: Cardiac transplantation as therapy for heart failure. Curr Probl Cardiol 164):219–305, 1991.
10. Anderson J, Baim D, Fein S: Efficacy of 48 hour infusion of milrinone in patients with severe congestive heart failure. J Am Coll Cardiol 9:711–722, 1987.

11. Kobashigawa J, Kirklin J, Naftel D, et al: Pretransplantation risk factors for acute rejection after heart transplantation: A multiinstitutional study. J Heart Lung Transplant 12:355–366, 1993.
12. Hammond E, Yowell R, Nunoda S, et al: Vascular (humoral) rejection in heart transplantation: Pathologic observations and clinical implications. J Heart Transplant :430–433, 1989.
13. Heroux A, Costanzo-Nordin M, Radvany R: Acute cardiac allograft dysfunction without cellular rejection: Clinical features and role of humoral immunity. Circulation 86:I-628, 1992.
14. Young JB, Naftel DC, Bourge RC, et al: Matching the heart donor and heart transplant recipient. Clues for successful expansion of the donor pool: A multivariable, multiinstitutional report. J Heart Lung Transplant 13:353–365, 1994.

Allograft Coronary Disease

Chapter 14

Leslie W. Miller, MD
Thomas Donohue, MD
Thomas L. Wolford, MD

The major limitation to long-term survival in heart transplant recipients is the development of an accelerated form of coronary artery disease. This disease has been reported since the original heart transplants were performed at Stanford in the late 1960s,[1] and its incidence has not decreased despite the advent of improved immunosuppression with cyclosporine.[2]

The incidence of this disease is approximately 5 to 10% per year posttransplant.[3] Because of the denervation that occurs at the time of transplantation, it has been though to be clinically "silent." Wilson has recently demonstrated, however, that many heart transplant recipients will in fact demonstrate reinnervation over time and develop typical symptoms of angina pectoris in response to development of coronary stenosis.[4] Patients who develop angina-like symptoms posttransplant should therefore be evaluated for the possible development of coronary artery disease.

The development of significant coronary stenosis in heart transplant recipients is associated with an adverse outcome (Fig. 1). The survival reported with 70% stenosis of even one major coronary vessel is approximately 60% at 2 years from the diagnosis and only 20% at 6 months if all 3 major vessels are involved.[5] A similar prognosis has also been reported for patients who develop angina, heart failure, or acute myocardial infarction regardless of coronary anatomy.[6]

The disease is presumed to be primarily immune-mediated.[7] This is derived from the following observations: (1) the vascular intimal thickening characteristic of this disease is confined to the allograft with sparing of other vascular beds and involves the entire vessel; (2) the disease may occur even in children or with donors less than 20 years of age in the absence of any apparent risk factors; and (3) the disease has been reproduced in a number of animal models of immune injury.[8]

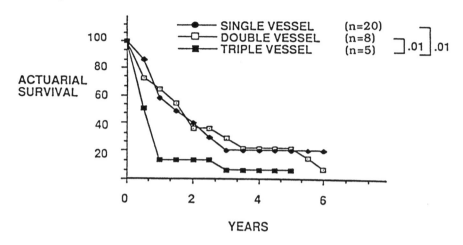

FIGURE 1.   Survival rates in heart transplant patients who develop coronary stenosis.

A number of theories have been advanced regarding the relative contribution of the humoral vs. cell-mediated components of the immune system to the pathogenesis of this disease. Libby[9,10] has described the similarity to a delayed hypersensitivity reaction based on the appearance of activated T cells subjacent to the endothelial cell layer which provide chronic stimulation for up-regulation of endothelial cells to express foreign donor class II antigens on their surface, thereby providing a continual stimulus for immune-mediated response at the level of the endothelium. Despite the preponderance of data suggesting a primary immune basis for this disease, the correlation with cellular rejection has been very poor.[11,12] This may partly result from increasingly conservative criteria used to initiate rejection therapy. Investigators have identified the presence of circulation human leukocyte antibodies (HLA) and the correlation of these antibodies with the development of allograft coronary disease.[13] The antibodies identified in these original reports were not donor-specific, but Rose[14] has subsequently demonstrated the correlation of allograft CAD with donor-specific circulating antibodies, which are often not directed against HLA antigens but against a family of endothelial cell antigens previously described by Cerilli.[15,16] Similarly, antibody-mediated rejection has also been shown to correlate with the development of this disease.[17]

Other nonimmune factors have been shown to correlate with ACAD (Table 1).[18] Although none of these factors have independently been shown to cause the development of this disease change, they may be important in providing an adverse environment or in accelerating the primarily immune-mediated basis for this disease. For example, animals fed a high-cholesterol diet can accelerate development of intimal thickening in immune-mediated arterial injury; diet alone causes only minimal progression of intimal thickening.[8] Plasma lipids, however, including both triglycerides and total cholesterol, have been shown to be statistically significant risk factors in most series of patients with allograft coronary artery disease.[19–21] More recently, cytomegalovirus (CMV), through

TABLE 1.   Nonimmune Factors

Cryo (thermal) injury	Cytomegalovirus infection
Ischemia/reperfusion	Obesity
Hyperlipidemia	Ischemic disease pretransplant

a variety of mechanisms, has been shown to be one of the other highly correlated non-immune risk factors,[22,23] suggesting that even mild illness with CMV may warrant more aggressive therapy.

Unfortunately, because of the diffuse nature of this disease, noninvasive tests have had poor correlation and predictive accuracy[24] and the diagnosis remains based on invasive techniques. Until recently, routine contrast coronary angiography has been the gold standard for the diagnosis. Gao[25] described the findings characteristic of this entity in transplant patients, which, in addition to routine proximal epicardial stenosis, include rapid rapid and abrupt stellate tapering or occlusion of third- and fourth-order branch vessels. This distal obliterative disease typically occurs in association with focal epicardial stenosis and is found much less frequently in the absence of epicardial stenosis. Contrast angiography, however, evidently is not a sensitive diagnostic tool because many patients have been found at autopsy to have significant diffuse epicardial stenoses within months of an apparently normal angiogram. The basis for this discrepancy between angiography and pathology is the reliance of measurement of luminal narrowing in angiography on the assumption that the neighboring vessel and origin of the vessel is entirely normal.[26] In fact, many patients have diffuse narrowing from the ostium distally that causes significant underestimation of stenosis severity when compared with actual measurement of cross-sectional area. Gao[27] demonstrated a statistically significant progression of intimal thickening between the angiogram performed early (< 4 weeks) after transplant and the previously routine initial study at 1 year posttransplant. This would be consistent with the immunologic basis of the disease and the preponderance of immune events (rejection) that occur during the first year. This has prompted many centers to perform the "baseline" study within 4 weeks of transplantation.

The recent development of intravascular ultrasound (IVUS),[28,29] which can directly measure intimal thickening using a Doppler ultrasound imaging system mounted onto a guiding catheter, promises to markedly enhance our ability to diagnose significant epicardial disease before it reaches the > 70% stenosis by angiography associated with a severe increase in mortality.[5] Preliminary data from serial studies with IVUS in cardiac transplant recipients suggest it may be even more accurate in predicting cardiac events than angiography.[30]

A second invasive technique used to investigate the physiologic importance of both epicardial stenosis and distal obliterative disease is measurement of coronary flow reserve (CFR).[31] This technique places an 0.018-inch Doppler guidewire down the coronary artery lumen. Baseline flow velocity is measured, and then intracoronary adenosine is given to provoke a maximal hyperemic response. This agent does not dilate epicardial vessels when given as a bolus, and therefore blood flow velocity serves as an accurate surrogate marker for volumetric blood flow. At peak hyperemia, coronary flow velocity is again measured. The CFR is calculated as the ratio of maximal coronary blood flow velocity to basal or resting blood flow velocity. Normal flow reserve is approximately ≥ 3.0.[32] Of interest, mean CFR was reported to be below normal (2.7 ± 0.4) in studies performed within 30 days of transplantation, but averaged 3.7 between 1 and 3 years posttransplant.[33] These findings support previous observations of early, reversible endothelial dysfunction,[34] perhaps related to nonimmune factors such as ischemia and reperfusion injury during organ preservation, as well as immune-mediated effects in the early posttransplant period that are reversible and recovered by the time of the first year examination.

One of the most critical observations made to date with CFR, which provides an assessment of the small vessel resistance, is the apparent maintenance of a "normal" flow reserve over time despite significant endoluminal thickening of the epicardial vessel.[35] It has been widely held that there is comparable severity of intimal thickening in proximal as well as distal coronary arteries,[36] thereby suggesting the presence of significant distal disease in all patients, especially those with epicardial stenosis. CFR data, however, suggest that the distal vasculature functionally remains relatively normal, with little or no loss of microvascular cross-sectional area in the majority of patients until late posttransplant, even in the presence of significant intimal thickening evidence by IVUS. This perhaps partly results from a compensatory increase in vessel diameter with development of epicardial stenosis as described by Glagov.[37] This finding has profound implications regarding possible therapeutic alternatives to retransplant for significant ACD, especially for patients who develop significant disease in proximal coronary arteries within the first 1 to 3 years posttransplant, including use of standard coronary bypass surgery, which has heretofore been considered nonapplicable in these patients because of the presumed uniform diffuse severe obliterative disease in the "run-off" vessels. Further follow-up will clearly be necessary to evaluate the potential role of this form of therapy.

Although prognosis without intervention is very poor if a 70% stenosis is evident angiographically, progression of this disease is clearly variable and not dissimilar to nontransplant coronary disease. Results with PTCA in transplant patients reported in a multicenter registry[38] were very similar to those in nontransplant patients and appear to offer an improvement in the natural history of the disease without intervention. Patients with angiographic evidence of significant distal disease have the worst outcome with angioplasty. Development of distal obliterative disease may be an independent adverse prognostic factor and so does not relate to the technical ability to perform angioplasty in these patients.

New immunosuppressive drugs being evaluated in cardiac transplantation include tacrolimus (FK506), micophenolate mofetil, and rapamycin. These drugs appear to inhibit markedly the smooth muscle proliferation characteristic of this disease in laboratory animals. They offer some hope of altering the natural history of this major obstacle to long-term survival in cardiac transplantation.

REFERENCES

1. Bieber CP, Hunt SA, Schwinn DA, et al: Complications in long-term survivors of cardiac transplantation. Transplant Proc 13:207–211, 1981.
2. Gao SZ, Schroeder JS, Alderman EL, et al: Prevalence of accelerated coronary artery disease in heart transplant survivors: Comparison of cyclosporine and azathioprine regimens. Circulation 80(Suppl III):100–105.
3. Miller LW: Long term complications of cardiac transplantation. Prog Cardiovasc Dis 33(4):242–248, 1991.
4. Wilson RF, Christensen BV, Olivari MT, et al: Evidence for structural sympathetic reinnervation after orthotopic cardiac transplantation in humans. Circulation 83:1210–1220, 1991.
5. Keogh AM: Proximal and mid-vessel coronary artery disease in the transplanted heart. J Heart Lung Transplant 11:S87, 1992.
6. Gao SZ, Schroeder JS, Hunt S, et al: Retransplantation for severe accelerated coronary artery disease in heart transplant recipients. Am J Cardiol 62:876–881, 1988.
7. Hosenpud JD, Shipley GD, Wagner CR: Cardiac allograft vasculopathy: Current concepts, recent developments, and future directions. J Heart Lung Transplant 11:9–23, 1992.
8. Kosek JC, Bieber C, Lower RR: Heart graft arteriosclerosis. Transplant Proc 3:512–514, 1971.
9. Libby P, Salomon RN, Payne DD, et al: Functions of vascular wall cells related to development of transplantation-associated coronary arteriosclerosis. Transplant Proc 21:3677–3684, 1989.
10. Salomon RN, Hughes CCW, Schoen FJ, et al: Human coronary transplantation-associated arteriosclerosis: Evidence for a chronic immune reaction to activated graft endothelial cells. Am J Pathol 38:791–798, 1991.
11. Costanzo-Nordin MR: Cardiac allograft vasculopathy: Relationship with acute cellular rejection and histocompatibility. J Heart Lung Transplant 11:S90–S103, 1992.
12. Gao SZ, Schroeder JS, Hunt SA, et al: Influence of graft rejection on incidence of accelerated graft coronary artery disease: A new approach to analysis. J Heart Lung Transplant 12:1029–1035, 1993.

13. Rose EA, Pepino P, Barr ML, et al: Relation of HLA antibodies and graft atherosclerosis in human cardiac allograft recipients. J Heart Lung Transplant 11:S120–S123, 1992.
14. Rose E: Antibody mediated rejection following cardiac transplantation. Transplantation Rev 7(3): 140–152, 1993.
15. Cerilli J, Brasile L, Galouzis T, et al: The vascular endothelial cell antigen system. Transplantation 39:268–289, 1985.
16. Cerilli J, Brasile L, Sosa J, et al: The role of autoantibody to vascular endothelial cell antigens in atherosclerosis and vascular disease. Transplant Proc 19(Suppl 5):47–49, 1987.
17. Hammond EH, Yowell RL, Price GD, et al: Vascular rejection and its relationship to allograft coronary artery disease. J Heart Lung Transplant 11:S111–S119, 1992.
18. Johnson MR: Transplant coronary disease: Nonimmunologic risk factors. J Heart Lung Transplant 11:S124–S132, 1992.
19. Ballantyne CM, Radovancevic B, Farmer JA, et al: Hyperlipidemia after heart transplantation: Report of a six year experience, with treatment recommendations. J Am Coll Cardiol 19:1315–1321, 1992.
20. Gao SZ, Schroeder JS, Alderman EL, et al: Clinical and laboratory correlates of accelerated coronary artery disease in the cardiac transplant patient. Circulation 76(Suppl V):56–61, 1987.
21. Winters GL, Kendall TJ, Radio SJ, et al: Posttransplant obesity and hyperlipidemia: Major predictors of severity of coronary arteriopathy in failed human heart allografts. J Heart Lung Transplant 9:364–371, 1990.
22. Grattan MT, Moreno-Cabral CE, Starnes VA, et al: Cytomegalovirus infection is associated with cardiac allograft rejection and atherosclerosis. JAMA 261:3561–3566, 1989.
23. Kendall TJ, Wilson JE, Radio SJ, et al: Cytomegalovirus and other herpesviruses: Do they have a role in the development of accelerated coronary arterial disease in human heart allografts? J Heart Lung Transplant 11:S14–S20, 1992.
24. Smart FW, Ballantyne CM, Cocanougher B, et al: Insensitivity of noninvasive tests to detect coronary artery vasculopathy after heart transplant. Am J Cardiol 167:334–340, 1988.
26. Dresser FA, Miller LW: Necropsy versus angiography: How accurate is angiography? J Heart Lung Transplant 11:56–59, 1992.
27. Gao SZ, Alderman EL, Schroeder JS, et al: Progressive coronary luminal narrowing after cardiac transplantation. Circulation 82(Suppl IV):269–275, 1990.
28. St. Goar FG, Pinto FJ, Alderman EL, et al: Intracoronary ultrasound in cardiac transplant recipients in vivo evidence of "angiographically silent" intimal thickening. Circulation 85:979–987, 1992.
29. Miller LW: The role of intracoronary ultrasound for the diagnosis of cardiac allograft vasculopathy. In press, Transplant Proceedings.
30. Mehra MR, Ventura HO, Stapleton DD, et al: Intimal hyperplasia predicts outcome in cardiac transplant recipients with allograft vasculopathy [abstract]. J Heart Lung Transplant 13(1, part 2):S49, 1994.
31. Tron C, Kern M, Donohue T, et al: Correlations between quantitative coronary angiography derived and directly measured translesional physiology. Eur Heart J 15:384(P2007), 1994.
32. Kern M, Aguirre F, Bach R, et al: Variations in normal coronary vasodilatory reserve by artery, sex, and status post-transplantation. Eur Heart J 15:353(1873), 1994.
33. Wolford T, Donohue T, Bach R, et al: Coronary flow reserve in angiographically normal coronary arteries varies with time post heart transplantation. Eur Heart J 15:605, 1994.
34. Yeung AC, Anderson T, Meredith I, et al: Endothelial dysfunction in the development and detection of transplant coronary artery disease. J Heart Lung Transplant 3:S69–S73, 1992.
35. Wolford R, Wolford T, Ast M, et al: Angiographic appearance of coronary arteries from transplant hearts predicts coronary flow reserve. Circulation 88(4)part 2:1–420, 1993.
36. Lin H, Wilson JE, Kendall TJ, et al: Comparable proximal and distal severity of intimal thickening and size of epicardial coronary arteries in transplant arteropathy of human cardiac allografts. J Heart Lung Transplant 13(5):824–833, 1994.
37. Glagov S, Weisenberg E, Zarins C, et al: Compensatory enlargement of human atherosclerotic coronary arteries. N Engl J Med 316:1371–1375, 1987.
38. Halle AA, Wilson RF, Massin EK, et al: Coronary angioplasty in cardiac transplant patients. Results of a multicenter trial. Circulation 86:458–462, 1992.

Futility of Routine Surveillance Endomyocardial Biopsy after Cardiac Transplantation

Chapter 15

Gulshan K. Sethi, MD
Sudhakar Kosaraju
Francisco A. Arabia, MD
Luis J. Rosado, MD
Michael S. McCarthy
Jack G. Copeland, MD

Since the introduction of cyclosporine in 1982, long-term survival of cardiac transplant patients has markedly improved; over 90% 1-year survival and about 80% 5-year survival has been reported by us and others.[1-3] During follow-up, routine surveillance endomyocardial biopsies at 3- to 12-month intervals to rule out unsuspected rejection have been recommended. Formerly, we performed routine endomyocardial biopsy at the time of annual evaluation. It was our impression that these "routine biopsies" rarely resulted in diagnosing an unsuspected rejection. To confirm our impression, a retrospective analysis of patients who underwent routine yearly biopsy was performed and has been reported elsewhere.[4] Based on the results of this study, starting in September 1989, we discontinued routine surveillance biopsies beyond 6 months following transplantation. Recently, a validity study was conducted to support our hypothesis that routine endomyocardial biopsies at the time of annual evaluations following heart transplantation in asymptomatic patients are not indicated. This report briefly reviews this retrospective study, presents data from the validity study, and reviews the literature dealing with this aspect of care of patients with heart transplant.

TABLE 1.   Endomyocardial Biopsy Protocol Following Heart Transplantation

1st month: twice a week	3 to 12 months: every other week
2nd month: once a week	12 months and beyond: yearly*
3rd month: every other week	

* Based on the results of our previous study, we no longer perform endomyocardial biopsies at 12 months postoperatively or during other annual evaluations.

RETROSPECTIVE STUDY

From March 1979 to September 1989, 211 patients underwent 216 heart transplantations. The endomyocardial biopsy protocol during this period is shown in Table 1. The data files of all patients who survived 1 or more years and in whom a routine heart biopsy was performed as part of their annual evaluation protocol were reviewed. Those evaluations in which heart biopsy was performed because of clinical suspicion of rejection were excluded from data analysis. During this period, three different protocols of immunosuppression were used. These included conventional immunosuppression (prednisone/azathioprine), steroids, and cyclosporine. All patients also received induction therapy with rabbit antithymocyte globulin (RATG). Results of this study have been previously published and are briefly discussed.[4] Overall mortality was 6.5%. One hundred and forty-eight patients qualified for at least first annual evaluation, and a total of 421 yearly clinical evaluations were performed. Three hundred and thirty-eight heart biopsies were performed as a part of routine yearly evaluation protocol. Pathologic abnormalities suggestive of acute rejection at routine biopsy were observed in only two specimens (0.5%). Both were asymptomatic, were in New York Heart Association Functional Class I, and had no clinical evidence of acute rejection. In the first patient, the biopsy at 2-year follow-up evaluation showed cardiac muscle fibers with multiple foci of degenerating fibers, accompanied by mononuclear infiltrates with occasional polynuclear leukocytes and nuclear debris. Masson's trichrome and methyl-green pyronine stain did not show definite evidence of necrotic myocardial fibers. These findings, although not pathognomonic, were consistent with acute rejection, and the patient was treated with intravenous methylprednisolone. Posttreatment biopsy was normal. The second patient also was asymptomatic and NYHA Class I. A routine biopsy performed at 3-year follow-up showed dense mononuclear infiltrate within the myocardium and mild myocardial fiber degeneration without definite evidence of myonecrosis. Because of focal myocytolysis and because the patient was noncompliant, he was treated with tapering dosages of prednisone. The posttreatment biopsy continued to show mild mononuclear infiltrates. Both these patients were doing well at 6- and 4-year follow-up: one was on CSA and steroids and the second on low-dose triple drug immunosuppressive therapy.

VALIDITY STUDY

To compare the results of this retrospective study with those of the validity study, only data from comparable patients must be analyzed. For this reason, only those patients who received low-dose triple drug therapy are considered for data analysis. The control group is considered to be those triple therapy patients who had a routine surveillance biopsy on at least one yearly evaluation. The validity group consisted of those triple therapy patients who had transplant after the use of yearly surveillance biopsies was discontinued.

Of the 211 patients described in the retrospective study, 119 (56%) were treated with low-dose triple drug therapy and qualify for the control group. Only one (0.8%) of the patients described in the earlier study with a positive surveillance biopsy belonged to this group. The operative (30-day) mortality was 2.6% (3 patients), and two additional patients died during the first year. In five patients the annual evaluations were performed elsewhere or the biopsy was not obtained. Thus 109 patients qualified in the control group. Because most patients survived through the change of protocol, they were censored at 1 year following their last surveillance biopsy for purposes of late rejection and late biopsy analysis. They were not censored for actuarial survival, however.

Based on our previous experience, we discontinued routine surveillance endomyocardial biopsies in September 1989. From then to July 1, 1994, we have performed 203 additional heart transplants. The 30-day operative mortality was 2% (4 patients) and an additional eight patients died during the first year. Forty-eight patients are not yet eligible for their 1-year follow-up. Thus 144 patients qualified for analysis as the validity group.

Late biopsy is defined as any biopsy not performed at the time of annual evaluation. biopsy in this group was usually unscheduled and performed for the diagnosis of suspected rejection. Similarly, late rejection is also defined as any rejection episode not diagnosed during annual evaluation and required treatment with augmentation with immunosuppressive therapy.

RESULTS

We have analyzed the actuarial survival rates, freedom from late rejections, and freedom from late biopsies for these two groups. Figure 1 compares the actuarial survival rates between patients in whom surveillance biopsies were performed with those of patients who did not undergo routine surveillance biopsies. No difference was shown in overall survival rates between the two groups (p = 0.94). Similarly, there was no difference in freedom from late rejection between these two groups (Fig. 2). Freedom from late unscheduled biopsies was significantly lower, however, in the group of patients in whom surveillance biopsies were performed (Fig. 3).

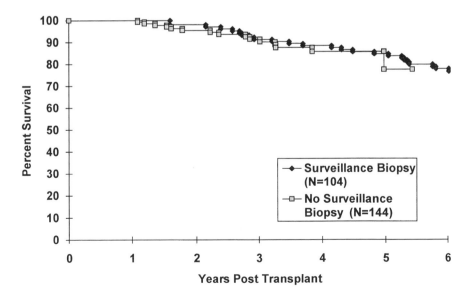

FIGURE 1.   Comparison of actuarial survival rates between patients who had routine surveillance endomyocardial biopsies and those who did not. P = 0.477.

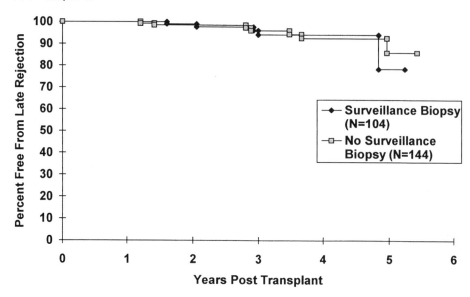

FIGURE 2.   Comparison of freedom from late rejections between surveillance and nonsurveillance biopsy groups. P = 0.988.

DISCUSSION

Despite improvements in immunosuppression therapy, infection and rejection continue to be the main causes of death after heart transplantation. Though various non-invasive assessment methods to detect rejection have been developed, endomyocardial biopsy remains the gold standard with which to diagnose rejection. During follow-up surveillance, endomyocardial biopsies at 3- to 12-month intervals and coronary arteriography at yearly intervals have been recommended.[5,6] Routine coronary arteriography appears to be necessary to evaluate the status of coronary arteries because development and progression of coronary artery disease in the transplanted heart is unpredictable. Furthermore, clinical diagnosis of coronary arteriosclerosis is difficult in these patients because they may not exhibit ischemic symptoms because of denervation of the transplanted heart.

Most rejections occur within the first 3 months of the transplant and only 5% of the rejections occur after the first year. These are usually associated with a decrease in immunosuppression initiated by the physician or by a noncompliant patient.[7] Late rejection in an asymptomatic patient is extremely rare. Sivathasan and coworkers reported that routine endomyocardial biopsy performed more than nine months postoperatively had a low yield of only 2.5%. In over a third of their patients, biopsy was clinically indicated to rule out rejection. Severity of rejection and details of management of these patients are not available[8] Surveillance endomyocardial biopsies were routinely performed at 3-month intervals in all heart-lung transplant patients at Stanford University; however, after reviewing their data they concluded that in long-term management phase (over 6 months) endomyocardial biopsies should be performed only for specific indications rather than as a routine surveillance procedure.[9] Our patient in the surveillance biopsy group, whose routine endomyocardial biopsy was suspicious for rejection, was treated because of special circumstances. He was seen earlier in our experience and was noncompliant. We doubt that under our current protocol we would treat such a patient for rejection.

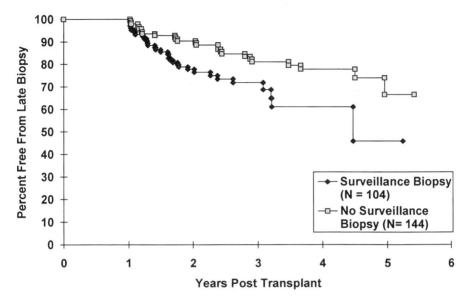

FIGURE 3.   Comparison of freedom from unscheduled late endomyocardial biopsies between surveillance and nonsurveillance biopsy groups. P = 0.012.

Treatment of late moderate rejection in asymptomatic patients who otherwise are adequately immunosuppressed is controversial.[10,11] Hutter and colleagues critically analyzed the outcome of patients whose endomyocardial biopsies showed moderate rejection. They treated only 29% of patients with moderate rejection that occurred between 3 to 12 months postoperatively, and most of them were symptomatic. They concluded that after 1 month postoperatively, it may not be necessary to augment immunosuppression when myonecrosis is observed at routine endomyocardial biopsy in an asymptomatic patient.[10] In the absence of a nonconfirmatory randomized trial to support their hypothesis, however, we are hesitant to take such a drastic approach.

We were surprised to observe the increased frequency of unscheduled biopsies in the surveillance group, because one would have expected otherwise. Patients who had surveillance biopsies were operated on between April 1985 and September 1989 and represent our earlier experience. We believe that during this period we were quite conservative and cautious and probably treated some borderline and suspicious rejections. Similarly, the more frequent incidence of unscheduled biopsies may also be explained by the function of the time of heart transplantation. The low frequency of late rejection in our patient population may reflect the stability, reliability, and compliance of these patients with their medications and the medical follow-up. Our current practice is to perform the last surveillance endomyocardial biopsy at 6 months postoperatively. After that, further heart biopsies are performed based upon clinical indications. These include sudden cardiac arrhythmias, decrease in exercise tolerance, dyspnea, congestive heart failure, presence of S3 gallop, and increase in heart size on chest roentgenogram.

In summary, based upon our experience, as well as that of others, we believe that routine surveillance endomyocardial biopsies in asymptomatic orthotopic heart recipients are not indicated. Biopsy should be performed if there is clinical suspicion of rejection or as a part of a research protocol. This will avoid unnecessary discomfort to the patients as well as prevent potential complications that may be associated with this procedure.[12,13] This may also decrease the cost of postoperative care of patients undergoing heart transplantation.

REFERENCES

1. Copeland JG, Icenogle TB, Williams RF, et al: Rabbit antithymocyte globulin: A 10-year experience in cardiac transplantation. J Thorac Surg 99:852–860, 1990.
2. Walwork J, Cory-Pearce R, English TAH: Cyclosporine for cardiac transplantation: VK trial. Transplant Proc 15:2559–2566, 1983.
3. Hosenpud JD, Novick RJ, Breen TJ, Daily OP: The registry of the International Society for Heart and Lung Transplantation: Eleventh official report—1994. J Heart Lung Transplant 13(4):561–570, 1994.
4. Sethi GK, Rosado LR, McCarty M, et al: Futility of yearly heart biopsies in patients undergoing heart transplantation. J Thorac Cardiovasc Surg 104:90–93, 1993.
5. Baughman KL: Monitoring of allograft rejection. In Baumgartner WA, Reitz BA, Achuff SC (eds): Heart and Heart-Lung Transplantation. Philadelphia, W.B. Saunders, 1990, pp 86–102.
6. Gao SZ, Alderman EL, Schroeder SS, et al: Accelerated coronary vascular disease in the heart transplant patient: Coronary arteriographic findings. J Am Coll Cardiol 12:334–340, 1988.
7. Copeland JG: Cardiac transplantation. Curr Probl Cardiol 13(3):157–224, 1988.
8. Sivathasan C, McDonald P, Keogh A, et al: The role of routine endomyocardial biopsy for monitoring the rejection after cardiac transplantation. J Heart Transplant 9:63, 1990.
9. Glanville AR, Imoto E, Baldwin JC, et al: The role of right ventricular endomyocardial biopsy in the long-term management of heart lung transplant recipients. J Heart Transplant 6:357–360, 1987.
10. Hutter JA, Wallwork J, English TAH: Management of rejection in heart transplant recipients: Does moderate rejection always require treatment? J Heart Transplant 9:87–91, 1990.
11. Crandall BG, Renlund DG, O'Connell JB, et al: Increased cardiac allograft rejection in female heart recipients. J Heart Transplant 7:419–423, 1988.
12. Bhat G, Burwig S, Walsh R: Morbidity of endomyocardial biopsy in cardiac transplant recipients. Am Heart J 125:1180–1181, 1993.
13. Aravot D, Fitzgerald M, Khaghani A, et al: Complications of endomyocardial biopsy of the transplanted human heart. A review of 6200 biopsies in 550 patients. J Am Col Cardiol 11:174, 1988.
14. United Network of Organ Sharing, personal communication.

Chapter 16

Management of Posttransplant Obesity and Hyperlipidemia

Kathleen D. Lake, PharmD, BCPS

HYPERLIPIDEMIA AND OBESITY

Hyperlipidemia and obesity are well-recognized complications following cardiac transplantation.[1-15] In patients surviving longer than 1 year, these conditions have been associated with development of accelerated graft atherosclerosis (AGAS).[1,16-34] Even though it is unlikely they are the sole or primary cause of this condition, both clinical and animal studies suggest that hyperlipidemia may accelerate the process.[1,19,24] Because the exact benefits of aggressive lipid-lowering strategies on the development or progression of graft atherosclerosis are not clear, the decision to treat must be based on the theoretic benefits vs. risks of drug therapy.[25] This article reviews incidence, risk factors, and etiology of these complications in the cardiac transplant recipient and discusses the risks vs. benefits of management strategies for these conditions.

Incidence

Hyperlipidemia occurs in 60 to 83% of heart transplant patients treated with triple-drug immunosuppression.[1-15] Elevations in total low-density lipoprotein (LDL) cholesterol and triglycerides typically develop within 3 to 18 months following transplantation. The magnitude of increase from pretransplant cholesterol is variable, ranging from 30 to 80 mg/dl.[26] My colleagues and I observed the greatest percentage increase in total cholesterol and LDL cholesterol in patients with no past history of hyperlipidemia, whereas patients with a positive history had a smaller percent rise. Those patients, who

TABLE 1.   Risk Factors for Hyperlipidemia in Transplant Recipients

Pretransplant hyperlipidemia[13,27,36–38]	Renal dysfunction[39,40,42,43,46,47]
Obesity[6,13,18,39–44]	Proteinuria[38,45,46,48]
Male[45]	Antihypertensive medications[45,46,48–50]
Diabetes[43,46]	Cyclosporine[51–53]
Age[13,41,43–45]	Prednisone dosage (cumulative, maintenance)[5,13,38–41,43,46,50,54,55]

already had elevated lipid levels, appeared to be less influenced by the drug-induced effects of cyclosporine (CsA) and prednisone following transplantation.[27]

Obesity has been reported to occur with an equally high prevalence following cardiac transplantation;[7,8,27–30] most patients gain between 5 and 10 kg (i.e., usually in excess of 10% actual body weight) during the first postoperative year.[27,28] Obesity has also been reported to be a predictive risk factor for development of AGAS[18] although others have found no association.[31,32]

Etiology and Risk Factors

The etiology of hyperlipidemia and obesity in the posttransplant period is multifactorial (Table 1).[1-15,27–30,33–38] It is not surprising that these factors have been associated with the development of posttransplant hyperlipidemia, because most have been related to hyperlipidemia in the general population. These conditions may also be exacerbated by immunosuppressants (e.g., CsA, prednisone) and other medications used commonly in these patients (Table 2).[56,67]

One of the most important determinants of posttransplant hyperlipidemia and obesity in the cardiac transplant recipient is that of a past history of either disorder.[27,58,59] Patients who have ischemic cardiomyopathy as their primary etiology for cardiac transplantation compared with idiopathic cardiomyopathy, have a higher prevalence of these complications.[7,12,36,37] At the time of transplantation these problems may be less evident. Serum cholesterol values may be depressed in the pretransplant period because of the pathophysiologic changes caused by severe congestive heart failure (e.g., cardiac

TABLE 2.   Effect of Posttransplant Medications on Lipoproteins

Medications	Effects
Thiazide diuretics	↑ 0–10% total LDL, triglycerides 30–50%
Beta-blockers (non-ISA)	↑ 15–50% triglycerides
Ethanol	↓ 5–15% HDL cholesterol
	↑ 50% triglycerides
Prazosin	↑ 0–15% cholesterol/triglycerides
Progestins	↑ 5–15% chylomicrons and VLDL cholesterol
Glucocorticoids	↑ 5–20% total, VLDL, and LDL cholesterol
Anabolic steroids	↑ 0–30% total cholesterol
	↓ 8–40% HDL cholesterol
Cyclosporine	↑ 20–30% total and LDL cholesterol
Isotretinoin	↑ 5–20% total cholesterol
	↓ 10–15% HDL cholesterol

(Data from Israel MK, McKenney JM: Hyperlipidemias. In Carter B, Angaran D, Lake K, Raekel M: Cardiovascular Module. Pharmacotherapy Self-Assessment Program (PSAP). Kansas City: American College of Clinical Pharmacy 2nd ed, 1995, pp 65–94, and from Henkin Y, Como JA, Oberman A: Secondary dyslipidemia inadvertent effects of drugs in clinical practice. JAMA 267(7):961–968, 1992.)

cachexia, passive congestion of the liver, elevated catecholamines, and altered gastrointestinal absorption patterns), and lipid profiles may not accurately reflect preexisting lipid abnormalities. One proposed mechanism for the high incidence of hyperlipidemia following cardiac transplantation is correction of severe congestive heart failure.

Another important contributing factor to posttransplant hyperlipidemia is the obesity that commonly develops following transplantation.[6,43,60,61] Obesity contributes to hyperlipidemia principally by causing excessive production of very-low-density lipoprotein (VLDL) particles and raised triglyceride levels. Excessive caloric consumption can increase VLDL and LDL production while decreasing HDL cholesterol concentrations. Patients gaining 5 kg or more during the first year following transplantation are more likely to have total serum cholesterol levels in excess of 240 mg/dl.[62] Weight gains of 15 to 20% total body weight have been associated with statistically significant elevations in cholesterol and triglycerides.[63]

Similarly, as regards obesity, patients may be at, or even below, their ideal body weight at the time of transplantation because of either prescribed or cachexia-induced weight loss during the waiting phase.[7] These factors can complicate analysis of weight gain following transplantation. An accurate assessment of the patient's true weight (i.e., prior to the onset of cardiac illness) is necessary to determine whether the patient has gained *new* weight or has simply regained a premorbid body habitus. In addition, assessment of weight gain alone may actually reflect a desirable return to normal body habitus in patients with cardiac cachexia.

Risk groups for weight gain among renal transplant recipients have included younger people, black people, and women. Other factors, such as increased sense of well-being associated with normal heart function, psychosocial stress, and, more important, a lack of compliance with exercise and dietary regimens, also contribute to posttransplant obesity.[7,64]

In addition, some of the agents listed in Table 2 may affect weight control following transplantation. Prednisone and oral contraceptives may increase weight gain by causing fluid retention, altering fat deposition, and increasing appetite.[65,66] Weight gain following transplantation has been reported to be statistically greater in patients who failed prednisone withdrawal (i.e., patients who experienced three rejection episodes during the first 4 months)[29] or in whom prednisone withdrawal was not attempted.[30] Hagan and associates[29] reported a significant weight gain in patients maintained on prednisone from the time of transplantation to 1 year postoperatively; however, when standardized to percentage change in ideal body weight, significance was not attained. Jones and associates[30] reported a significant difference in body mass index at 1 year between patients on and off prednisone but did not report the baseline weight status of these patients nor the change in weight over time. Our research in heart recipients and that of Hricik and coworkers in renal transplant patients found no difference in weight gained, when standardized to ideal body weight, in patients weaned from prednisone compared with those maintained on steroid therapy.[27,67] Interestingly, if prednisone was the sole culprit in transplant-induced obesity, one could speculate that patients in whom prednisone is tapered or discontinued should lose weight, yet this has not been reported.

Alcohol provides excess "empty" calories and may also stimulate appetite. Other medications reported to cause weight gain include antidepressants,[68] antipsychotics including lithium and clozapine,[69–73] and anticonvulsants such as carbamazepine and valproic acid.[74,75]

Significance

Studies in the general population have established hyperlipidemia as a risk factor for premature atherosclerosis and have demonstrated the value of lowering serum cholesterol in reducing cardiovascular morbidity and mortality.[76-78] If experience in the general population can be extrapolated to cardiac transplant recipients, there could be a speculated causal relationship between posttransplant hyperlipidemia and development of AGAS.

In one of the earliest analyses of this problem in the precyclosporine era, cholesterol was not found to be an important risk factor for the development of AGAS.[60] In a subsequent retrospective multivariate analysis, only two factors were identified as being significantly related to the development of AGAS, an older donor age (23.5 vs. 21.3 years) and higher fasting plasma triglyceride levels (236 mg/dl vs. 170 mg/dl)[79] (neither of which were considerably high). In this study, neither cholesterol nor its subfractions were related to the development of AGAS. In another retrospective analysis, an association between hyperlipidemia and AGAS was made in which high-risk cholesterol values at 6 months predicted the development of coronary artery disease after the third year.[19] An unusual finding in this study was that all patients under 20 years of age developed coronary artery disease by 3 years after transplantation. In addition to these studies, several others support at least a contributory role of hyperlipidemia to the development of AGAS,[16-18, 21-23,80] whereas a few have not.[31,81]

Other factors associated with the development of AGAS, and quite distinct from risk factors for nontransplant coronary artery disease, include a higher incidence of cellular rejection,[60,82] a previous history of ischemic heart disease,[31] older donor hearts,[16,22,79] HLA incompatibility,[83-85] and high cytotoxic antibody titers.[1] Posttransplant cytomegalovirus infection has been associated with the development of AGAS in a number of series.[86-88] Traditional risk groups such as older people, men, hypertensives, diabetics, and smokers have not been found to be risk groups for AGAS.[20]

Those opposed to treating hyperlipidemia feel there are no compelling data to suggest that lowering lipid levels provides any real benefit in the development of AGAS and that, before widespread adoption of empiric treatment protocols occurs, large multicenter trials should be conducted.[89] Several series have demonstrated clinical efficacy using lipid-lowering drugs but have not yet shown a difference on the ultimate outcome of AGAS.[3,90,91] Second, based on the premise that AGAS is different from native coronary artery disease,[92] in its distribution and morphology, histology, and associated risk factors, it might not warrant aggressive lipid-lowering strategies but may require other therapies, such as augmented or alternative immunosuppression.

DRUG-INDUCED HYPERLIPIDEMIA

Conflicting data exist regarding the exact mechanisms of immunosuppressant-induced hyperlipidemia, but it is generally agreed that CsA and prednisone independently, and perhaps synergistically, promote development of hyperlipidemia.[52,93,94] Azathioprine does not contribute to the posttransplant hyperlipidemia.

CsA

With the introduction of CsA to most immunosuppressive regimens, lower prednisone dosages were anticipated. This was expected to have a salutary effect on the hyperlipidemia seen in transplant recipients treated with conventional immunosuppression. Ironically, patients maintained on CsA continued to have hyperlipidemia, with even more significant elevations of serum cholesterol than those reported previously.[9,35,42,43,52,93-96]

Cyclosporine causes a 20 to 30% increase in total and LDL-cholesterol and can also cause hypertriglyceridemia.[2,9,52,64,97] These findings have also been confirmed in nontransplant patients with psoriasis and amyotrophic lateral sclerosis receiving CsA as monotherapy.[52,98,99] One possible mechanism for cyclosporine-induced hyperlipidemia may be related to its binding of lipoproteins in plasma.[100] By binding to the LDL receptor, CsA possibly changes the binding kinetics in a manner that could alter those feedback mechanisms that control cholesterol synthesis.[101,102] Impairment of LDL clearance may result in an accumulation of LDL and total cholesterol (i.e., a more atherogenic lipoprotein profile).[9,52] CsA may also inhibit metabolic conversion of cholesterol to bile acids[102] and like steroids, it may induce peripheral insulin resistance and hyperinsulinemia.[103] Other proposed mechanisms include a direct effect on lipoprotein lipase activity,[104] an interaction with renal function, or alteration of the function of apolipoprotein C-II.[14] Lipoprotein lipase activity has been reported to be inversely related to CsA levels and low levels of activity may lead to increases in plasma triglycerides.[14]

It is not clear whether the lipid-elevating effects induced by CsA are dose- or concentration-dependent. Winters and coworkers[18] reported a high correlation (r = 0.96, p < 0.01) with mean cyclosporine levels and posttransplant total blood cholesterol levels; others, however, have not found a similar association.[43,45] Based on these observations, some practitioners have recommended empirically decreasing the CsA dose to lower lipid levels.

Withdrawal of cyclosporine from kidney transplant recipients has resulted in improved lipid profiles despite continued treatment with steroids.[51,53] Whether this is related to elimination of CsA's direct effect or improved prednisone clearance or better renal function is unclear. Other investigators have found no benefit from withdrawing CsA.[43–45,105]

Prednisone

Corticosteroids have been reported to increase cholesterol levels by 5 to 10% and that of triglycerides by 15 to 20% in nontransplant patients.[65,106] A substantial amount of evidence, much of which was gained during the precyclosporine era, exists documenting the contributor role of prednisone to the development of hyperlipidemia following transplantation.[13,38–43,46,50,54,55,107,108–110]

Corticosteroids may induce insulin resistance[111] and a state of hyperinsulinemia, which may lead to increased synthesis of VLDL. This may explain the hypertriglyceridemia commonly seen during steroid therapy. Steroids also may increase hepatic synthesis of VLDL by enhancing the activities of rate-limiting enzymes involved in lipogenesis.[42,50,111] The bulk of evidence suggests that corticosteroids increase total cholesterol by increasing triglycerides and HDL cholesterol with either no effect or a lowering effect on LDL cholesterol.[3,5,11,12] Even though prednisone's primary effects are on HDL cholesterol and triglycerides, a few studies have also reported increases in LDL-cholesterol.[4,5]

The hyperlipidemic effect of prednisone can be seen as early as 3 to 6 weeks postoperatively.[3] Most reports support a dose-dependent effect based on total daily dose; however, a few studies have implicated the cumulative dose.[11,112,113] Conflicting data exist regarding the impact of lower dose regimens[12] and this may result from the narrow dosage range currently used by most centers.

Withdrawal of corticosteroids has been associated with cholesterol levels 20 to 26% lower than in patients maintained on prednisone;[11] however, Renlund and colleagues did not differentiate the incidence of patients with a past medical history of hyperlipidemia. Similar benefits of steroid withdrawal have been reported in renal transplant recipients.[67,114,115] Other investigators found no correlation with prednisone use and hyperlipidemia.[9,14,52] The effect of alternate day steroids has proved beneficial in some patients[108,109,116] but not in others.[40,41,50]

Some conflicting data in the literature may be related to the presence or absence of other risk factors commonly seen in cardiac transplant recipients (Table 1). Certainly those patients with multiple risk factors would be expected to have higher lipid levels than those with only drug-induced hyperlipidemia. Similarly, the benefit of withdrawing immunosuppressant therapy may be more apparent in patients with only drug-induced processes compared with those with multiple risk factors.

Reports implicating either cyclosporine or prednisone as the causative agent for posttransplant hyperlipidemia may actually support the premise that an additive or synergistic lipid-elevating effect exists with use of these drugs. This interaction may result from an inhibition of each's metabolism by the other's.[117,118] Even though this mechanism is attractive, until recently it would have been difficult to prove, because few centers would have considered withdrawing both cyclosporine and prednisone from their hyperlipidemic transplant recipients. Now, however, with the availability of tacrolimus, it is possible to convert these patients to determine if their hyperlipidemia improves. Most important, it will be interesting to observe whether the incidence of AGAS changes with use of newer immunosuppressive regimens that lack lipid-elevating effects.

Tacrolimus (formerly FK506)

One of the purported advantages of tacrolimus is a lower incidence of hyperlipidemia.[119,120] Tacrolimus is similar to CsA in many pharmacokinetic aspects. It is highly lipophilic and distributes well throughout the body, but a major difference is that in plasma it binds to alpha 1-acid glycoprotein and albumin rather than lipoproteins. If CsA's mechanism for inducing hyperlipidemia is related to its binding of LDL, this may explain why tacrolimus does not increase cholesterol levels. Another pharmacokinetic difference with tacrolimus is that bile is not necessary to facilitate its absorption; this may be clinically beneficial if bile acid resins or probucol are used.[121]

Other factors contributing to the lower incidence of hyperlipidemia include that tacrolimus has been reported to be steroid-sparing[122] and this may also account for a lower incidence of hyperlipidemia, especially in patients completely weaned from steroids. In addition, most initial reports of a lower incidence of hyperlipidemia with the use of tacrolimus are based on the multicenter trials in liver transplant patients, who in general have a somewhat lower incidence of hyperlipidemia.[64,123]

Tacrolimus has been reported to cause glucose intolerance and to induce diabetes in up to 18% of patients;[124,125] thus, as with CsA and steroids, it may cause insulin resistance and hyperinsulinemia leading to hypertriglyceridemia. Trials assessing its efficacy in autoimmune disorders should provide insight on its actual hyperlipidemic effects. Until the drug is more widely used in renal and heart transplant recipients, who have a much higher incidence of hyperlipidemia, we will not be able to assess its true merits.

Other Drugs

Various other drugs including certain diuretics,[126,127] non-ISA containing beta-adrenergic blockers,[48,128–130] certain vasodilators,[128,131] sympatholytics,[132,133] oral contraceptives,[65,106] isotretinoin,[134] and ethanol[135] have also been reported to increase serum lipids (Table 2).[56,57]

TABLE 3.   NCEP Dietary Recommendations

Initial classification based on total and HDL cholesterol

Total cholesterol

Under 200 mg/dl	Desirable
200–239 mg/dl	Borderline-high
240 and over	High

HDL cholesterol

Under 35 mg/dl	Low

Treatment based on LDL cholesterol

Diet Therapy	Initiation Level	LDL Goal
Without CHD and without 2 risk factors	160 mg/dl or over	Under 160 mg/dl
Without CHD and with 2 or more risk factors	Over 130 mg/dl	Under 130 mg/dl
With CHD	Over 100 mg/dl	100 mg/dl or under
Drug Treatment	Initiation Level	LDL Goal
Without CHD and without 2 risk factors	190 mg/dl or over	Under 160 mg/dl
Without CHD and with 2 or more risk factors	160 mg/dl or over	Under 130 mg/dl
With CHD	130 mg/dl or over	100 mg/dl or under

(Data from Expert Panel on Detection, Evaluation, and Treatment of High Blood Cholesterol in Adults: Summary of the second report of the National Cholesterol Education Program (NCEP) Expert Panel on Detection, Evaluation, and Treatment of High Blood Cholesterol in Adults (Adult Treatment Panel II). JAMA 269(23):3015–3023, 1993.)

NONPHARMACOLOGIC MANAGEMENT STRATEGIES

Even though the benefits of dietary intervention have not proved to alter the course of AGAS, it seems prudent to follow the recommendations of the National Cholesterol Education Program (NCEP) for the nonpharmacologic treatment of cardiac transplant recipients (Tables 3 and 4).[136] Other nondrug approaches, including weight loss, exercise, and smoking cessation, should be instituted at the same time.[136] Caloric restriction reduces triglyceride concentrations and increases HDL concentrations. Exercise has been found to decrease VLDL and LDL cholesterol as well as to increase HDL cholesterol concentrations.

Because dietary indiscretion has been associated with a rise in cholesterol of 40 to 50 ml/dl, the first step, and one of the safest methods of treating hyperlipidemia, is to

TABLE 4.   American Heart Association Diet

Step I	Step II
8–10% of calories from saturated fat	Less than 7% of calories from saturated fat
30% or fewer calories from total fat	30% or fewer calories from total fat
Fewer than 300 mg of cholesterol a day	Fewer than 200 mg of cholesterol a day

(Data from Expert Panel on Detection, Evaluation, and Treatment of High Blood Cholesterol in Adults: Summary of the second report of the National Cholesterol Education Program (NCEP) Expert Panel on Detection, Evaluation, and Treatment of High Blood Cholesterol in Adults (Adult Treatment Panel II). JAMA 269(23):3015–3023, 1993.)

have patients follow the Step I diet initially and then advance to Step II (Table 4).[137–141] Step II diets will be necessary in most patients because only a 0 to 4% reduction in cholesterol has been reported with the Step I diet vs. a 6.5 to 15% reduction with Step II.[142] Progress should be assessed at 4 to 6 weeks, again at 3 months, and on an ongoing basis to reinforce compliance. Little information is available on the efficacy of diet alone in heart transplant recipients, but statistically significant decreases in cholesterol, triglycerides, and LDL have been reported in renal transplant recipients.[138,139,151,143,144]

If the response to diet therapy is inadequate and the patient has been diligent in efforts with nondrug interventions, then pharmacologic therapy should be instituted. It needs to be emphasized to the patient that drug therapy is being added to the nonpharmacologic strategies rather than replacing them.

Other global strategies include the development of new drugs or drug combinations that do not adversely affect lipid metabolism and establishment of better matching of organs and recipients, thus allowing for less overall immunosuppression.

RECOMMENDATIONS FOR DRUG THERAPY

The decision whether to apply the NCEP Guidelines to heart transplant recipients is based on whether the theoretic benefits of lowering serum lipids are greater than the individual or collective toxicities of the various treatments.[3,25] Once the decision to treat is made, a number of other questions arise.

When should you initiate drug therapy?

NCEP guidelines recommend initiating pharmacologic therapy after a minimum of 6 months of intensive dietary therapy and other nonpharmacologic interventions (e.g., weight loss, smoking cessation, exercise). Shorter periods can be considered in patients with severe elevations of LDL cholesterol and in patients who have already demonstrated compliance with the AHA Step II diet before transplantation but have experienced minimal benefit. Generally, this period should coincide with lower immunosuppressive dosages, but it might be prudent to wait until the immunosuppressant dosages are at a maintenance level, unless the total plasma cholesterol concentrations remain consistently above 300 mg/dl.

However, if the cause of AGAS is immunologic damage in the presence of even modestly elevated lipid levels, it may be more appropriate to initiate therapy at 3 months or sooner. This type of therapeutic plan coincides with the occurrence of the most significant immunologic challenges (i.e., acute rejection and CMV infection) facing the patient. The typical delay in treating patients may also explain the lack of evidence supporting input of lipid-lowering agents on the development of AGAS. Kobashigawa and associates have recently reported that administration of pravastatin starting 1 to 2 weeks posttransplant is not only associated with lower cholesterol levels but may also decrease incidence of severe rejection either directly through its immunosuppressive properties[145,146] or indirectly by altering the lipoprotein binding of CsA. Preliminary analysis of data also showed less AGAS in the treatment group, but longer follow-up is necessary. Even though the authors did not suggest it,[145] it is possible that aggressive lipid-lowering strategies employed very early posttransplant, in addition to the proposed immunologic benefit, may have a long-term benefit on the development of AGAS.

At what cholesterol levels should therapy be initiated?

NCEP guidelines call for initiating drug treatment at an LDL cholesterol level > 160 mg/dl in patients with two or more risk factors vs. > 190 mg/dl in patients with fewer than two risk factors. Because many cardiac transplant recipients initially had ischemic cardiomyopathy, they typically would be considered as having a sufficiently high risk to warrant therapy. One could also argue that any recipient, regardless of gender or traditional risk factors, should be considered at high risk for developing AGAS and should be treated for hyperlipidemia. In fact, as suggested by a recent retrospective study, it may be necessary to initiate drug therapy at even lower LDL cholesterol levels (e.g., more than 115 mg/dl) to achieve a positive impact on the occurrence of AGAS.[80] It is possible that preventing hyperlipidemia in the cardiac recipient is more important than treating it after it reaches some arbitrary level.

Because little evidence supports that isolated hypertriglyceridemia is an important factor in the pathogenesis of AGAS,[19,21,23,31,79] diet, weight loss, and avoidance of alcohol are usually sufficient unless triglyceride concentrations are in excess of 400 mg/dl.

What is the lipid-lowering drug of choice for cardiac transplant recipients?

No one drug of choice exists for all patients, however, low-dose hydroxy-methyl-gluteryl coenzyme-A (HMG-CoA) reductase inhibitors are preferred by many transplant centers.[3,90,91,147,148]

Decisions regarding drug selection should be individualized with each transplant recipient and should be based on the type of hyperlipidemia, the presence of other concomitant illnesses that can be exacerbated by additional drug therapy, and whether other life-sustaining medications are being administered that can interact with the lipid-lowering agents and cause serious consequences (Table 5).[3,33–35] Being aware of the indications, contraindications, and relative toxicities of the individual agents allows the practitioner to select the optimal agents and minimize the risk of adverse consequences.

Bile Acid Sequestrants

In the general population, bile acid resins or sequestrants (e.g., cholestyramine, colestipol) are considered a first-line therapy because they have been shown to decrease the incidence of coronary artery disease and to have a relatively low incidence of side effects.[136] These agents are not absorbed systemically and act by binding bile acids in the intestinal lumen. Cholestyramine (20 g daily) and colestipol (15 g daily) decrease cholesterol and LDL by 15 to 25%, cholesterol in a dose-dependent manner and with concurrent small increase in HDL. Efficacy of higher doses is limited only by patient compliance because constipation and gastrointestinal complaints (abdominal pain,

TABLE 5.   Special Considerations in the Use of Lipid-Lowering Drugs after Heart Transplantation

Drug	Possible Side Effects	Interactions with Immunosuppressants
Bile acid sequestrant (cholestyramine, colestipol)	May prevent absorption of fat-soluble drugs: poor compliance because of constipation and bloating	May inhibit absorption of cyclosporine, which is extremely fat soluble
Nicotinic acid	Elevation of liver function tests, increased uric acid levels, decreased glucose tolerance, exacerbation of peptic ulcer disease, flushing-poor compliance	Cyclosporine may cause elevation of liver function tests and uric acid levels; prednisone decreases glucose tolerance and may predispose to peptic ulcer disease
Fibric acid derivative (gemfibrozil)	Gallstones, myositis, nausea, potentiation of warfarin	Increased myositis with concomitant lovastatin and immunosuppressive drugs; decreased metabolism in renal failure
HMG-CoARIs (lovastatin)	Elevation of transaminase levels, myositis, sleep disturbances	Cyclosporine may increase liver function tests; greatly increased myositis risk with lovastatin and immunosuppressive drugs (cyclosporine)

(Data from Ballantyne CM, Radovancevic B, Farmer JA, et al: Hyperlipidemia after heart transplantation: Report of a 6-year experience, with treatment recommendations. J Am Coll Cardiol 19(6):1315–1321, 1992.)

belching, bloating, gas, heartburn, nausea) are the dose-limiting side effects. In addition, these agents may transiently increase triglycerides (about 7% acutely, and 2 to 3% after prolonged therapy); this is not; however, of major importance unless the patient already has a significantly elevated triglyceride level.

Another important consideration with these agents is that they may alter the absorption of fat-soluble drugs (e.g., CsA) and vitamins (A, D, E, and K). Because absorption of CsA depends on the presence of bile, its absorption may decrease as these agents act by binding bile in the small intestine. A study evaluating this interaction in five patients reported highly variable effects with CsA levels being both increased and decreased.[149] Obviously, further work is needed to clarify the true impact of this interaction. Other medications that may exhibit decreased bioavailability in the presence of cholestyramine include amiodarone, digoxin, thiazide diuretics, thyroid hormones, warfarin, and nonsteroidal anti-inflammatory agents.[150] Based on the theoretical risk, it is best not to administer CsA or any other medication 1 hour before to 4 to 6 hours after administration of the bile acid resin. This schedule may increase the complexity of the transplant patient's drug regimen because most patients are already receiving multiple medications throughout the day. As the new formulations of CsA (Neoral CsA)[151] and tacrolimus do not require the presence of bile for absorption,[120] drug interactions between these agents and the bile acid resins may be less problematic.

Nicotinic Acid

Niacin, or nicotinic acid, is recognized for its efficacy in lowering total and LDL cholesterol and in decreasing the morbidity and mortality of coronary artery disease in the general population; however, it must be used very cautiously in transplant recipients. Because both cyclosporine and niacin can increase liver function tests and increase serum uric acid,[152] concomitant administration of these agents requires close monitoring and avoidance in patients with hepatotoxicity or gout. Niacin can also increase glucose, as can prednisone and tacrolimus, so it should be avoided in diabetic transplant patients. In one series, 65% of patients discontinued niacin therapy because of new onset or exacerbation of hyperglycemia.[153] Other annoying side effects related to the drug's prostaglandin-associated vasodilatory action (headache, palpitations, tachycardia, flushing and itching) have been alleviated somewhat with the sustained-release formulation, but the trade-off has been a higher incidence of hepatotoxicity and inferior efficacy with this product.[154,155] Alternatively, the use of aspirin 30 minutes before each dose has been found to be useful in decreasing the prostaglandin-mediated vasodilation. In addition, niacin in combination with CsA, lovastatin and/or gemfibrozil can cause myositis and rhabdomyolysis, so concomitant administration of three or more of these agents should be avoided if at all possible.

Fibric Acid Derivatives

The fibric acid derivatives (clofibrate, gemfibrozil, and fenofibrate) are best reserved for transplant patients with hypertriglyceridemia, because they have only a modest effect on LDL cholesterol.[136,156] As these agents act by increasing excretion of cholesterol into the bile, they can cause gallstones. This can be a concern because an increased incidence of cholelithiasis requiring cholecystectomy has been reported among transplant recipients.[157] Other adverse effects include increased creatine kinase and myopathy, gastrointestinal discomfort, and impotence. Also of concern are reports suggesting higher than expected incidence of malignancy in patients receiving these drugs.[158,159] In addition to drug interactions with lovastatin and CsA leading to rhabdomyolysis,[160,161–165] these agents interact with insulin and sulfonylureas, so they should be used cautiously in diabetic patients. Elevated creatine kinase levels and an increased incidence of musculoskeletal pain have been reported with pravastatin and gemfibrozil.[166] Gemfibrozil may also potentiate the effects of warfarin.

HMG-CoA Reductase Inhibitors

HMG-CoA reductase inhibitors (e.g., lovastatin, pravastatin, simvastatin, fluvastatin) are considered the treatment of choice for mixed hyperlipidemias commonly seen in transplant recipients, because they effectively decrease LDL cholesterol and triglycerides while increasing HDL.[136] The worrisome feature of these agents (especially lovastatin) is their dose-related propensity to elevate creatine kinase levels and to cause myositis and rhabdomyolysis, especially in patients receiving other medications metabolized by the cytochrome P450 enzyme system (e.g., erythromycin, niacin, gemfibrozil, cyclosporine).[3,160–171] Incidence of these complications is decreased by limiting the dose of lovastatin to 20 to 40 mg/day during concomitant therapy.[3,91,148,172,173] This dosage provides lovastatin levels and/or HMG-CoA reductase activity comparable with (or higher than) those obtained in control subjects receiving higher doses because CsA inhibits the metabolism of lovastatin.[3,173] In patients administered more than two drugs metabolized by the cytochrome P450 enzyme system, it seems prudent to limit lovastatin dosage to 10 to 20 mg/day. Other HMG-CoA reductase inhibitors appear to be as efficacious but to have fewer problems with myositis and rhabdomyolysis associated with their use.[90,147,166,174–178] Altered pharmacokinetic disposition of pravastatin and simvastatin have been reported during concomitant CsA therapy.[179,180] Elevations in creatine kinase levels have occurred during concomitant administration of these agents with CsA, and a case of rhabdomyolysis has been attributed to simvastatin in a heart transplant recipient.[175,181] If transaminase levels increase beyond three time the upper limit of normal, the medication should be discontinued.

Miscellaneous Agents

Probucol is only modestly efficacious in decreasing total and LDL cholesterol and can adversely decrease HDL. Thus, it is considered a first line agent neither in the general population nor in transplant recipients. It also has a number of worrisome side effects (e.g., syncope, arrhythmias) and should be used only when other agents fail or when combination therapy is necessary.[182] Because probucol decreases bile secretion, it may decrease cyclosporine absorption.[183,184] We observed a 50% decrease in CsA whole blood concentrations in one patient taking probucol doses of 1000 mg/day but were unable to demonstrate a change in area under the curve at lower (500 mg/day) dosages (unpublished findings).

Other agents have been used to decrease serum lipids (e.g., soluble fibers, activated charcoal, neomycin, fish oil, dextrothyroxine, and estrogens); however, there is limited or no experience with these agents in heart transplant recipients.

SUMMARY

Because aggressive strategies to decrease lipids have not proved to have any salutary effect on development of accelerated graft atherosclerosis, one must weigh the theoretic benefits vs. risks of lipid-lowering agents in these patients, and also take into consideration not only the cost of drug therapy but also the cost of additional monitoring required during concomitant therapy.

Before initiating drug therapy, nonpharmacologic strategies should be optimized and maintained throughout the course of therapy. If possible, other drugs known to elevate lipid levels (Table 2) should be replaced by alternative agents.

Because most cardiac transplant recipients have multiple risk factors for hyperlipidemia (Table 1), it is unlikely that any single lipid-lowering agent will sufficiently decrease cholesterol levels to the desired range. Because of the risks associated with concomitant administration of HMG-CoA reductase inhibitors, other lipid-lowering agents (e.g., niacin, gemfibrozil) and other drugs metabolized through the cytochrome P450 system (e.g.,k cyclosporine, cimetidine, erythromycin, and possibly calcium channel blockers, among others), the preferred lipid-lowering combination is an HMG-CoA reductase inhibitor and a bile acid resin. In addition, because of the lower incidence of side effects, the other HMG-CoA reductase inhibitors (e.g., pravastatin, simvastatin, fluvastatin) may be preferred over lovastatin. In the event that additional interacting lipid-lowering agents (e.g., niacin, gemfibrozil) are deemed necessary, the dosage of lovastatin (and possibly the other HMG-CoA reductase inhibitors) should be limited to 20 mg/day in CsA-treated patients. In addition, because these patients are receiving other medications (e.g., diuretics, antihypertensive agents, antiinfective agents, and other agents metabolized by the cytochrome P450 system, and so forth), it is necessary to remember that many of these agents interact with CsA and the lipid-lowering drugs.

Finally, because AGAS remains the primary cause of long-term morbidity and mortality in the cardiac transplant recipient, and because newer immunosuppressive agents have had minimal impact on its incidence, multicenter, prospective, randomized clinical trials are needed to determine whether aggressive lipid-lowering strategies can alter development and progression of AGAS.

REFERENCES

1. Hess ML, Hastillo A, Mohanakumar T, et al: Accelerated atherosclerosis in cardiac transplantation: role of cytotoxic B cell antibodies and hyperlipidemia. Circulation 68(Suppl II):94–101, 1983.
2. Ballantyne CM, Jones PH, Payton-Ross C, et al: Hyperlipidemia following heart transplantation: Natural history and intervention with mevinolin (lovastatin). Transplant Proc 19(4 Suppl 5):60–62, 1992.
3. Ballantyne CM, Radovancevic B, Farmer JA, et al: Hyperlipidemia after heart transplantation: Report of a 6-year experience, with treatment recommendations. J Am Coll Cardiol 196):1315–1321, 1992.
4. Becker DM, Marakis M, Sension M, et al: Prevalence of hyperlipidemia in heart transplant recipients. Transplantation 44(2)323–325, 1987.
5. Becker DM, Chamberlain B, Swank R, et al: Relationship between corticosteroid exposure and plasma lipid levels in heart transplant recipients. Am J Med 85:632–638, 1988.
6. Keogh A, Simons L, Spratt P, et al: Hyperlipidemia after heart transplantation. J Heart Transplant 7(3):171–175, 1988.
7. Grady KL, Herold LS: Comparison of nutritional status in patients before and after heart transplantation. J Heart Transplant 7:123–127, 1988.
8. Grady K, Costanzo-Nordin M, Herold L, et al: Obesity and hyperlipidemia after heart transplantation. J Heart Lung Transplant 10:449–454, 1991.
9. Stamler JS, Vaughan DE, Rudd MA, et al: Frequency of hypercholesterolemia after cardiac transplantation. Am J Cardiol 62(17):1268–1272, 1988.
10. Stamler JS, Vaughan DE, Loscalzo J: Immunosuppressive therapy and lipoprotein abnormalities after cardiac transplantation. Am J Cardiol 6:389–391, 1991.
11. Renlund DG, Bristow MR., Crandall BG, et al: Hypercholesterolemia after heart transplantation: Amelioration by corticosteroid-free maintenance immunosuppression. J Heart Transplant 8:214–220, 1989.
12. Taylor DO, Thompson JA, Hastillo A, et al: Hyperlipidemia after clinical heart transplantation. J Heart Transplant 8(3):209–213, 1989.
13. Rudas L, Pflugfelder PW, McKenzie FN, et al: Serial evaluation of lipid profiles and risk factors for development of hyperlipidemia after cardiac transplantation. Am J Cardiol 66:1135–1138, 1990.

14. Superko HR, Haskell WL, DiRicco CD: Lipoprotein and hepatic lipase activity and high-density lipoprotein subclasses after cardiac transplantation. Am J Cardiol 66:1131–1134, 1990.

15. Farmer JA, Ballantyne CM, Frazer OH, et al: Lipoprotein(a) and apolipoprotein changes after cardiac transplantation. J Am Coll Cardiol 18:926–930, 1991.

16. Bieber CP, Hunt SA, Schwinn DA, et al: Complications in long-term survivors of cardiac transplantation. Transplant Proc 13:207–211, 1981.

17. Bilodeau M, Fitchett DH, Guerraty A Sniderman AD: Dyslipoproteinemias after heart and heart-lung transplantation: Potential relation to accelerated graft arteriosclerosis. J Heart Transplant 8(6)454–459, 1989.

18. Winters GL, Kendall TJ, Radio SJ, et al: Posttransplant obesity and hyperlipidemia: Major predictors of severity of coronary arteriopathy in failed human heart allografts. J Heart Transplant 9:364–371, 1990.

19. Eich D, Thompson JA, Daijin K, et al: Hypercholesterolemia in long-term survivors of heart transplantation: An early marker of accelerated coronary artery disease. J Heart Lung Transplant 10:45–49, 1991.

20. Johnson MR: Transplant coronary disease; nonimmunologic risk factors. J Heart Lung Transplant 11:S124–S132, 1992.

21. Gao SZ, Schroeder JS, Hunt S, Stinson EB: Retransplantation for severe accelerated coronary artery disease in heart transplant recipients. Am J Cardiol 62:876–881, 1988.

22. Sharples LD, Caine N, Mullins P, et al: Risk factor analysis for the major hazards following heart transplantation—rejection, infection, and coronary occlusive disease. Transplantation 52:244–252, 1991.

23. Heroux AL, O'Sullivan EJ, Liao Y, et al: Early and late cardiac allograft arteriopathy: Are they different entities? [abstract]. J Am Coll Cardiol 19:174A, 1992.

24. Alonso DR, Staret PK, Minick CR: Studies on the pathogenesis of arteriosclerosis induced in rabbit cardiac allografts by the synergy of graft rejection and hypercholesterolemia. Am J Pathol 87:415–442, 1977.

25. Butman SM: Hyperlipidemia after cardiac transplantation: Be aware and possibly wary of drug therapy for lowering serum lipids. Am Heart J 121:1585–1590, 1991.

26. Miller LW, Schlat RC, Kobashigawa J, et al: Task Force 5: Complications. J Am Coll Cardiol 22(1):41–53, 1993.

27. Lake KD, Reutzel TJ, Pritzker MR, et al: The impact of steroid withdrawal on the development of lipid abnormalities and obesity in cardiac transplant recipients. J Heart Lung Transplant 12(4):580–590, 1990.

28. Baker AM, Levine TB, Goldberg AD, Levine AB: Natural history and predictors of obesity after orthotopic heart transplantation. J Heart Lung Transplant 11:1156–1159, 1992.

29. Hagan ME, Holland CS, Herrick CM, Rasmussen LG: Amelioration of weight gain after heart transplantation by corticosteroid-free maintenance immunosuppression. J Heart Transplant 9:382–384, 1990.

30. Jones BM, Taylor FJ, Wright OM, et al: Quality of life after heart transplantation in patients assigned to double- or triple-drug therapy. J Heart Transplant 9:392–396, 1990.

31. Olivari MT, Homans DC, Wilson RF, Kubo SH, Ring WS: Coronary artery disease in cardiac transplant patients receiving triple-drug immunosuppressive therapy. Circulation 80(Suppl III):111–115, 1989.

32. Pahl E, Fricker FJ, Armitage J, et al: Coronary arteriosclerosis in pediatric heart transplant survivors: Limitation of long-term survival. J Pediatr 116:177–183, 1990.

33. Hricik DE: Posttransplant hyperlipidemia: The treatment dilemma. Am J Kidney Dis 23(5):768–771, 1994.

34. Pirsch JD, D'Alessandro AM, Sollinger HW, et al: Hyperlipidemia and transplantation: Etiologic factors and therapy. J Am Soc Nephrol 2(12 Suppl):S238–S242, 1992.

35. Pirsch JD, Friedman R: Primary care of the renal transplant patient. J Gen Intern Med 9(1):29–37, 1994.

36. Kubo SH, Peters JR, Knutson KR, et al: Factors influencing the development of hypercholesterolemia after cardiac transplantation. Am J Cardiol 70:520–526, 1992.

37. Laufer G, Grablowitz V, Laczkovics A, et al: The determinants of elevated total plasma cholesterol levels in cardiac transplant recipients administered low dose cyclosporine for immunosuppression. J Thorac Cardiovasc Surg 104:241–247, 1992.

38. Kasiske BL, Umen AJ: Persistent hyperlipidemia in renal transplant patients. Medicine 66:309–316, 1987.

39. Ibels LS, Stewart JH, Mahony JF, et al: Occlusive arterial disease in uraemic and haemodialysis patients and renal transplant recipients: A study of the incidence of arterial disease and of the prevalence of risk factors implicated in the pathogenesis of arteriosclerosis. Q J Med 46:197–214, 1977.

40. Ibels LS, Alfrey AC, Weil III R: Hyperlipidemia in adult, pediatric and diabetic renal transplant recipients. Am J Med 64:634–642, 1978.

41. Saldanha F, Hurst KS, Amend WJC, et al: Hyperlipidemia after renal transplantation in children. Am J Dis Child 130:951–953, 1976.
42. Chan MK, Vargese Z, Moorhead JF: Lipid abnormalities in uremia, dialysis, and transplantation. Kidney Int 19:625–637, 1981.
43. Vathsala A, Weinberg RB, Schoenberg L, et al: Lipid abnormalities in renal transplant recipients treated with cyclosporine. Transplant Proc 21:3670–3673, 1989.
44. Isoniemi H, Tikkanen M, Hayry P, et al: Lipid profiles with triple drug immunosuppressive therapy and with double drug combinations after renal transplantation and stable graft function. Transplant Proc 23:1029–1031, 1991.
45. Bittar AE, Ratcliffe PJ, Richardson AJ, et al: The prevalence of hyperlipidemia in renal transplant recipients: Associations with immunosuppressive and antihypertensive therapy. Transplantation 50:987–992, 1990.
46. Lowry RP, Soltys G, Mangel R, et al: Type II hyperlipoproteinemia hyperapobetalipoproteinemia and hyperalphalipoproteinemia following renal transplantation: Prevalence and precipitating factors. Transplant Proc 19:2229–2232, 1987.
47. Nicholls AJ, Cumming AM, Catto GRD, et al: Lipid relationships in dialysis and renal transplant patients. Q J Med 50:149–150, 1981.
48. Jackson JM, Lee HA: The role of propranolol therapy and proteinuria in the etiology of post renal transplantation hyperlipidemia. Clin Nephrol 18:95–100, 1982.
49. Chatterjee SN, Chin HP, Azen SP, et al: Abnormal serum lipid patterns in primary renal allograft recipients. Surgery 82:655–659, 1977.
50. Chan MK, Varghese Z, Persaud JW, et al: The role of multiple pharmacotherapy in the pathogenesis of hyperlipidemia after renal transplantation. Clin Nephrol 15:309–313, 1981.
51. Harris KPG, Russell GI, Parvin SD, et al: Alterations in lipid and carbohydrate metabolism attributable to cyclosporin A in renal transplant recipients. Br Med J 292:16, 1986.
52. Ballantyne CM, Podet EJ, Patsch WP, et al: Effects of cyclosporine therapy on plasma lipoprotein levels. JAMA 262(1):53–56, 1989.
53. Versluis DJ, Wenting GJ, Derkx FHM, et al: Who should be converted from cyclosporine to conventional immunosuppression in kidney transplantation, and why. Transplantation 44:387–389, 1987.
54. Pennisi AJ, Heuser ET, Mickey MR, et al: Hyperlipidemia in pediatric hemodialysis and renal transplant patients. Am J Dis Child 130:957–961, 1976.
55. Ponticelli C, Barbi GL, Cantaluppi A, et al: Lipid disorders in renal transplant recipients. Nephron 20:189–195, 1978.
56. Israel MK, McKenney JM: Hyperlipidemias. In Carter B, Angaran D, Lake K, Raekel M: Cardiovascular (Module 1) Pharmacotherapy Self-Assessment Program (PSAP). 2nd ed. Kansas City, American College of Clinical Pharmacy, 1995, pp 65–94.
57. Henkin Y, Como JA, Oberman A: Secondary dyslipidemia inadvertent effects of drugs in clinical practice. JAMA 267(7):961–968, 1992.
58. Rubin S, Dale J, Santamaria C, Tomalty J: Weight change in cardiac transplant patients. Can J Cardiovasc Nurs 2(2):9–13, 1991.
59. Palmer M, Schaffner F, Thung SN: Excessive weight gain after liver transplantation. Transplantation 51(4):797–800, 1991.
60. Griepp RB, Stinson EB, Bieber CP, et al: Control of graft atherosclerosis in human heart transplant recipients. Surgery 81:262–269, 1977.
61. Johnson CP, Gallagher-Lepak S, Zhu YR, et al: Factors influencing weight gain after renal transplantation. Transplantation 56(4):822–827, 1993.
62. Gonyea JE, Anderson CF: Weight change and serum lipoproteins in recipients of renal allografts. Mayo Clin Proc 67:653–657, 1992.
63. Sims EAH, Goldman RF, Gluck CM, et al: Experimental obesity in man. Trans Assoc Am Physicians 81:153–169, 1968.
64. Munoz SJ, Deems RO, Moritz MJ, et al: Hyperlipidemia and obesity after orthotopic liver transplantation. Transplant Proc 23:1480–1483, 1991.
65. Bagdade JD, Porte D Jr, Bierman EL: Steroid-induced lipemia. Arch Intern Med 125:129–134, 1970.
66. Kaunitz AM: Combined oral contraception with desogestrel/ethinyl estradiol: Tolerability profile. Am J Obstet Gynecol 168(3 Pt2):1028–1033, 1993.
67. Hricik DE, Mayes JT, Schulak JA: Early vs. late withdrawal of steroid therapy following renal transplantation. Dialysis Transplant 19:131–132, 137, 1990.
68. Szarek BL, Brandt DM: A comparison of weight changes with fluoxetine, desipramine, and amitriptyline: A retrospective study of psychiatric inpatients. J Nerv Ment Dis 181(11):702–704, 1993.
69. Chen Y, Silverstone T: Lithium and weight gain. Int Clin Psychopharmacol 5(3):217–225, 1990.
70. Coxhead N, Silverstone T, Cookson J: Carbamazepine versus lithium in the prophylaxis of bipolar affective disorder. Acta Psychiatr Scand 85(2):114–118, 1992.

71. Leadbetter R, Shutty M, Pavalonis D, et al: Clozapine-induced weight gain: Prevalence and clinical relevance. Am J Psychiatry 149(1):68–72, 1992.
72. Weibe EJ: Weight gain with clozapine treatment [letter]. Can J Psychiatry 38(1):70, 1993.
73. Lamberti JS, Bellnier T, Schwarzkopf SB: Weight gain among schizophrenic patients treated with clozapine. Am J Psychiatry 149(5):689-690, 1992.
74. Breum L, Astrup A, Gram L, et al: Metabolic changes during treatment with valproate in humans: Implication for untoward weight gain. Metabolism 41(6):666–670, 1992.
75. Lampl Y, Eshel Y, Rapaport A, Sarova-Pinhas I: Weight gain, increased appetite, and excessive food intake induced by carbamazepine. Clin Neuropharmacol 14(3):251–255, 1991.
76. The Lipid Research Clinics Coronary Primary Prevention Trial Results II: The relationship of reduction in incidence of coronary heart disease to cholesterol lowering. JAMA 251:365–374, 1984.
77. Frick MH, Elo O, Haapa K, et al: Helsinki heart study: Primary-prevention trial with gemfibrozil in middle-aged men with dyslipidemia. Safety of treatment, changes in risk factors, and incidence of coronary heart disease. N Engl J Med 317:1237–1245, 1987.
78. Blankenhorn DH, Nessim SA, Johnson RL, et al: Beneficial effects of combined colestipol-niacin therapy on coronary atherosclerosis and coronary venous bypass grafts. JAMA 257:3323–3340, 1987.
79. Gao SZ, Schroeder JS, Alderman EL, et al: Clinical and laboratory correlates of accelerated coronary artery disease in the cardiac transplant patient. Circulation 76(Suppl V):V56–V61, 1987.
80. Carrier M, Pelletier GB, Genest J Jr, et al: Cholesterol-lowering intervention and coronary artery disease after cardiac transplantation. Ann Thorac Surg 57(2):353–356, 1994.
81. Uretsky BF, Murali S, Reddy PS, et al: Development of coronary artery disease in cardiac transplant patients receiving immunosuppressive therapy with cyclosporine and prednisone. Circulation 76:827–834, 1987.
82. Narrod J, Kormos R, Armitage J, et al: Acute rejection and coronary artery disease in long-term survivors of heart transplantation. J Heart Transplant 8:418–421, 1989.
83. Costanzo-Nordin MR: Cardiac allograft vasculopathy: Relationship with acute cellular rejection and histocompatibility. J Heart Lung Transplant 11:S90–S103, 1992.
84. Petrossian GA, Nicohols AB, Marboe CC, et al: Relations between survival and development of coronary artery disease and anti-HLA antibodies after cardiac transplantation. Circulation 80(Suppl III):122–125, 1989.
85. Zerbe T, Uretsky B, Kormos R, et al: Graft atherosclerosis: Effects of cellular rejection and human lymphocyte antigen. J Heart Lung Transplant 11:S104–S110, 1992.
86. Grattan MT, Moreno-Cabral CE, Starnes VA, et al: Cytomegalovirus infection is associated with cardiac allograft rejection and atherosclerosis. JAMA 261:3651–3656, 1989.
87. McDonald K, Rector TS, Braunlin EA, et al: Association of coronary artery disease in cardiac transplant recipients with cytomegalovirus infection. Am J Cardiol 64:359–362, 1989.
88. Cameron DE, Greene PS, Alejo D, et al: Postoperative cytomegalovirus (CMV) infection and older donor age predispose to coronary atherosclerosis after heart transplantation [abstract]. Circulation 80(Suppl II):II-526, 1989.
89. Grant SC, Brooks NH: Accelerated graft atherosclerosis after heart transplantation. Br Heart J 69(5):469–470, 1993.
90. Barbir M, Rose M, Kushwaha S, et al: Low-dose simvastatin for the treatment of hypercholesterolemia in recipients of cardiac transplantation. Int J Cardiol 33:241–246, 1991.
91. Kuo PC, Kirshenbaum JM, Gordon J, et al: Lovastatin therapy for hypercholesterolemia in cardiac transplant recipients. Am J Cardiol 64:631–635, 1989.
92. Billingham ME: Cardiac transplant atherosclerosis. Transplant Proc 19(4 Suppl 5):19–25, 1987.
93. Hricik DE, Mayes JT, Schulak JA: Independent effects of cyclosporine and prednisone on posttransplant hypercholesterolemia. Am J Kidney Dis 18:353–358, 1991.
94. Kasiske BL, Tortorice KL, Heim-Duthoy KL, et al: The adverse impact of cyclosporine on serum lipids in renal transplant recipients. Am J Kidney Dis 6:700–707, 1991.
95. Markell MS, Brown CD, Butt KMH, Friedman EA: Prospective evaluation of changes in lipid profiles in cyclosporine-treated renal patients. Transplant Proc 21:1497–1499, 1989.
96. Markell MS, Armenti V, Danovitch G, Sumrani N: Hyperlipidemia and glucose intolerance in the post-renal transplant patient. J Am Soc Nephrol 4:S37–S47, 1994.
97. Raine AEG, Carter R, Mann JI, et al: Increased plasma LDL cholesterol after renal transplantation associated with cyclosporine immunosuppression. Transplant Proc 19:1820–1821, 1987.
98. Ellis CN, Gorsulowsky DC, Hamilton TA, et al: Cyclosporine improves psoriasis in a double-blind study. JAMA 256:3110–3116, 1986.
99. Stiller MJ, Grace HP, Kenny C, et al: Elevation of fasting serum lipids in patients treated with low-dose cyclosporine for severe plaque-type psoriasis. J Am Acad Dermatol 27:434–438, 1992.
100. Sgoutas D, MacMahon W, Love A, Jerkunica I: Interaction of cyclosporin A with human lipoproteins. J Pharm Pharmacol 583–588, 1986.

101. DeGroen P: Cyclosporine, low-density lipoprotein and cholesterol. Mayo Clin Proc 63:1012–1021, 1988.
102. Princen HMG, Meijer P, Hofstee B, et al: Effects of cyclosporin A on LDL receptor activity and bile acid synthesis in hepatocyte monolayer cultures and in vivo in the rat. Hepatology 7:1109, 1987.
103. Ost L, Tyden G, Fehrman I: Impaired glucose tolerance in cyclosporine-prednisolone-treated renal graft recipients. Transplantation 46(3):370–372, 1988.
104. Leunissen KML, Teule J, Degenaar CP, et al: Impairment of liver synthetic function and decreased liver flow during cyclosporin A therapy. Transplant Proc 19:1822–1824, 1987.
105. Gonwa TA, Atkins C, Velez RL, et al: Metabolic consequences of cyclosporine-to-azathioprine conversion in renal transplantation. Clin Transplant 2:91–96, 1988.
106. Hazzard WR, et al: Studies on the mechanism of increased plasma triglyceride induced by oral contraceptives. N Engl J Med 280:471–474, 1969.
107. Ghose P, Evans DB, Tomlinson SA, Calne RY: Plasma lipids following renal transplantation. Transplantation 15:521–522, 1973.
108. Cattran DC, Steiner G, Wilson DR, Fenton SSA: Hyperlipidemia after renal transplantation: Natural history and pathophysiology. Ann Intern Med 91:554–559, 1979.
109. Curtis JJ, Galla JH, Woodford SY, et al: Effect of alternate-day prednisone on plasma lipids in renal transplant recipients. Kidney Int 22:42–47, 1982.
110. Zimmerman J, Fainaru M, Eisenberg S: The effects of prednisone therapy on plasma lipoproteins and apolipoproteins: A prospective study. Metabolism 33:521–526, 1984.
111. Hays AP, Hill RB: Enzymes of lipid synthesis in the liver of the cortisone treated rat. Biochim Biophys Acta 98:646–655, 1965.
112. Ratkovec RM, Wray RB, Renlund DG, et al: Influence of corticosteroid-free maintenance immunosuppression on allograft coronary artery disease after cardiac transplantation. J Thorac Cardiovasc Surg 100:6–12, 1990.
113. Ettinger JD, Goldberg AP, Applebaum-Bowden D, Hazaard WR: Dyslipoproteinemia in systemic lupus erythematosus. Effect of corticosteroids. Am J Med 83:503–508, 1987.
114. Pirsch JD, Armbrust MJ, Knechtle SJ, et al: Effects of steroid withdrawal on hypertension and cholesterol levels in living-related recipients. Transplant Proc 23:1363–1364, 1991.
115. Kupin W, Venkat KK, Oh HK, Dienst S: Complete replacement of methylprednisolone by azathioprine in cyclosporine-treated primary cadaveric renal transplant recipients. Transplantation 45:53–55, 1988.
116. Beaumont JE, Galla JH, Luke RG, et al: Normal serum-lipids in renal-transplant patients. Lancet 1:599–601, 1965.
117. Ost L: Impairment of prednisolone metabolism by cyclosporine treatment in renal graft recipients. Transplantation 44(4):533–535, 1987.
118. Ost L, Klintmalm G, Ringden O: Mutual interaction between prednisolone and cyclosporine in renal transplant patients. Transplant Proc 17:1252, 1985.
119. Fung JJ, Alessiana M, Abu-Elmagd K, et al: Adverse effects associated with the use of FK506. Transplant Proc 23:3105–3108, 1991.
120. McDiarmid SV, Gornbein JA, Fortunat M, et al: Serum lipid abnormalities in pediatric liver transplant patients. Transplantation 53:109–115, 1992.
121. Peters DH, Fitton A, Plosker GL, Faulds D: Tacrolimus: A review of its pharmacology, and therapeutic potential in hepatic and renal transplantation. Drugs 46(4):746–794, 1993.
122. Klintmalm G: A review of FK506: A new immunosuppressant agent for the prevention and rescue of graft rejection. Transplant Rev 8(2):53–63, 1994.
123. Mathe D, Adam R, Malmendier C, et al: Prevalence of dyslipidemia in liver transplant recipients. Transplantation 54(1):167–170, 1992.
124. European FK506 Study Group: A European multicentre randomized study to compare the efficacy and safety of FK506 with that of cyclosporine in patients undergoing primary liver transplantation. Abstract. Presented at The American Society of Transplant Surgeons 19th Annual Scientific Meeting, Houston, Texas, May 1993.
125. US Multicenter FK506 Liver Study Group: Use of Prograf (FK506) as rescue therapy for refractory rejection after liver transplantation. Transplant Proc 25:679–688, 1993.
126. Ames RP: Metabolic disturbances increasing the risk of coronary heart disease during diuretic-based antihypertensive therapy: Lipid alteration and glucose intolerance. Am Heart J 106:1207–1214, 1983.
127. Grimm RH, Leon AS, Hunninghake DB, et al: Effects of thiazide diuretics on plasma lipids and lipoproteins in mildly hypertensive patients: A double-blind controlled trial. Ann Intern Med 94:7–11, 1981.
128. Leren P, Eide I, Foss OP, et al: Antihypertensive drugs and blood lipids: the Oslo study. Br J Clin Pharmacol 13:441S–444S, 1982.
129. Lasser NL, Grandits G, Caggiula AW, et al: Effects of antihypertensive therapy on plasma lipids and lipoproteins in the Multiple Risk Factor Intervention Trial. Am J Med 76(2A):52–66, 1984.

130. Chait A: Effect of antihypertensive agents on serum lipids and lipoproteins. Am J Med 86:5–7, 1989.
131. Lowenstein J: Effects of prazosin on serum lipids in patients with essential hypertension: A review of the findings presented at the Satellite Symposium on coronary heart disease: hypertension and other risk factors, Milan, 1983. Am J Cardiol 53:21A–23A, 1984.
132. Dujovne CA, DeCoursey S, Krehbiel P, et al: Serum lipids in normo- and hyperlipidemics after methyldopa and propranolol. Clin Pharmacol Ther 36:157–162, 1984.
133. Ames RP, Hill P: Antihypertensive therapy and the risk of coronary heart disease. J Cardiovasc Pharmacol 4(Suppl 2):S206–S212, 1982.
134. Bershad S, Rubinstein A, Paterniti JR, et al: Changes in plasma lipids and lipoproteins during isotretinoin therapy for acne. N Engl J Med 313(16):981–985, 1985.
135. Ginsberg H, Olefsky J, Farquhar JW, Reaven GM: Moderate ethanol ingestion and plasma triglyceride levels. A study in normal and hypertriglyceridemic persons. Ann Intern Med 80:143–149, 1974.
136. Expert Panel on Detection, Evaluation, and Treatment of High Blood Cholesterol in Adults: Summary of the second report of the National Cholesterol Education Program (NCEP) Expert Panel on Detection, Evaluation, and Treatment of High Blood Cholesterol in Adults (Adult Treatment Panel II). JAMA 269(23):3015–3023, 1993.
137. Disler PB, Goldberg RB, Kuhn L, et al: The role of diet in the pathogenesis and control of hyperlipidemia after renal transplantation. Clin Nephrol 16:29–34, 1981.
138. Moore RA, Callahan MF, Cody M, et al: The effect of the American Heart Association step one diet on hyperlipidemia following renal transplantation. Transplantation 49:60–62, 1990.
139. Nelson J, Beauregard H, Gelinas M, et al: Rapid improvement of hyperlipidemia in kidney transplant patients with a multifactorial hypolipidemic diet. Transplant Proc 20:1264–1270, 1988.
140. Perez R: Managing nutrition problems in transplant patients. Nutr Clin Pract 8(1):28–32.
141. Shen SY, Lukens CW, Alongi SV, et al: Patient profile and effect of dietary therapy on posttransplant hyperlipidemia. Kidney Int Suppl 24(Suppl 15):147–152, 1983.
142. Ramsey L, Yeo W, Jackson P: Dietary reduction of serum concentrations: Time to think again. Br J Med 303:953–957, 1991.
143. Divakar D, Bailey RR, Price M, et al: Effect of diet on post-transplant hyperlipidemia. N Z Med J 105:79–80, 1992.
144. Gokal R, Mann JI, Moore RA, Morris PJ: Hyperlipidaemia following renal transplantation. Q J Med 48:507–517, 1979.
145. Kobashigawa JA, Gleeson M, Stevenson LW, et al: Pravastatin lowers cholesterol and may prevent severe cardiac transplant rejection: A randomized trial. J Heart Lung Transplant 13(1, Pt 2):S75, 1994.
146. Katznelson S, Kobashigawa JA, Wang XM, et al: Pravastatin lowers natural killer cell activity in heart transplant patients and may prevent severe allograft rejection. Proceedings from the American Society of Transplant Physicians 13th Annual Meeting May 16–18, 1994.
147. Castelao AM, Grino JM, Andres E, et al: HMGCoA reductase inhibitors lovastatin and simvastatin in the treatment of hypercholesterolemia after renal transplantation. Transplant Proc 25(1 Pt 2):1043–1046, 1993.
148. Kasiske BL, Tortorice KL, Heim-Duthoy KL, et al: Lovastatin treatment of hypercholesterolemia in renal transplant recipients. Transplantation 49:95–100, 1990.
149. Keogh A, Day R, Critchley L, et al: The effect of food and cholestyramine on the absorption of cyclosporine in cardiac transplant recipients. Transplant Proc 20:27–30, 1988.
150. Knodel LC, Talbert RL: Adverse effects on hypolipidemic drugs. Med Toxicol 2:10–32, 1987.
151. Mueller EA, Kovarik JM, van Bree JB, et al: Pharmacokinetics and tolerability of a microemulsion formulation of cyclosporine in renal allograft recipients—A concentration-controlled comparison with the commercial formulation. Transplantation 57:1178–1182, 1994.
152. Lin HY, Rocher LL, McQuillan MA, et al: Cyclosporine-induced hyperuricemia and gout. N Engl J Med 321:287–292, 1989.
153. Henkin Y, Oberman A, Hurst DC, Segrest JP: Niacin revisited: Clinical observations on an important but under utilized drug. Am J Med 91:239–246, 1991.
154. Rader JI, Calvert RJ, Hathcock JN: Hepatic toxicity of unmodified and time-release preparation of niacin. Am J Med 92:77–81, 1992.
155. Stern RH, Freeman D, Spence JD: Differences in metabolism of time-release and unmodified nicotinic acid: Explanation of the differences in hypolipidemic action? Metabolism 41:879–881, 1992.
156. Knight RJ, Vathsala A, Schoenberg L, et al: Treatment of hyperlipidemia in renal transplant patients with gemfibrozil and dietary modification. Transplantation 53:224–225, 1992.
157. Sekela ME, Hutchins DA, Young JB, Noon GP: Biliary surgery after cardiac transplantation. Arch Surg 126:571–573, 1991.
158. WHO Cooperative Trial on primary prevention of ischaemic heart disease using clofibrate to lower serum cholesterol: Mortality follow-up report of the committee of principal investigators. Lancet 2:379–383, 1980.

159. Thomas DB: Steroid hormones and drugs that alter cancer risk. Cancer 62(Suppl):1755–1767, 1988.
160. East C, Alivizatos PA, Grundy SM, et al: Rhabdomyolysis in patients receiving lovastatin after cardiac transplantation [letter]. N Engl J Med 318:47–48, 1988.
161. Tobert JA: Letter to the editor. N Engl J Med 318:48, 1988.
162. Wirebaugh SR, Shapiro ML, McIntyre TH, Whitney EJ: A retrospective review of the use of lipid-lowering agents in combination, specifically, gemfibrozil and lovastatin. Pharmacotherapy 12(6): 445–450, 1992.
163. Pierce LR, Wysowski DK, Gross TP: Myopathy and rhabdomyolysis associated with lovastatin-gemfibrozil combination therapy. JAMA 264:71–75, 1990.
164. Marais G, Larson KK: Rhabdomyolysis and acute renal failure induced by combination lovastatin and gemfibrozil therapy. Ann Intern Med 112:338–230, 1990.
165. Tobert JA: Efficacy and long-term adverse effect pattern of lovastatin. Am J Cardiol 62:28–30, 1988.
166. Wiklund O, Angelin B, Bergman M, et al: Pravastatin and gemfibrozil alone and in combination for the treatment of hypercholesterolemia. Am J Med 94:13–20, 1993.
167. Corpier CL, Jones PH, Suki WN, et al: Rhabdomyolysis and renal injury with lovastatin use; report of two cases in cardiac recipients. JAMA 260:239–241, 1988.
168. de Alava E, Sola JJ, Lozano MD, Pardo-Mindan FJ: Rhabdomyolysis and acute renal failure in a heart transplant recipient treated with hypolipemiants. Nephron 66(2):242–243, 1994.
169. Norman DJ, Illingworth DR, Nunson J, Hosenpud J: Myolysis and acute renal failure in a heart transplant recipient receiving lovastatin [letter]. N Engl J Med 318:46–47, 1988.
170. Ayanian JZ, Fuchs CS, Stone RM: Lovastatin and rhabdomyolysis. Ann Intern Med 109:682–683, 1988.
171. Reaven P, Witztum JL: Lovastatin, nicotinic acid, and rhabdomyolysis. Ann Intern Med 109:597–598, 1988.
172. Kobashigawa JA, Murphy FL, Stevenson LW, et al: Low-dose lovastatin safely lowers cholesterol after cardiac transplantation. Circulation 82:281–283, 1990.
173. Cheung AK, DeVault GA Jr, Gregory MC: A prospective study on treatment of hypercholesterolemia with lovastatin in renal transplant patients receiving cyclosporine. J Am Soc Nephrol 3(12):1884–1891, 1993.
174. Kainuma O, Asano T, Ochiai T, Isono K: Lipid disorders in renal transplant recipients. Transplant Proc 24:1585–1587, 1992.
175. Vanhaecke J, Cleemput JV, Lierde JV, et al: Safety and efficacy of low dose simvastatin in cardiac transplant recipients treated with cyclosporine. Transplantation 58:42–45, 1994.
176. Martinez-Hernandez BE, Persaud JW, Varghese Z, Moorhead JF: Low-dose simvastatin is safe in hyperlipidaemic renal transplant patients. Nephrol Dial Transplant 8(7):637–641, 1993.
177. Wenke K, Thiery J, Arndtz N, et al: Treatment of hypercholesterolemia and prevention of coronary artery disease after heart transplantation by combination of low-dose simvastatin and HELP-LDL-asphersis. Transplant Proc 24(6):2674–2676, 1992.
178. Yoshimura N, Oka T, Okamoto M, Ohmori Y: The effects of pravastatin on hyperlipidemia in renal transplant recipients. Transplantation 53:94–99, 1992.
179. Regazzi MB, Iacona I, Campana C, et al: Altered disposition of pravastatin following concomitant drug therapy with cyclosporin A in transplant recipients. Transplant Proc 25(4):2732–2733, 1993.
180. Arnadottir M, Eriksson LO, Thysell H, Karkas JD: Plasma concentration profiles of simvastatin 3-hydroxy-3-methyl-glutaryl-coenzyme A reductase inhibitory activity in kidney transplant recipients with and without ciclosporin. Nephron 65(3):410–413, 1993.
181. Blaison G, Weber JC, Sachs D, et al: Rhabdomyolysis caused by simvastatin in a patient following heart transplantation and cyclosporine therapy. Rev Med Interne 13(1):61–63, 1992.
182. Anderson JL, Schroeder JS: Effects of probucol on hyperlipidemic patients with cardiac allografts. J Cardiovasc Pharmacol 1:353_365, 1975.
183. Sundararajan V, Cooper DKC, Muchmore J, et al: Interaction of cyclosporine and probucol in heart transplant patients. Transplant Proc 23(3):2028–2032, 1991.
184. Galego C, Sanchez P, Plannels C, et al: Interaction between probucol and cyclosporine in renal transplant patients. Ann Pharmacother 2:940–943, 1994.

Chapter 17

Malignancies Following Transplantation

Luis J. Rosado, MD
Francisco A. Arabia, MD

Malignancies are a well-recognized complication of chronic immunosuppressive therapy.[1-3] the pharmacologic agents currently used for immunosuppression are contributing factors for the higher incidence of malignancies observed in series of patients with transplanted organs. With the markedly improved results following thoracic organ transplantation observed during the past decade,[4,5] the incidence of malignant neoplasias will probably increase and could become a significant limiting factor for long-term survival. This study was undertaken to evaluate the clinical impact of malignant neoplasias in our thoracic organ recipients managed with a triple-drug immunosuppressive regimen.

MATERIALS AND METHODS

From April 1985 to June 1993, 305 patients (247 male, 58 female) underwent 274 heart, 21 heart-lung, and 17 lung transplants (six patients had heart retransplantation and one required a second heart-lung transplant during this period). Mean age at the time of transplantation was 48 years for heart, 36 years for hear-lung, and 48 years for lung recipients.

Diagnosis resulting in heart transplantation was ischemic cardiomyopathy in 145 patients (53%) and nonischemic cardiomyopathy in 129 patients (47%). For heart-lung transplant recipients, the diagnosis leading to transplantation was primary pulmonary hypertension in 12 patients (57%), Eisenmenger's in 4 patients (19%), cystic fibrosis in 2 patients (10%), obliterative bronchiolitis in 2 patients (10%), and alpha-1 antitrypsin deficiency in one patient (5%). Single lung transplantation was performed in 8 patients with emphysema (47%), 3 patients with alpha-1 antitrypsin deficiency

TABLE I.   Immunosuppression Protocol Used at the University of Arizona Cardiothoracc Transplant Program

	Cyclosporine A	Imuran	Prednisone	Solu-Medrol	RATG
Preoperative	4 mg/kg	4 mg/kg	—	—	—
Intraoperative	—	—	—	500 mg	—
Postoperative	4 mg/kg	200 mg/day	—	125 mg BID	200 mg/day
Day 1	4 mg/kg	200 mg/day	—	125 mg BID	200 mg/day
Day 2	5 mg/kg	200 mg/day	1.5 mg/kg	—	200 mg/da
> Day 2	250–300 ng/ml*	WBC > 3,5	$1.5 \rightarrow 0.5$ mg/kg†	—	—
Rejection	—	—	—	1 g/day × 3	—

RATG = rabbit antithymocyte globulin; WBC = white blood cell count.
* Measured in whole blood
† Gradual reduction during first week.

(18%), and 1 patient with obliterative bronchiolitis (6%). One patient had a bilateral single-lung transplant for cystic fibrosis (6%).

All patients who received transplants during this period received induction therapy with rabbit antithymocyte globulin (RATG) and a triple-drug immunosuppressive regimen of cyclosporine (CSA), prednisone, and azathioprine according to the protocol defined in Table 1. Acute rejection episodes were managed with intravenous administration of methylprednisolone at the dose of 1 g/day for 3 consecutive days. In rare instances a prednisone taper was used following the administration of methylprednisolone. No patient received monoclonal antibodies (OKT3).

Rejection surveillance for heart transplant recipients was performed according to a protocol of endomyocardial biopsies performed twice a week for 4 weeks, once a week for 4 weeks, every 2 weeks for 4 weeks, and at 6 months posttransplantation. During the initial period, routine yearly biopsies were performed, but this practice was discontinued in 1989.[6] Grading of the biopsy specimens was done according to a modified Billingham's criteria of none, mild, moderate, or severe rejection.[7] Heart-lung transplant recipients did not have heart biopsies. Heart-lung and lung transplant recipients underwent lung biopsies only when indicated for differential diagnosis between infection and rejection in the presence of fever and/or lung infiltrates.

Patients were followed in our outpatient clinic at weekly intervals during the first 3 months, then at 6, 9, and 12 months posttransplantation. After the first year posttransplantation, most patients were followed by their primary care physician and by one of the members of our transplant program at least once per year at the time of routine yearly posttransplant evaluation.

Occurrence of any kind of malignant neoplasms, treatment, and clinical outcome after treatment were recorded and kept in our computerized data base by direct communication among the transplant coordinators, the primary care physician, the physician managing the treatment, the patient, or any of the patient's relatives. Follow-up is 100% complete up to the time of the revision for the present report. Closing date was July 31, 1994.

RESULTS

Of 305 patients included in the present study, 235 did not develop any malignancy and 70 (65 heart recipients, 3 heart-lung recipients, and 2 lung recipients) developed malignant neoplasias during the follow-up. There were 95 kinds of malignancies among these 70 patients. Skin carcinomas were the most frequently observed (67 patients), followed by hematologic (8), respiratory tract (7), genitourinary (6), and gastrointestinal

TABLE 2.   Distribution of Malignancies and Type of Organ Recipients

Site of Malignancy	Heart	Heart-Lung	Lung	Total
Skin	62	4	1	67
Hematologic	7	0	1	8
Respiratory tract	6	0	1	7
Genitourinary	5	1	0	6
Gastrointestinal	5	0	0	5
Other	2	0	0	2
Total	87	5	3	95

neoplasias (5). Distribution of the neoplasias and the type of organ recipients is summarized in Table 2. Fifty patients had only one malignancy, 15 patients had two, 4 patients had three, and one patient had four different malignancies.

Cutaneous Malignancies

Of 67 skin neoplasias, squamous cell carcinoma was observed in 39 patients (38 heart and 1 heart-lung recipients), basal cell carcinoma was observed in 24 patients 21 heart, 2 heart-lung and 1 lung recipients) and melanoma in four patients (3 heart and 1 heart-lung recipients). Squamous and basal cell carcinomas were frequently recurrent lesions; 29 patients presented with only one skin lesion, 12 patients with 2 lesions, 6 patients with 3 lesions, 3 patients with 4 lesions, 2 patients with 5 lesions, 2 patients with 8 lesions, and 3 patients with 10 or more lesions. All basal cell carcinomas have been localized to the skin and completely resected. In 2 of 39 patients with squamous cell carcinoma, clinical evidence of invasion to lymph nodes and deep structures was observed. Local invasion to intracranial structures was the direct cause of death in one of these two patients despite aggressive deep resection and adjuvant radiation therapy. Three melanomas have been successfully resected in 3 heart transplant recipients without evidence of recurrence 16 to 70 months later. One heart-lung transplant recipient who had a melanoma resected from his back in November 1991, presented with axillary lymph node recurrence 21 months later and died of multiple lung metastasis 28 months after resection of the primary lesion.

Hematologic Malignancies

Hematologic neoplasias were observed in 8 patients. Two heart transplant recipients who developed multiple myeloma were treated with melfalan. Both died of this disease at 20 and 46 months posttransplantation. B-cell lymphoma developed in 5 heart and 1 single lung transplant recipients. The lung transplant recipient had two nodular lesions in the transplanted lung diagnosed by CT scan guided core needle biopsy compatible with B-cell lymphoma 4 months after her transplant. CSA was discontinued and the patient was switched to a conventional immunosuppressive regimen of prednisone and azathioprine. In addition, she was placed on acyclovir, 1200 mg/day. With this modification, complete resolution of the pulmonary lesions was observed and the patient remains disease-free 2 years later. Four heart transplant recipients had B-cell lymphoma. This was an incidental finding in the small bowel at postmortem examination in two patients. The other two patients developed multiple pulmonary lesions diagnosed as lymphoma on open lung-biopsy specimens. Chemotherapy was given; however, the malignancy eventually became disseminated, causing their deaths 16 and

17 months after the initial diagnosis. One heart transplant recipient developed a T-cell lymphoma of the frontal sinus 6 months after his transplant. He was successfully treated with discontinuation of CSA, high doses of acyclovir, and a multiple drug regimen of chemotherapy agents; the patient remains disease free 25 months later.

Respiratory Malignancies

Respiratory tract neoplasias developed in 7 patients (6 lung carcinomas and 1 carcinoma of the larynx). Of the patients with lung carcinoma, 2 were small-cell neoplasias, 2 adenocarcinomas, 1 squamous carcinoma, and 1 bronchoalveolar carcinoma. Five of these patients died of lung cancer. The patient with bronchoalveolar carcinoma was a single lung transplant recipient who underwent a native lung resection for extensive aspergillosis. The bronchoalveolar carcinoma was an incidental finding in the resected specimen. The patient developed aplastic anemia as a complication of antifungal therapy and eventually died of complications of thrombocytopenia. The patient with carcinoma of the larynx was a heavy smoker who continued to smoke after his transplant. His carcinoma of the larynx was successfully treated with radiation therapy but the patient later developed a transitional cell carcinoma of the bladder and eventually died of metastatic bladder carcinoma 8 months after a radical cystectomy.

Genitourinary Malignancies

Genitourinary malignancies were observed in 6 patients (prostate, 3; cervix, 2; kidney, 1; and bladder, 1). Of the 3 patients with prostatic carcinoma, 1 was an incidental finding at postmortem examination in a heart transplant recipient who died of pancreatic carcinoma; the other 2 were diagnosed by physical examination and prostate specific antigen determination, and both patients have been conservatively managed with hormonal manipulation. Two women with cervical carcinoma and a man with renal cell carcinoma have been successfully treated with surgical resection.

Gastrointestinal Tract Malignancies

Two patients died of pancreatic carcinoma that presented with extensive liver metastasis 7 and 33 months after their heart transplant. One patient developed colon carcinoma 9 months after his heart transplant and underwent complete surgical resection but eventually died of metastatic disease 54 months later. One patient with liver carcinoma and another with esophageal adenocarcinoma remained alive but terminally ill at the time of last follow-up.

One patient has had a low grade sarcoma of the pharynx resected twice. He is still alive without evidence of recurrence but with significant graft atherosclerosis. Another patient had a low grade retroperitoneal sarcoma resected 5 years after his heart transplant; he is disease-free one year later.

Freedom from any kind of malignancy in this group of patients is shown in Figure 1. Overall actuarial survival of patients without malignant neoplasia is similar to the survival of patients who have developed any kind of malignancy during the posttransplant period (Fig. 2); however, when we excluded all skin neoplasias, the survival of patients with other kinds of malignancies is significantly worse (Fig. 3).

DISCUSSION

The risk of developing malignancies after transplantation has been estimated to be approximately 100 times higher than in the general population.[3] This increased risk

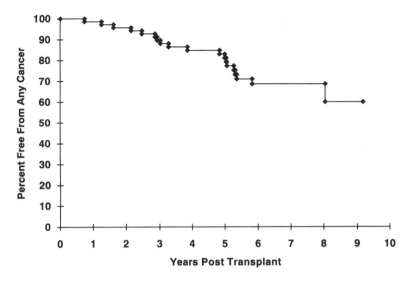

FIGURE 1.   Freedom from malignancy after cardiothoracic organ transplantion.

seems to be related to the side effects of the agents commonly used in current immunosuppressive protocols. The overall incidence of malignant neoplasias in our patient population managed with RATG and a triple-drug regimen of CSA, prednisone, and azathioprine is approximately 23%. The majority of the tumors observed have been skin carcinomas, neoplasias that are commonly found in patients living in areas of intense sunlight exposure, such as our area, Arizona. The cumulative dosage of immunosuppression also appears to have an impact in the incidence of malignancies. This incidence is higher in heart transplant recipients than in renal transplant recipients, where the immunosuppressive therapy is less intense.[1]

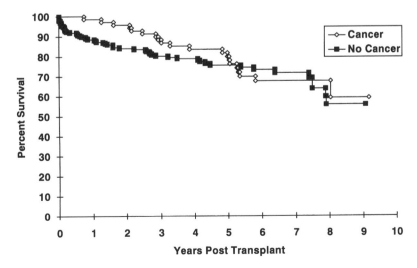

FIGURE 2.   Actuarial survival of patients with and without malignancy after cardiothoracic organ transplantation.

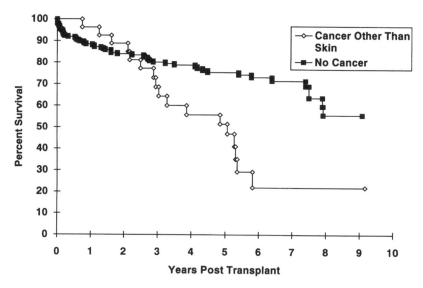

FIGURE 3. Comparison of actuarial survival of patients without malignancy and patients who developed malignant neoplasias different from skin carcinomas.

The incidence of lymphomas is low (2%) in our patient population. This low incidence in a group of patients receiving RATG as immunosuppressive induction contrasts with the significant increase on lymphoproliferative disorders reported by other transplants groups that routinely use OKT3 for induction therapy. In addition, the incidence of lymphoproliferative disorders associated with OKT3 appears to increase sharply after cumulative doses greater than 75 mg.[8] We are not aware of any prospective randomized study comparing these two different antithymocyte agents to draw any conclusions regarding the possible reasons for the observed difference in the incidence of lymphomas.

Even though the number of patients in our study is too small to draw any definitive conclusions regarding the potential role of other known factors for the development of malignancies (other than the required chronic immunosuppression), it would seem advisable for this group of patients to avoid intensive sunlight exposure as much as possible, to decrease the amount of ultraviolet radiation, and to completely avoid the use of tobacco and other well-known carcinogenic substances

Overall, the survival of patients with any malignant neoplasia developed after transplantation when compared with the survival rate observed in patients without malignancy seems to be similar in both groups. This lack of a statistically significant difference is probably related to the fact that most malignant neoplasias observed were skin carcinomas that were successfully resected. These types of neoplasia usually carry a good prognosis. When we excluded from the analysis all those patients with skin malignancies, however, a significant difference in survival was observed.

In conclusion, incidence of malignancies in cardiothoracic transplant recipients is approximately 23%. The most common type of malignant neoplasias observed is either squamous cell or basal cell carcinoma of the skin with a reasonably benign prognosis if surgically resected. Overall actuarial survival of patients of any kind of malignancy is similar to the survival of the patients without malignant neoplasias, but patients who develop malignancies other than skin carcinomas have a very high mortality rate that has a significant impact on the chances of long-term survival after cardiothoracic transplantation.

REFERENCES

1. Penn I, Hammond W, Brettschneider L, Starzl TE: Malignant lymphomas in transplantation patients. Transplant Proc 1:106–112, 1969.
2. Cole W: The increase in immunosuppression and its role in the development of malignant lesions. J Surg Oncol 30:139–144, 1985.
3. Penn I: Cancers complicating organ transplantation. N Engl J Med 323:1767–1768, 1990.
4. Rosado LJ, Copeland JG: Drug therapy after cardiac transplantation. In Ewy GA, Bressler R (eds): Cardiovascular Drugs and Management of Heart Disease. New York, Raven Press, 1992, pp 441–453.
5. Hosenpud JD, Novick RJ, Breen TJ, Daily OP: The registry of the international society for heart and lung transplantation: Eleventh official report. J Heart Lung Transplant 13:561–570, 1994.
6. Sethi GK, Rosado LJ, McCarthy M, et al: Futility of yearly heart biopsies in patients undergoing heart transplantation. J Thorac Cardiovasc Surg 104:90–93, 1992.
7. Billingham ME: Diagnosis of cardiac rejection by endomyocardial biopsy. Heart Transplant 1:25–30, 1981.
8. Swinnen LJ, Costanzo-Nordin MR, Fisher SG, et al: Increased incidence of lymphoproliferative disorder after immunosuppression with monoclonal antibody OKT3 in cardiac transplant recipients. N Engl J Med 323:1723–1728, 1990.

Chapter 18

Drug Interactions in Transplant Patients

Kathleen D. Lake, PharmD, BCPS

Several drugs have been reported to interact with cyclosporine (CsA) and the other immunosuppressive agents (Tables 1–12).[1-7] The clinical implications of drug interactions in the transplant patient may vary from a minor disturbance requiring more frequent drug level monitoring and dosage modification to more significant consequences, including graft rejection or nephrotoxicity.[8-10]

Although drug interactions are usually thought of as detrimental, they are common in the transplant patient and are dealt with on a fairly routine basis. In the transplant patient, the inherent possibility of a drug interaction is magnified not only by the multitude of drugs prescribed for these patients but also by the unintended side effects of these medications, thus necessitating further drug therapy. In addition to drug–drug interactions, medications can interact with food or alcohol; a drug's pharmacokinetics can also be altered by the effects of various coexisting disease states seen in transplant.[11]

Because it is impossible to be familiar with all potential interactions, the practitioner must have a thorough understanding of the fundamental mechanisms of these interactions. Anticipation of potential problems allows for early detection and/or avoidance of troublesome regimens whenever possible. However, not all drug interactions are bad; in fact, some interactions may be beneficial therapeutically or lower costs.

DRUG INTERACTIONS

In general, drug interactions can alter the pharmacokinetic and/or the pharmacodynamic parameters of the interacting drugs. *Pharmacokinetic* interactions are classified based on changes in absorption, distribution, metabolism, or excretion of the drug, thus increasing or decreasing the measured drug concentration. Changes in drug concentrations may or may not correspond with an altered physiologic effect. *Pharmacodynamic* interactions alter the pharmacologic or toxicologic effect of the agent. In this setting, altered response may be observed even though the drug concentration appears to be within the therapeutic range. Pharmacodynamic interactions are seen clinically when drugs with either additive or antagonistic properties are administered concomitantly. In general, pharmacodynamic interactions are more difficult to assess and thus are also more difficult to predict.

CsA

Many medications have been reported to interact with CsA (Tables 1, 2, and 3). Some interactions have been confirmed with detailed pharmacokinetic studies, whereas others have been described only in case reports, in which CsA levels were observed to increase or decrease.

Although the mechanism for most CsA drug interactions cannot be determined from clinical studies because of deficiencies in study design, most interacting drugs are either inducers, inhibitors, or substrates for enzymes in the CYP3A[12] (formerly called cytochrome P450-IIIA) gene family (see Table 2). Thus, when considering CsA's pharmacokinetic interactions, clinically significant interactions usually result from changes in its absorption and metabolism rather than distribution and excretion. The most prominent CYP3A enzyme (CYP3A4) and at least one other enzyme (CYP3A5) have been shown to be responsible for CsA's metabolism.[13] Drugs metabolized by the other two gene families, CYP1 (e.g., phenacetin, caffeine, theophylline) and CYP2 (e.g., propranolol, quinidine, ethanol, haloperidol, desipramine) do not appear to interact with CsA (see Table 4).

TABLE 1. Cyclosporine Drug Interactions*

Increase CsA Concentrations	Decrease CsA Concentrations	Alter CsA Nephrotoxicity
Increase CsA's Absorption	**Decrease CsA's Absorption**	**Increase Nephrotoxicity**
Erythromycin[23–25]	Phenytoin[29]	Aminoglycosides[163,164]
Metoclopramide[42,43]	Rifampin[26,27]	Amphotericin B[165]
Grapefruit juice[30–36]	Cholestyramine(?)[44]	Nonsteroidal antiinflammatory agents[167–170]
	Octreotide[47,48]	Tacrolimus[253]
	Probucol[45,46]	
Decrease CsA's Metabolism†	**Increase CsA's Metabolism†**	**Decrease Nephrotoxicity**
Diltiazem,[89–93] nicardipine,[94–96] verapamil[87,88,93,97–101]	Nafcillin[138]	Diltiazem[196–199] verapamil[192–195]
Ketoconazole,[56–63] itraconazole[64–68] fluconazole[69–73]	Phenytoin[123–125]	
Erythromycin,[23–25,74–81] josamycin[82,83] clarithromycin[84]	Phenobarbital[126,127] Carbamazepine[128,129] Primidone[127,130]	
Oral contraceptives[109,110]	Rifampin, isoniazid[26–28,130–135]	
Danazol[110]	Sulfadimidine[136,137]	
Tacrolimus[85,86]		

* A comprehensive listing of CsA's drug interactions is provided in Table 12.
† Many of the interactions reported to affect the hepatic metabolism of CsA may also alter CsA's absorption by either inhibiting or enhancing its intestinal (presystemic) metabolism.

TABLE 2.   Commonly Used Medications that Affect the Rate of CsA Metabolism in Cultured Hepatocytes

CYP3A Inhibitors	CYP3A Inducers	No CYP3A Effect
Triacetyloleandomycin	Rifampicin*	Cimetidine*
Erythromycin*	Phenobarbital*	Ranitidine
Ketoconazole*	Phenytoin*	Omeprazole
Miconazole	Phenylbutazone	Norfloxacin
Midazolam	Dexamethasone	Isoniazid
Nifedipine	Sulfinpyrazone	Sulfamethoxazole
Diltiazem*	Carbamazepine*	Trimethoprim
Verapamil*		Quinidine
Nicardipine*		Aspirin
Ergotamine		Imipramine
Dihydroergotamine		Valproic acid
Ethinyl estradiol		Doxycycline*
Progesterone		Captopril
Bromocriptine		
Cortisol		
Prednisone		
Prednisolone		
Methylprednisolone		

* Substantiated interaction based on clinical reports.
(Modified from Watkins PB: The role of cytochrome P450 in cyclosporine metabolism. J Am Acad Dermatol 23:1301–1311, 1990; Pichard L, Fabre I, Fabre G, et al: Cyclosporin A drug interactions. Drug Metab Dis 18(5):595–606, 1990.)

Absorption

Absorption of CsA from the gastrointestinal tract is slow and incomplete, with a mean bioavailability of approximately 30%.[14] Several factors, including bile flow,[15,16] presence and type of food,[17–19] duration of therapy,[20] gastrointestinal dysfunction (e.g., diarrhea),[21] and concurrent administration of other drugs, influence both its absorption and bioavailability.

TABLE 3.   Miscellaneous Drug Interactions with Cyclosporine

Signs and Symptoms	Drug
Pharmacodynamic	
Gingival hyperplasia[214,217,218]	Nifedipine*[219,221,224–226]
	Other calcium channel blockers[215,216] (verapamil,[223] diltiazem,[221] nitrendipine[220] felodipine[222])
	Phenytoin*
Hirsutism, hypertrichosis	Minoxidil
	Phenytoin
	Prednisone
Hyperlipidemia[213]	Beta-blockers
	Ethanol
	Isotretinoin
	Prednisone
	Progestins
	Thiazide diuretics
Pharmacokinetic	
Myositis, rhabdomyolysis[139–149]	Lovastatin* (CsA increases lovastatin levels)

* Substantiated

TABLE 4. Hepatic Drug Metabolizing Enzymes

Substrates

CYP1A[C,O,S]	CYP2A[B]	CYP2C[B,R]	CYP2D[C,Q,R]	CYP2E1[E,I]	CYP3A[B,G,K,R]
Caffeine	Coumarin	Diazepam	Alprenolol	Ethanol	Cortisol
Phenacetin	Nicotine	Hexobarbital	Amitriptyline		CsA
Tacrolimus		Methylpheno-	Clomipramine		Dapsone
Theophylline		barbital	Codeine		Erythromycin
			Debrisoquine		Ethinyl estradiol
			Desipramine		Lidocaine
			Dextromethorphan		Lovastatin
			Encainide		Methylprednisolone
			Flecainide		Midazolam
			Imipramine		Nifedipine
			Metoprolol		Progesterone
			Nortriptyline		Tacrolimus
			Propaphenone		Tamoxifen
			Propranolol		Terfenadine
			Timolol		Triazolam

B: Induced by barbiturates and phenytoin
C: Nonselective inhibition by cimetidine
E: Induced by ethanol
G: Inhibited by grapefruit juice
I: Induced by isoniazid
K: Inhibited by ketoconazole
O: Induced by omeprazole (CYP1A2)
Q: Selective inhibition by quinidine
R: Nonselective induction by rifampin
S: N—demethylation induced by smoking (CYP1A1)

This table lists the cytochrome P450 gene families responsible for the hepatic (and probably intestinal) metabolism of various compounds. Competitive inhibition may occur between drugs metabolized at the same site; however, other factors (e.g., binding affinity, dosage of the competing agent, genetic polymorphism) determine whether a clinically significant drug interaction will occur. Drugs metabolized by the other gene families listed above do not appear to interact with CsA by competitively inhibiting its metabolism at the CYP3A. Tacrolimus is metabolized primarily by the CYP4501A and 3A subtypes.

The liver is probably the major site of CsA's metabolism; however, high concentrations of the specific CYP450 enzymes responsible for metabolizing CsA have been identified in rat and human intestinal mucosa.[22] It is therefore probable that presystemic metabolism in the intestinal mucosa is responsible in large part for the poor oral bioavailability of CsA and may explain alterations in CsA's bioavailability observed during concomitant erythromycin,[23–25] rifampin,[26–27] or phenytoin[28] therapy. Erythromycin decreases the intestinal metabolism of CsA, allowing for increased absorption of CsA,[232–25] whereas phenytoin[28] and rifampin[26–27] increase CsA's intestinal metabolism, decreasing its bioavailability.

An example of a "drug–food" interaction has been reported with grapefruit juice and CsA. Grapefruit juice increases the bioavailability of CsA[29–35] and a number of other drugs[36] including felodipine,[37] nisoldipine,[38] and terfenadine,[39] metabolized by the CYP450 enzyme system. Components of grapefruit juice (e.g., flavonoids including naringin) are capable of inhibiting the CYP450 enzymes in the gut wall, resulting in increased drug absorption. Occasional consumption of grapefruit juice may contribute to the intra- and interpatient variability seen with CsA. Consistent use of grapefruit juice has resulted in an average increase in CsA trough concentrations of 32%.[29–32] Based on these preliminary findings, routine administration of grapefruit juice with CsA appears to be an exploitable interaction; patients must be educated, however, on the importance of compliance to reap the benefits of this drug–food interaction.

Another consideration is that interactions involving absorption (i.e., altered CYP450 activity in the small intestine) are more problematic when two interacting agents are administered simultaneously rather than at different dosing intervals.[40,41] This may also account for some of the intra- and interpatient variability seen when patients alter the timing of their medication administration to accommodate lifestyle changes.

In addition to the agents mentioned above, other drugs have been reported to alter CsA's absorption by various mechanisms. Metoclopramide facilitates gastric emptying, possibly allowing for increased absorption time in the small intestine.[43,43] Cholestyramine may decrease CsA's absorption by binding bile acids in the intestinal lumen, although conflicting results have been reported.[44] Probucol has also been reported to decrease the absorption of CsA.[45,46] Octreotide, a somatostatin analogue, acts by a similar mechanism and impairs intestinal absorption of CsA by inhibiting the secretion of bile acids.[47,48]

A "drug–disease" interaction has been observed in patients with gastrointestinal dysfunction (e.g., greater than 500 ml of diarrhea over a 72-hour period) who have impaired CsA absorption. Theoretically, agents (e.g., drugs or enteral feedings) or conditions (e.g., pseudomembranous colitis) capable of inducing diarrhea of a similar magnitude may also impair the absorption of CsA through this mechanism.[21]

Distribution

No drugs have been reported to displace CsA from lipoprotein binding sites;[49] however, an association between hypocholesterolemia and CsA-induced neurotoxicity has been reported.[50,51] A few drugs (e.g., erythromycin,[52] ketoconazole,[53] acetazolamide[54]) may alter the distribution characteristics of CsA, but other mechanisms seem more plausible.

Metabolism

Drugs that Increase CsA Levels

Most drugs capable of increasing CsA concentrations do so by inhibiting its hepatic (and probably intestinal) metabolism. This inhibition usually results from competition of two drugs with affinity for the same binding site on the CYP450 isoenzymes. Onset of enzyme inhibition occurs more rapidly (i.e., within the first 24 hours) than does enzyme induction. Inhibition of this enzyme system is dose-dependent, with higher doses producing greater inhibition. The new half-life of the affected drug may be significantly prolonged, and it may take a week or more to reach a new steady state. Because of the toxicity associated with elevated CsA levels, dosage modification is usually necessary before a new steady state is reached.

Drugs known to inhibit the metabolism of CsA include the "azole" antifungal agents[55] (ketoconazole,[56–63] itraconazole,[64–68] fluconazole[69–73]), the macrolide antibiotics (erythromycin,[23–25,74–81] josamycin,[82,83] clarithromycin,[84] tacrolimus,[85,86] and possibly rapamycin) and the calcium antagonists[87,88] (diltiazem,[89–93] nicardipine,[94–96] and verapamil[87,88,93,97–101]). Of note, the calcium antagonists nifedipine,[88,102,103] isradipine,[104] amlodipine,[105] and nitrendipine[106] do not interact with CsA. Dosage reductions of CsA initially from 50% to 15 to 20% with concomitant ketoconazole[57,107,108] and to at least 45 to 50% with erythromycin and diltiazem have been reported.[74–81,89–93] Oral contraceptive hormones and other steroidal agents also decrease CsA's metabolism.[109,110]

On the basis of structure alone, it is not possible to predict which drugs will interact with CsA. If, however, data are available describing the specific CYP450 gene family responsible for metabolism of a given drug it is possible to make at least an intelligent guess as to whether an interaction may occur. It is known that although specific CYP450 enzymes may metabolize many different drugs, any single agent may be metabolized in vivo by only a single CYP450 enzyme. Studies performed in cultured human hepatocytes measuring the rate of CsA metabolism and microsomal content of immunoreactive CYP3A have confirmed or disproved many of the reported interactions with CsA (Table 2).[86,111] It is possible, however, that some of these agents may interact with CsA or its metabolites by other mechanisms.

Even though some of the interactions appear to be related to specific classes of drugs (e.g., macrolides, azole antifungals, calcium channel blockers), factors other than chemical structure determine the magnitude of interaction. Studies have demonstrated the importance of the relative binding affinity between a drug and the CYP3A site. Even though two chemically related drugs are metabolized by the same enzyme gene family, it does not necessarily mean that a clinically significant interaction occurs at dosages of the medication used routinely. Ketoconazole has a high binding affinity for CYP3A, and even subtherapeutic doses of ketoconazole dramatically impair CsA's metabolism. During concomitant therapy with ketoconazole, CsA dosage must be reduced to 20 to 30% of the previous steady-state dose. By contrast, itraconazole is only half as potent as ketoconazole, and fluconazole is even less potent (doses of 200 mg/day are needed before the metabolism of CsA is altered), so interactions with these agents and CsA are less problematic. Another example demonstrating the importance of binding affinity can be seen with chemically unrelated compounds. Nifedipine's binding affinity is approximately 10% that of ketoconazole; thus at clinical doses nifedipine does not interact with CsA. At the much higher doses used in in vitro studies, however, it interacts with CsA.

Because significant dosage reductions of CsA are necessary during concomitant ketoconazole,[56–63,107,108,112,113] diltiazem,[89–93,114–116] or erythromycin therapy,[74–81] a few centers have advocated intentionally administering these agents to reduce the overall cost of CsA therapy.[57,108,112–118] Coadministration of ketoconazole necessitates a 70 to 80% reduction in CsA dosage,[47,107] whereas diltiazem or erythromycin result in only a 40–50% reduction in CsA dosage.[114–118] Even though significant cost savings may be achieved with these regimens,[57,107,113–118] further studies are needed to document long-term safety and efficacy of such strategies.[58,108,119,120] In addition, cost–benefits of these interactions may be reduced by the addition of other interacting drugs (e.g., alkalinization through antacids or H2-antagonists reduces absorption of ketoconazole, which leads to lower CsA levels).[121,122] It may be easier to rationalize the use of diltiazem for its cost-savings potential when the agent is also used to treat hypertension rather than intentionally administering another agent (e.g., ketoconazole) only to save money. When ketoconazole is used, prophylactic antifungal therapy (e.g., miconazole, nystatin) can be discontinued; however, development of resistance during chronic antifungal therapy has been raised as a theoretic concern. Other concerns with intentional use of enzyme-inhibiting agents include the need for compliance of both interacting drugs, toxicity of the interacting agent and possible enhanced toxicity of CsA, other drug interactions with the interacting agent (see Table 9), and, ultimately, the long-term impact of chronic enzyme inhibition.

Drugs that Decrease CsA Levels

Drugs that decrease CsA drug concentrations by inducing hepatic (and probably intestinal) CYP450 enzymes include the anticonvulsants—phenytoin,[123–125] phenobarbital,[126,127] carbamazepine,[128,129] and primidone.[127,130] Valproic acid may be an effective alternative in CsA-treated patients because it does not alter metabolism of CsA at routine doses.[128] Other agents, such as rifampin,[26-28,130-135] sulfadimidine and trimethoprim,[136,137] and nafcillin,[138] have also been reported to decrease CsA levels by this mechanism.

Onset of enzyme induction is less rapid than enzyme inhibition because induction requires activation of enzymes. The induction period may last from 2 to 4 weeks; however, more rapid induction may occur with larger doses of the interacting agent. A similar period or even longer is required to reverse the effect following discontinuation of the offending agent. The clinical significance of enzyme induction is substantial because rifampin and most anticonvulsants decrease CsA concentrations to levels at or below the limit of detection for most assays.[8-10] Dosage increases of up to two- to threefold for CsA may be necessary during concomitant rifampin or phenytoin therapy.[8-10,26-28,124,125,130-135]

CsA-Induced Alterations in Drug Metabolism

Lovastatin has been reported to cause myositis and elevated serum creatinine phosphokinase levels in less than 0.5% of patients. When administered concomitantly with immunosuppressive therapy (e.g, CsA) or other drugs metabolized by CYP450 (e.g., erythromycin, niacin, gemfibrozil), the incidence is higher (30%).[139-141] Signs and symptoms may progress to myalgias, rhabdomyolysis, and acute renal failure.[142-149] Incidence of these complications decreases by limiting the dose of lovastatin to 20 to 40 mg/day during concomitant therapy.[140,150-152] This dosage provides lovastatin levels and/or HMG-CoA reductase activity comparable with (or higher than) those obtained in control subjects receiving higher doses because CsA inhibits metabolism of lovastatin.[140,152] Other HMG-CoA reductase inhibitors have fewer problems with myositis and rhabdomyolysis associated with their use.[153-155] Altered pharmacokinetic disposition of pravastatin and simvastatin has been reported during concomitant therapy with CsA.[156,157] Elevations in creatine kinase levels have occurred during concomitant administration of these agents with CsA. A case of rhabdomyolysis has been attributed to simvastatin in a heart transplant recipient.[158,159]

CsA Pharmacodynamic Interactions

Nephrotoxicity is the primary side effect observed in all patients maintained on CsA.[160-162] Theoretically, any drug capable of causing nephrotoxicity may exacerbate the nephrotoxicity of CsA. Whether the effect of administering two or more nephrotoxic agents is additive or synergistic remains to be elucidated. Several drugs, including the aminoglycosides,[163,164] amphotericin B,[165] acyclovir,[5,160] ganciclovir,[166] diclofenac,[167] indomethacin,[168] sulindac,[168-170] melphalan,[60,171] and others[172-175] have been reported to increase CsA nephrotoxicity.

Acute CsA nephrotoxicity is concentration-dependent and is usually reversible following reduction in dosage.[176] Chronic nephrotoxicity is irreversible and may be a consequence of persistent renal vasoconstriction and mesangial cell proliferation with resultant glomerulosclerosis.[177] Vasoconstriction appears to be mediated by increased production of thromboxane A_2 and endothelin.[178,179] Agents including captopril,[180] enisoprostil,[181] misoprostil,[182-184] pentoxifylline,[185] cilastatin,[186,187] urodilatin,[188] and others[189-191] have been studied for their potentially beneficial renal protective effects; however, the calcium channel antagonists[192,192] (e.g., verapamil,[194,195] diltiazem,[196-199] filodipine,[200] nifedipine,[201] nicardipine,[96] isradipine[202,203]) appear to be most promising. These agents may block endothelin-induced constriction of smooth muscle cells dependent on the influx of calcium.[204] This mechanism may also explain, at least in part, the efficacy of calcium antagonists for the treatment of CsA-induced hypertension.[205]

Increased serum creatinine levels may occur in patients treated with trimethoprim,[206-208] disopyramide,[209] and cimetidine[210] without an apparent change in renal function or CsA level. Trimethoprim[206,207] and cimetidine[174] have been reported to inhibit renal tubular secretion of creatinine competitively.

In addition to observing a decrease in glomerular filtration rate (GFR) and an increase in serum creatinine levels and BUN, other CsA-induced laboratory abnormalities include hypomagnesemia, hyperkalemia, and hyperuricemia. CsA-treated patients commonly require aggressive magnesium supplementation to maintain serum Mg^{++} levels at the lower end of the normal range.[211] In addition, other medications used concomitantly in CsA-treated patients may exacerbate these fluid and electrolyte derangements (e.g., diuretics—hyperuricemia and gout, hypomagnesemia, enhanced nephrotoxicity with volume depletion). K^+-sparing diuretics (e.g., spironolactone, amiloride, triamterene), beta-blockers, and angiotensin-converting enzyme inhibitors may exacerbate hyperkalemia.

Other complications of CsA that are difficult to manage include hypertension and hyperlipidemia.[212,213] Again, both these conditions can be complicated by administration of other drugs in CsA-treated patients (e.g., corticosteroids—hypertension and hyperlipidemia; diuretics—hyperlipidemia; beta-blockers—hyperlipidemia). These disorders require aggressive strategies including multi-drug regimens, dietary interventions, and, if necessary, either reducing CsA concentrations or discontinuing therapy.

CsA has also been associated with certain benign, but troublesome, dose-related side effects such as hirsutism, neurotoxicity, and gingival hyperplasia (Fig. 1). (see Table 3).[214-217] Gingival hyperplasia has been reported as an adverse effect of certain drugs (e.g., phenytoin, CsA, nifedipine, and the other calcium channel blockers).[214-226] Concomitant administration of nifedipine and CsA resulted in an increased rate of this condition (51%) compared with that for CsA alone (8%).[224-226] The mechanism by which these drugs cause this disorder may be related to calcium channel inhibition; however, a direct local effect may also occur with the liquid form vs. capsules.[227] Based on these observations, concurrent administration of drugs capable of inducing gingival hyperplasia should be avoided whenever possible. Plaque control and removal of local irritants have been of some benefit[218] and a recent four-patient case report suggests that metronidazole therapy may be useful.[228] Surgery and discontinuation of CsA may be necessary in patients who do not respond to these modalities.

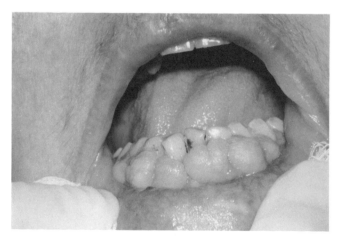

FIGURE 1.   Gingival hyperplasia in a patient receiving CsA. [Photo courtesy of Dr. Si Pham, University of Pittsburgh.]

Summary.   Management of confirmed CsA drug interactions requires proactive measures such as altering CsA dose either upon initiation or during concomitant administration of the interacting agent; measuring CsA drug levels and, when available, those of the offending agents; and monitoring other parameters such as renal function tests, creatinine phosphokinase levels, and any other tests indicative of pharmacologic or toxic response.

When dealing with unknown interactants, the interactive potential of the new agent must be assessed based on current experience. Examples of important chemical classes of drugs which may interact with CsA include macrolide antibiotics, azole antifungal drugs, calcium channel blockers, nonsteroidal antiinflammatory agents, and any nephrotoxic drug. In this setting, drug concentrations must be measured more frequently when another drug is added or discontinued, and the overall clinical condition of the patient must be monitored to ensure efficacy and prevent toxicity.

TACROLIMUS

Tacrolimus, formerly known as FK506, was approved in 1994 for use in solid organ transplantation, and studies are under way in a variety of autoimmune disorders.[229] To date, only a few drug interactions have been reported with tacrolimus (Table 5); however, because it is metabolized primarily by the CYP3A and also by the 1A enzyme systems,[85,230–236] tacrolimus is suspected to have a drug interaction profile similar to, if not identical with, CsA.

Pharmacokinetic Interactions

Drugs that Increase Tacrolimus Levels

Elevated trough tacrolimus concentrations have been observed in transplant recipients receiving concomitant CYP4503A4 enzyme inhibitors including erythromycin,[237]

TABLE 5.   Drug Interactions with Tacrolimus (FK506)

Drug Name	Mechanism	Species
Drugs that increase Tacrolimus concentration		
Erythromycin[237,247]	Inhibition of intestinal and hepatic metabolism	Liver/kidney transplant patients, rats
Fluconazole[238,239,247]	Inhibition of metabolism	Liver transplant patients, rats
Clotrimazole[240]	Inhibition of intestinal metabolism	One liver transplant patient, rats
Danazol[241]	Inhibition of metabolism	Transplant patients, rats
Methylprednisolone[239,241]	Inhibition of metabolism	Transplant patients
Diltiazem[239,247]	Inhibition of metabolism	Rats
Verapamil[246]	Inhibition of metabolism	Rats
Cimetidine[239]	Inhibition of metabolism	Rats
Itraconazole[246]	Inhibition of metabolism	Rats
Ketoconazole[239,247]	Inhibition of metabolism	Rats
Drugs that decrease Tacrolimus concentration		
Dexamethasone[230,235]	Induction of metabolism	Rats
Rifampin[245,256]	Induction of metabolism	One liver transplant patient, rats
Antacids[244]	Degradation/adsorption of tacrolimus by antacids	In vitro
Effect of Tacrolimus on other drugs		
Cyclosporine[231,232,243,251]	Increased bioavailability (decreased presystemic metabolism) Additive nephrotoxicity	Dogs

fluconazole,[238,239] clotrimazole,[239,240] and danazol.[241] In the case of clotrimazole, the authors speculated that clotrimazole competes with tacrolimus for the binding sites of the CYP450 enzyme system in the small intestine, resulting in decreased metabolism by the intestinal mucosa and increased bioavailability of tacrolimus. Conflicting results have been reported for the interaction between tacrolimus and methylprednisolone.[239,242] Because tacrolimus is also metabolized by the CYP1A system, it may exhibit some unique interactions with compounds that do not interact with CsA (Table 4).

Drugs that Decrease Tacrolimus Levels

One unique difference between the pharmacokinetic profiles of CsA and tacrolimus is that absorption of tacrolimus does not depend on the presence of bile.[239,243] Thus, unlike CsA, agents that alter bile secretion and/or bind to bile salts, such as probucol,[45,46] cholestyramine,[44] and octreotide,[47,48] should not interact with tacrolimus and decrease its absorption. An in vitro study suggested that antacids containing magnesium oxide and aluminum hydroxide gel impair absorption of tacrolimus;[244] however, this has not been confirmed in patients.

It is assumed, but not yet confirmed, with the exception of rifampin,[245,246] that the other enzyme inducers such as phenytoin, phenobarbital, and carbamazepine will induce the metabolism of tacrolimus resulting in decreased levels. Tacrolimus levels should be monitored closely because they may decline precipitously during concomitant enzyme inducer therapy.

In Vitro and In Vivo Studies

Laboratory studies have confirmed that tacrolimus is susceptible to enzyme inhibition and induction.[230] Increased tacrolimus concentrations have been reported in rats with the enzyme inhibitors erythromycin, ketoconazole, diltiazem, fluconazole, and cimetidine.[247] Studies using hepatic microsomes have shown inhibition of tacrolimus metabolism by a number of agents (Table 6).[230,248]

Tacrolimus-Induced Alterations in Drug Metabolism

Tacrolimus may also inhibit the oxidation of other drugs known to be substrates for the CYP4503A4, including troleandromycin, erythromycin, midazolam, nifedipine, ethinylestradiol, diltiazem, cortisol, and progesterone.[232] The inhibitory action of tacrolimus may be related to its strong affinity for the CYP4503A4 active site because it appears to be the most potent of all macrolides tested thus far.[232] Tacrolimus has been reported to inhibit metabolism of CsA resulting in increased CsA concentrations in humans,[249,250] but it may not result from altered clearance.[243] Studies in dogs suggest that tacrolimus may inhibit intestinal metabolism of CsA, resulting in increased absorption and a corresponding increase in CsA concentration.[251] Combined use of these two agents results in synergistic immunosuppression[252] and increased nephrotoxicity[253]

TABLE 6.   Inhibitors of FK506 Metabolism in Human Liver Microsomes

Bromocriptine	Josamycin	Nifedipine
Corticosterone	Ketoconazole	Omeprazole
Cyclosporine	Methylprednisolone	Troleandomycin
Erythromycin	Miconazole	Verapamil
Ergotamine	Midazolam	
Ethinyl estradiol		

(Data from Christians[230] and Iwasaki.[248])

TABLE 7.   Tacrolimus

Pharmacodynamic interactions	
Aminoglycosides Amphotericin B Cisplatin Cyclosporine[261,262] NSAIDs (ibuprofen)[260]	Increased nephrotoxicity
K⁺-sparing diuretics	Enhanced hyperkalemia
Acyclovir Ganciclovir Imipenem Quinolone antibiotics	Enhanced neurotoxicity

Because tacrolimus is a macrolide, it may interact with other drugs known to interact with erythromycin, including theophylline, terfenadine, and CsA.[254,255] Cimetidine, which is known to inhibit metabolism of these compounds through the CYP4501A site, may also impair the metabolism of tacrolimus.[256,257]

Pharmacodynamic Interactions

Because clinical studies indicate that the incidence of nephrotoxicity is approximately equivalent with use of tacrolimus or CsA,[253,258,259] similar concern should be exhibited for the concomitant administration of tacrolimus and other nephrotoxic agents (e.g., aminoglycosides, amphotericin B, cisplatin). Additive nephrotoxicity has been reported with therapy using concomitant tacrolimus and ibuprofen[260] or cyclosporine.[261,262] Patients should be monitored closely when receiving concomitant nephro- and neurotoxins (Table 7).

Summary.   Based on available data, tacrolimus is susceptible to CYP450 enzyme inhibition and induction. Because of its metabolism through the CYP1A and CYP3A isoenzymes,[85,230-236] agents known to interact with CsA and erythromycin should be considered as potential interactants for tacrolimus until proved otherwise.

AZATHIOPRINE (AzA)

Only a few drugs interact with Aza (Table 8). The most clinically significant interaction occurs between azathioprine and allopurinol, a xanthine-oxidase inhibitor used to treat gout.[263,264] Allopurinol blocks intestinal metabolism of Aza and

TABLE 8.   Azathioprine Drug Interactions

Interacting Agents	Effect
Allopurinol[263-266]	Decreased azathioprine intestinal metabolism resulting in a 2–3-fold increase in azathioprine absorption
Cyclophosphamide, vincristine, methotrexate, etc.	Enhanced bone marrow toxicity metabolism
Ganciclovir[166]	Enhanced bone marrow toxicity
Pancuronium[281,282]	Increased pancuronium clearance
Succinylcholine[282,283]	Enhanced activity of succinylcholine
Trimethoprim-sulfamethoxazole	Enhanced bone marrow toxicity
Warfarin (interaction reported with mercapto-purine, may possibly occur with azathioprine)[284]	Decreased hypoprothrombinemic effect

causes a 2- to 3-fold increase in its bioavailability.[265,266] When these agents are used concomitantly, the Aza dosage must be reduced to 25 to 33% of the previous maintenance dose. If the Aza is not reduced, life-threatening pancytopenia and its associated complications (e.g., opportunistic infections, bleeding, and so forth) will occur. This interaction is especially worrisome in that many patients are prescribed allopurinol on an outpatient basis for treatment of gout and they may be instructed to return to clinic after 3 to 6 months. Signs and symptoms of Aza toxicity may develop rather insidiously over 4 to 6 weeks, and the patient may not return until profound pancytopenia develops.

The primary toxicity of Aza is its dose-related bone marrow suppression characterized by leukopenia, thrombocytopenia, macrocytic anemia, pure red blood cell aplasia, and reticulocytopenia. Administration of other myelotoxic agents (Table 8) may exacerbate Aza's marrow toxicity. Other adverse effects include hepatotoxicity, alopecia, stomatitis, acute pancreatitis, and an increased risk of infection and malignancy.

CORTICOSTEROIDS

Oral contraceptives decrease clearance of prednisone.[267,268] Other drug interactions involving prednisolone that have been reported in healthy subjects are also expected to occur in transplant patients.[269] A 25% reduction in the total body clearance of prednisolone and an increase in the half-life from 2.9 to 4.3 hours was observed in renal transplant patients receiving cyclosporine when compared with patients receiving azathioprine.[270,272] Ketoconazole appears to decrease the clearance of methylprednisolone;[273,274] however, its effects on prednisolone clearance are conflicting.[275,276]

Many of the drugs that increase the metabolism of CsA (phenytoin, phenobarbital, rifampin) also increase the metabolism of prednisone and may adversely affect the status of the graft (Table 9).[10,136,277] Rifampicin has also been reported to reduce the bioavailability of prednisolone in healthy subjects.[278]

The effect of steroids on the kinetics of other drugs used in transplant patients must also be recognized. Steroids are known to induce metabolism of salicylic acid and to increase urinary excretion of metronidazole.[279,280] The use of pancuronium with prednisone causes rapid termination of the muscular blockade.[281]

In addition, a variety of prednisone's known side effects may be potentiated by the concomitant administration of other drugs (Table 9).

TABLE 9.   Corticosteroid Drug Interactions[268,269]

Pharmacokinetic	Effect
CsA[110,270,272]	Decreased CsA and/or prednisone metabolism
Estrogens[267]	Decreased prednisolone metabolism (conflicting reports)
Ketoconazole[273-276]	Decreased methylprednisolone metabolism (conflicting reports)
Metronidazole[278]	Increased urinary excretion of metronidazole
Phenytoin phenobarbital	Increased prednisone metabolism
Rifampin[8,9,10,135,277,278]	Increased prednisone metabolism
Salicylic acid[280]	Increased salicylic acid metabolism
Pharmacodynamic	
Amphotericin-B, diuretics	Enhanced K+ depletion
Hypoglycemic agents	Decreased efficacy
Nonsteroidal antiinflammatory agents	Increased gastritis
Pancuronium[281]	Rapid termination of muscular blockade

TABLE 10.   Alternative Noninteractive Agents for Use with Cyclosporine

Interacting Agents	Substitute
Anticonvulsants[123-130] Phenytoin, phenobarbital, carbamazepine, primidone	Valproic acid[128]
Calcium channel blockers[87-101] Diltiazem, verapamil, nicardipine	Nifedipine,[88,94,102-103] isradipine,[104] amlodipine[105] nitrendipine[106]
Macrolide antibiotics[255] Erythromycin,[23-25,52,74-81] josamycin,[82,83] clarithromycin[84]	Azithromycin,[185] spiramycin[286-288]
Nephrotoxins NSAIDs[168-170]	Acetaminophen

SUMMARY

Management of drug interactions in the transplant recipient depends on a number of factors:

Whether alternative noninteracting but equally efficacious agents are available (Table 10) (i.e., in a critical care setting it is necessary to manage a patient's life-threatening problem with the most appropriate drug first and then when the patient is stabilized, either deal with the drug interaction or switch to a noninteracting agent).

Whether therapy is prescribed for an acute vs. chronic process (i.e, it is probably not worth the time and effort it takes to adjust the patient's CsA or tacrolimus dosage if he or she will require only 7 to 14 days of therapy—in this situation it is preferable to use a noninteracting agent).

Whether the patient is compliant with other medications.

Whether the patient is available for more frequent drug concentration monitoring to allow for dosage adjustments (i.e., it is easier to adjust concomitant therapy in a hospitalized patient than in one who has returned to work and is not scheduled to return to clinic again for 2 to 3 months.

Whether the patient is receiving other drugs (i.e., it is reasonably easy to manage an interaction between CsA and one or even two other agents, but it is far more complex to deal with four or five interacting agents such as CsA, ketoconazole, phenytoin, and erythromycin).

Drug interactions of other agents used commonly in transplant patients are summarized in Table 11 and a comprehensive listing of cyclosporine interactions is provided in Table 12.

TABLE 11.   Drug Interactions of Other Agents Commonly Used in Transplant Recipients

Drug	Interactant	Possible Effect
Alternative immunosuppressants		
Cyclophosphamide (Cytoxan—CTX)	Allopurinol	Enhanced bone marrow toxicity
	Cotrimoxazole	Enhanced bone marrow toxicity
	Ganciclovir	Enhanced bone marrow toxicity
	Anticonvulsants (phenytoin, phenobarbital)	Enhanced metabolism (decreased efficacy of CTX)
Methotrexate (MTX)	Azathioprine	Enhanced bone marrow toxicity
	Cotrimoxazole	Enhanced bone marrow toxicity
	NSAIDs	Enhanced bone marrow toxicity (inhibit renal elimination of MTX)

(Table continued on following page.)

TABLE 11. Drug Interactions of Other Agents Commonly Used in Transplant Recipients *(Cont.)*

Drug	Interactant	Possible Effect
Alternative immunosuppressants *(cont.)*		
Methotrexate (MTX) *(cont.)*	Sulfonamides	Enhanced bone marrow toxicity
Rapamycin	Unknown at this time	May have interactions similar to tacrolimus
Anti-infective agents		
Cotrimoxazole	Cyclophosphamide	Enhanced bone marrow toxicity
	Ganciclovir	Enhanced bone marrow toxicity
	Methotrexate	Enhanced bone marrow toxicity
	Oral hypoglycemic agents	Enhanced hypoglycemia
	Warfarin	Enhanced hypoprothrombinemic effect
Ganciclovir (GCV)[166]	Cotrimoxazole	Enhanced bone marrow toxicity
	Dapsone	Enhanced bone marrow toxicity
	Pentamidine	Enhanced bone marrow toxicity
	Vincristine	Enhanced bone marrow toxicity
	Imipenem-Cilastatin	Increased risk of seizures
	Probenecid	Increased GCV levels (reduced renal clearance GVC)
Azole-antifungals[55]		
Fluconazole[289]	Antacids, H_2-antagonists	No effect
	Cyclosporine (CsA)	Fluconazole > 200 mg/day inhibits CsA metabolism
	Oral hypoglycemics[290]	Enhanced hypoglycemia
	Phenytoin	Inhibits phenytoin's metabolism (increased phenytoin levels)
	Rifampin	Enhanced metabolism of fluconazole
	Tacrolimus[238,239,247]	Inhibits tacrolimus metabolism
Itraconazole	Antacids, H_2-antagonists	No effect
	Cyclosporine	Inhibits CsA's metabolism
	Oral hypoglycemics[290]	Enhanced hypoglycemia
	Phenytoin	Inhibits phenytoin's metabolism (increased phenytoin levels)
	Rifampin	Enhanced metabolism of itraconazole
Ketoconazole (KTZ)[289]	Antacids, H_2-antagonists (cimetidine, ranitidine, sucralfate)[121,122,291,292,293]	Reduced absorption of KTZ (decreased efficacy), and if in combination with CsA see decreased CsA levels
	Anticoagulants (warfarin)[294]	Enhanced hypoprothrombinemic effect (KTZ inhibits warfarin's metabolism)
	Corticosteroids,[273–276] methyl-prednisolone, prednisolone	Inhibits metabolism of methylpredniso-lone (conflicting data)
	Cyclosporine	Inhibits CsA's metabolism
	Chlordiazepoxide (Librium)	Inhibits Librium's metabolism
	Ethanol	Disulfiram-like reaction
	Food[295–297]	No effect (conflicting reports)
	Isoniazid[41,297–299]	Induces metabolism of KTZ
	Phenytoin	Altered metabolism of one or both drugs
	Quinidine[300]	Inhibits quinidine's metabolism
	Rifampin[41,298,299]	Induces metabolism of KTZ and variable effect on rifampin
	Terfenadine	Inhibits metabolism of terfenadine (torsades de pointes)
	Theophylline[301]	Inhibits metabolism
Metronidazole	Anticoagulants (warfarin)	Inhibits metabolism of warfarin
	Ethanol	Disulfiram reaction
	Phenobarbital	Enhanced metabolism of metronidazole
	Phenytoin	Impaired metabolism of phenytoin
	Antibiotics	Increased estrogen levels and diminished efficacy
Oral contraceptives		
	Anticonvulsants (phenytoin, phenobarbital)	Enhanced metabolism and diminished efficacy

TABLE 12. Cyclosporine (CsA) Drug Interactions

Drug	Proposed Mechanism	Possible Effects	References
Anticonvulsants			
Carbamazepine*	Increased CsA metabolism	Decreased CsA blood concentrations	128,129
Mesuximide	As above	As above	5
Phenobarbital*	As above	As above	126,127
Phenytoin*	As above	As above	10,123–125
	Decreased CsA absorption	As above	29
		Increased gingival hyperplasia	214
Primidone	Increased CsA metabolism	Decreased CsA blood concentrations	127,130
Valproic acid	—	No effect	128
Anti-infective agents			
Acyclovir	Nephrotoxic agent	Increased nephrotoxicity	160
Aminoglycosides*	As above	Increased nephrotoxicity	162–164
Amphotericin B*	As above	Increased nephrotoxicity	165
Azithromycin	—	No effect	285
Cephalosporin	—	No effect (animal studies)	163
Ciprofloxacin	—	No effect	302–305
Clarithromycin	Decreased CsA metabolism	Increased CsA concentrations	84
Doxycycline*	Unknown	Increased CsA concentrations	5
Erythromycin*	Decreased CsA metabolism	Increased CsA blood concentrations with and without nephrotoxicity	52,74–81,255
	Decreased biliary excretion	As above	79
	Increased absorption	As above	23–25
Fluconazole	Decreased CsA metabolism	Increased CsA concentrations (conflicting data)	69–73
Ganciclovir	Unknown	Increased nephrotoxicity	166
Imipenem/Cilastatin	Increased CsA metabolism	Decreased CsA blood concentrations (animal studies)	187
	Unknown	Enhanced neurotoxicity(?)	306
	Unknown	Possible renal protectant	186
Itraconazole	Decreased CsA metabolism	Increased CsA blood concentrations (conflicting data) with nephrotoxicity	64–68
Josamycin*	Decreased CsA metabolism	Increased CsA blood concentrations with and without nephrotoxicity	82,83
Ketoconazole*	Decreased CsA metabolism	Increased CsA blood concentrations with and without nephrotoxicity	53,56–63,107,108 112,113,118–120 307
Miconazole	Decreased CsA metabolism	Increased CsA blood concentrations	55
Nafcillin*	Increased CsA metabolism	Decreased CsA blood concentrations	138
Norfloxacin	Decreased CsA metabolism	Increased CsA concentrations (conflicting data)	308
Pristinamycin	Decreased CsA metabolism	Increased CsA concentrations	5
Spiramycin	—	No effect	286–288
Sulfamethoxazole* (sulfadimidine) and/or Trimethoprim IV*	Unknown	Decreased CsA blood concentrations with associated rejection episodes	136,137
PO	Altered tubular secretion of creatinine	Increased serum creatinine	206–208
Ticarcillin	Unknown	Increased CsA concentrations	5

---

* Substantiated interaction[1]

(Table continued on following page.)

TABLE 12.   Cyclosporine (CsA) Drug Interactions *(Cont.)*

Drug	Proposed Mechanism	Possible Effects	References
Antituberculous agents			
Isoniazid	Increased CsA metabolism (?)	Decreased CsA blood concentrations with concomitant rifampin therapy	133
Rifampin*	Increased CsA metabolism	As above	8,9,131–135
	Enhanced CsA intestinal metabolism	Decreased bioavailability	26–27
Cardiovascular agents			
Amlodipine	—	Conflicting data	105
Diltiazem*	Decreased CsA metabolism	Increased CsA blood concentrations	87–92, 114–117
			309–310
		Increased risk gingival hyperplasia	221
		Protective renal effort	196,199
Disopyramide	Unknown	Increased serum creatinine	209
Enalapril	Unknown	Protective renal effect	170
Felodipine		Protective renal effect	200
		Increased risk gingival hyperplasia	222
Isradipine	—	No effect	104
Nicardipine*	Decreased CsA metabolism	Increased CsA blood concentrations	94–96
		Protective renal effect	201
Nifedipine	Unknown	No effect on CsA	87,102,103
		Increased gingival hyperplasia	214–219,221,224–226
Nitrendipine	—	No effect on CsA	106
		Increased risk gingival hyperplasia	220
Prazosin	Improved renal blood flow	Protective renal effect (animal studies)	191
Propranolol	Unknown	Antagonistic immunosuppressive effect (animal studies)	170
Verapamil*	Decreased metabolism	Increased CsA concentrations	87,88,93,97–101
		Increased gingival hyperplasia	223
		Protective renal effect	194,195,198
	Inhibits lymphocyte activation	Enhanced immunosuppression	311–313
Warfarin	Altered CsA metabolism in combination with phenobarbital	Decreased CsA concentrations and increased prothrombin activity	314
Diuretics			
Acetazolamide	Increased absorption Decreased metabolism Altered distribution	Increased CsA concentrations	54
Furosemide	Sodium depletion	Increased nephrotoxicity (animal studies)	175
		Protective renal effect	189
Mannitol	Unknown	Increased nephrotoxicity (animal studies)	172
Metolazone	Unknown	Protective renal effect (animal studies)	170
Spironolactone	Unknown		
Gastrointestinal agents			
Antacids	Decreased or increased absorption	Unknown—may be similar to food (conflicting data)	17,18

* Substantiated interaction[1]

(Table continued on following page.)

TABLE 12. Cyclosporine (CsA) Drug Interactions *(Cont.)*

Drug	Proposed Mechanism	Possible Effects	References
Gastrointestinal agents *(cont.)*			
Cholestyramine	Altered CsA absorption	Variable CsA concentrations or no effect	44
Cimetidine	Decreased CsA metabolism(?)	Increased CsA blood concentrations and/or nephrotoxicity (conflicting data)	256,315–317
	Altered tubular secretion of creatinine	Elevated serum creatinine	174
Enisoprostil	—	No beneficial renal protective effect	181
Famotidine	—	No effect	318
Lovastatin	Decreased lovastatin metabolism	Myositis, increased creatine phosphokinase, rhabdomyolysis	139–152
Metoclopramide	Increased CsA absorption	Increased CsA blood concentrations with nephrotoxicity	42,43
Misoprostil	—	—	183,184
Octreotide	Decreased CsA absorption	Decreased CsA concentrations	47,48
Omeprazole	Increased CsA metabolism	Decreased CsA concentrations	5
Pravastatin	Decreased pravastatin metabolism	Increased pravastatin concentrations	157
Probucol	Decreased CsA absorption	Decreased CsA concentrations	45,46
Ranitidine	—	No effect	210,256,316,317
Simvastatin	Decreased simvastatin metabolism	Increased simvastatin concentrations and rhabdomyolysis	156,158,159
Nonsteroidal and other anti-inflammatory agents			
Colchicine	—	Increased CsA concentrations with nephrotoxicity	190
Diclofenac	Decreased prostaglandin production	Increased nephrotoxicity	167
Indomethacin	Prostaglandin depletion	Increased nephrotoxicity	170
Sulfinpyrazone	Assay interference	Decreased CsA concentrations	5
Sulindac		Increased CsA concentrations(?)	169
Sex hormones			
Danazol*	Decreased CsA metabolism	Increased CsA blood concentration with nephrotoxicity	110
Methyltestosterone*	As above	Increased CsA blood concentrations with nephrotoxicity and hepatotoxicity	319
Noresthisterone*	As above	Increased CsA blood concentrations with nephrotoxicity	110
Oral contraceptives	As above	As above	109,110
Steroids			
Methylprednisolone*	Unknown	Increased CsA plasma concentrations (RIA) but not HPLC	321,322
		Decreased CsA blood concentrations (HPLC)	322
		Convulsions	323,324
Prednisolone*	Competitive inhibition of cytochrome P-450	Reduced clearance and elevated prednisone concentrations	270–272
Miscellaneous			
Alcohol (heavy intake)	Decreased CsA metabolism Altered CsA absorption	Increased CsA concentrations	325
Atracurium	Unknown	Enhanced neuromuscular blockade (animal studies)	326
Doxorubicin	Unknown	Enhanced cytotoxicity	327

* Substantiated interaction[1]

(Table continued on following page.)

TABLE 12. Cyclosporine [CsA] Drug Interactions *(Cont.)*

Drug	Proposed Mechanism	Possible Effects	References
Miscellaneous *(cont.)*			
Etoposide	Unknown	Enhanced cytotoxicity	327
Fentanyl	Unknown	Enhanced analgesia (animal studies)	328
Food	Fatty foods may stimulate bile secretion and increase CsA absorption	Increased bioavailability (conflicting data)	18,19
Grapefruit juice	Decreased CsA intestinal metabolism	Increased bioavailability	29–35
Melphalan*	Unknown	Increased nephrotoxicity	61,171
Metamizole	Unknown	Decreased CsA concentrations	5
Mizoribine	Unknown	Enhanced immunosuppression	327
Pentazocine	Unknown	Increased CsA concentrations	5
Pentoxifylline		Possible renal protective effect	185
Tamoxifen	Unknown	Increased CsA concentrations	5
Urodilatin	Unknown	Possible renal protectant	188
Vecuronium	Unknown	Enhanced neuromuscular blockade (animal studies)	326

* Substantiated interaction[1]

REFERENCES

1. Lake KD: Cyclosporine drug interactions: A review. Cardiac Surgery: State of the Art Reviews 2(4):617–630, 1988.
2. Lake KD: Management of drug interactions with cyclosporine. Pharmacotherapy 11(5):110S–118S, 1991.
3. Lake KD, Canafax DM: Important interactions of drugs with immunosuppressive agents used in transplant recipients. J Antimicrob Chemother 35:August–September Supplement, 1995.
4. Baciewicz AM, Baciewicz FA: Cyclosporine pharmacokinetic drug interactions. Am J Surg 157:264–271, 1989.
5. Cockburn IT, Krupp P: An appraisal of drug interactions with Sandimmune. Transplant Proc 21(5):3845–3850, 1989.
6. Yee GC: Pharmacokinetic interactions between cyclosporine and other drugs. Transplant Proc 22(3):1203–1207, 1990.
7. Yee GC, Mcguire TR: Pharmacokinetic drug interactions with cyclosporine (Parts I & II) Clin Pharmacokinet 19:319–332, 400–415, 1990.
8. Modry DL, Stinson EB, Oyer PE, et al: Acute rejection and massive cyclosporine requirements in heart transplant recipients treated with rifampin. Transplantation 39:313–314, 1985.
9. Offermann G, Keller F, Molzahn M: Low cyclosporine A blood levels and acute graft rejection in a renal transplant recipient during rifampin treatment. Am J Nephrol 5:385–387, 1985.
10. Wassner SJ, Pennisi AJ, Malekzadeh MH, Fine RN: The adverse effect of anticonvulsant therapy on renal allograft survival. J Pediatr 88(1):134–137, 1976.
11. Venkataramanan R, Habucky K, Burckart GJ, Ptachcinski RK: Clinical pharmacokinetics in organ transplant patients. Clin Pharmacokinet 16(3):134–161, 1989.
12. Nelson DR, Kamataki R, Waxman DJ, et al: The P450 superfamily: Update on new sequences, gene mapping, accession numbers, early trivial names of enzymes, and nomenclature. DNA Cell Biol 112(1):1–51, 1993.
13. Kronbach T, Fischer V, Meyer UA: Cyclosporine metabolism in human liver: Identification of a cytochrome P-450III gene family as the major cyclosporine-metabolizing enzyme with other drugs. Clin Pharmacol Ther 43:630–635, 1988.
14. Ptachcinski RJ, Venkataramanan R, Burckart GJ: Clinical pharmacokinetics of cyclosporine. Clin Pharmacokinet 11:107–132, 1986.
15. Venkataramanan R, Starzl TE, Yang S, et al: Biliary excretion of cyclosporine in liver transplant patients. Transplant Proc 17:286–289, 1985.
16. Tredger JM, Naoumov NV, Steward CM, et al: Influence of biliary T tube clamping on cyclosporine pharmacokinetics in liver transplant recipients. Transplant Proc 20(2 Suppl 2):512–515, 1988.
17. Keown PA, Stiller CR, Sinclair NR, et al: The clinical relevance of cyclosporine blood levels as measured by radioimmunoassay. Transplant Proc 4:2438–2441, 1983.

18. Ptachcinski R, Venataramanan R, Rosenthal JT, et al: The effect of food on cyclosporine absorption. Transplantation 40:174–176, 1985.
19. Gupta SK, Benet IZ: Food increases the bioavailability of cyclosporine in healthy volunteers. Clin Pharmacol Ther 45:148, 1989.
20. Tufveson G, Frodin L, Lindberg A, et al: Why can we reduce the dose of cyclosporine with time after transplantation and how can we predict its clearance? Transplant Proc 18:1264–1625, 1986.
21. Atkinson K, Biggs JC, Britton K, et al: Oral administration of cyclosporine A for recipients of allogeneic marrow transplants: Implications of clinical gut dysfunction. Br J Haematol 56(2):223–231, 1984.
22. Watkins PB, Wrighton SA, Schuetz EG, et al: Identification of glucocorticoid-inducible cytochromes P-450 in the intestinal mucosa of rats and man. J Clin Invest 80(4):1029–1036, 1987.
23. Wadhwa NK, Schroeder TJ, O'Flaherty E, et al: Pharmacokinetics and drug interactions of cyclosporine and erythromycin. Clin Res 34:638A, 1986.
24. Wadhwa NK, Schroeder TJ, O'Flaherty E, et al: Interaction between erythromycin and cyclosporine in a kidney and pancreas allograft recipient. ther Drug Monit 9(1):123–125, 1987.
25. Gupta SK, Bakran A, Johnson RWG, Rowland M: Cyclosporine-erythromycin interaction in renal transplant patients. Br J Clin Pharmacol 27:475–481, 1989.
26. Hebert MF, Roberts JP, Preuksaritanont T, Benet LZ: Pharmacokinetics and drug disposition: Bioavailability of cyclosporine with concomitant rifampin administration is markedly less than predicted by hepatic enzyme induction. Clin Pharmacol Ther 52:453–457, 1992.
27. Van Buren D, Wideman CA, Ried M, et al: The antagonistic effect of rifampin upon cycosporine bioavailability. Transplant Proc 16:1642–1645, 1984.
28. Rowland M, Gupta SK: Cyclosporine-phenytoin interaction: Reevaluation using metabolite data. Br J Clin Pharmacol 24:329–334, 1987.
29. Ducharme MP, Provenzano R, Dehoorne-Smith M, Edwards DJ: Trough concentrations of cyclosporine in blood following administration with grapefruit juice. Br J Clin Pharmacol 36:457–459, 1993.
30. Ducharme MP, Warbasse LH, Edwards DJ: Grapefruit affects oral but not IV cyclosporine disposition in man. Presented at the Sixth North American International Society on the Study of Xenobiotics, Raleigh, NC, October 23, 1994.
31. Ducharme MP, Warbasse LH, Edwards DJ: Disposition of intravenous and oral cyclosporine following administration with grapefruit juice. Clin Pharmacol Ther 1995 (in press).
32. Yee G, Stanley DL, Ruiz J, et al: Effect of grapefruit juice on oral cyclosporine pharmacokinetics. Pharmacotherapy 14(3):37, 1994.
33. Rooij JV, Hollander AAMJ, Arbouw F, et al: The effect of grapefruit juice on the pharmacokinetics of cyclosporine A (CyA) in renal transplantation patients. Br J Clin Pharmacol 37:497P, 1994.
34. Herlitz H, Edgar B, Hedner T, et al: Grapefruit juice: A possible source of variability in blood concentration of cyclosporin A. Nephrol Dial Transplant 8(4):375, 1993.
35. Edwards DJ, Ducharme MP, Provenzano R, Dehoorne-Smith M: Effect of grapefruit juice on blood concentrations of cyclosporine. Clin Pharmacol Ther 53(2):237, 1993.
36. Lee YS, Lorenzo BA, Reidenberg MM: Grapefruit juice inhibits 11-ß-hydroxysteroid dehydrogenase. Clin Pharmacol Ther 55(2):139, 1994.
37. Bailey DG, Arnold JMO, Tran LT, et al: Marked effects of both erythromycin and grapefruit on felodipine pharmacokinetics. Clin Pharmacol Ther 55(2):165, 1994.
38. Bailey DG, Arnold MO, Strong HA, et al: Effect of grapefruit and naringin on nisoldipine pharmacokinetics. Clin Pharmacol Ther 54(6):589–594, 1993.
39. Benton R, Honig P, Zamani K, et al: Grapefruit juice alters terfenadine pharmacokinetics resulting in prolongation of QTc. Clin Pharmacol Ther 5592):146, 1994.
40. Doble N, Hykin P, Shaw R, Keal EE: Pulmonary mycobacterium tuberculosis in acquired immune deficiency. Br Med J 291:849–850, 1985.
41. Abadie-Kemmerly S, Pankey GA, Dalovisio JR: Failure of ketoconazole treatment of blastomyces dermatitidis due to interaction of isoniazid and rifampin. Ann Intern Med 109:844–845, 1988.
42. Wadhwa NK, Schroeder TJ, O'Flaherty E, et al: The effect of oral metoclopramide on the absorption of cyclosporine. Transplantation 43(2):211–213, 1989.
43. Wadhwa NK, Schroeder TJ, O'Flaherty E, et al: The effect of oral metoclopramide on the absorption of cyclosporine. Transplant Proc 19:1730–1733, 1989.
44. Keogh A, Day R, Critchly L, et al: The effect of food and cholestyramine on the absorption of cyclosporine in cardiac transplant recipients. Transplant Proc 20:27–30, 1988.
45. Sundararajan V, Cooper DKC, Muchmore J, et al: Interaction of cyclosporine and probucol in heart transplant patients. Transplant Proc 23(3):2028–2032, 1991.
46. Gallego C, Sanchez P, Planells C, et al: Interaction between probucol and cyclosporine in renal transplant patients. Ann Pharmacother 28:940–943, 1994.
47. Landgraf R, Landgraf-Leurs MMC, Nusser J, et al: Effect of somatostatin analogue (SMS201-995) on cyclosporine levels. Transplantation 445):724–725, 1987.

48. Rosenberg L, Dafoe DC, Schwartz R, et al: Administration of somatostatin analogue (SMS 201-995) in the treatment of a fistula occurring after pancreas transplantation. Transplantation 43(5):764–766, 1987.
49. LeMaire M, Tillement JP: Role of lipoprotein and erythrocytes in the vitro binding and distribution of cyclosporin A in the blood. J Pharm Pharmacol 34:715–718, 1993.
50. Bhatt B, Meriano FV, Buchwald D: Cyclosporine-associated central nervous system toxicity after liver transplantation: The role of cyclosporine and cholesterol. N Engl J Med 317:861–866, 1987.
52. Aoki FY, Yatscoff R, Jeffery J, et al: Effects of erythromycin on cyclosporine A kinetics in renal transplant patients. Clin Pharmacol Ther 41:221, 1987.
53. Smith J, Hows J, Donnelly P, et al: Interaction of cyclosporin A and ketoconazole. Exp Hematol 11(Suppl 13):177–178, 1983.
54. Keogh A, Esmore D, Spratt P, et al: Acetazolamide and cyclosporine. Transplantation 46:478–479, 1988.
55. Horton CM, Freeman CD, Nolan PE Jr, Copeland JG: Cyclosporine interactions with miconazole and other azole-antimycotics: A case report and review of the literature. J Heart Lung Transplant 11(6):1127–1132, 1992.
56. Daneshmend TK: Ketoconazole-cyclosporine interaction. Lancet 2:1342–1243, 1982.
57. Dieperink H, Moller J: Ketoconazole and cyclosporine. Lancet 2:1217, 1982.
58. First MR, Schroeder TJ, Weiskittel P, et al: Concomitant administration of cyclosporine and ketoconazole in renal transplant patients. Lancet 2(8673):1198–1201, 1989.
59. Frey FJ: Concomitant cyclosporine and ketoconazole. Lancet 335:109, 1990.
60. Gumbleton M, Brown JE, Hawsworth G, Whiting PH: The possible relationship between hepatic drug metabolism and ketoconazole enhancement of cyclosporine nephrotoxicity. Transplantation 40:454–455, 1985.
61. Morgenstern CR, Powles R, Robinson B, McElwain TJ: Cyclosporine interaction with ketoconazole and melphalan. Lancet 2:1342, 1982.
62. Schroeder TJ, Melvin DB, Clardy CW, et al: Use of cyclosporine and etoconazole without nephrotoxicity in two heart transplant recipients. J Heart Transplant 6:84–89, 1987.
63. White DJ, Blatchford R, Canwenbergh G: Cyclosporine and ketoconazole. Transplantation 37:214–215, 1984.
64. Kramer MR, Marshall SE, Denning DW, et al: Cyclosporine and itraconazole interaction in heart and lung transplant recipients. Ann Intern Med 113(4):327–329, 1990.
65. Trenk D, Brett W, Jahnchen E, Birnbaum D: Time course of cyclosporine/itraconazole interaction. Lancet 2:1335–1336, 1987.
66. Kwan JT, Foxall PJ, Davidson DG, et al: Interaction of cyclosporine and itraconazole. Lancet 2:282, 1987.
67. Novakova I, Donnelly P, DeWitte T, et al: Itraconazole and cyclosporine nephrotoxicity. Lancet 2:920–021. 1098/
68. Shaw MA, Gumbleton M, Nicholls PJ: Interaction of cyclosporine and itraconazole. Lancet 6:637, 1987.
69. Canafax DM, Graves NM, Hilligoss DM, et al: Interaction between cyclosporine and fluconazole in renal allograft recipients. Transplantation 51(5):1014–1018, 1991.
70. Sugar AM, Saunders C, Idelson BA, Bernard DB: Interaction of fluconazole and cyclosporine. Ann Intern Med 110:844, 1989.
71. Kruger HU, Schuler U, Zimmermann R, Ehninger G: Absence of significant interaction of fluconazole with cyclosporine. J Antimicrob Chemother 24:781–796, 1989.
72. Lopez-Gil JA: Fluconazole-cyclosporine interaction: A dose-dependent effect? Ann Pharmacother 27(4):427–430, 1993.
73. Graves NM, Matas AJ, Hilligoss DM, Canafax DM: Fluconazole/cyclosporine interaction. Clin Pharmacol Ther 47:208A, 1990.
74. Freeman DJ, Martell R, Carruthers SG, et al: Cyclosporine-erythromycin interaction in normal subjects. Br J Clin Parmacol 23:776–778, 1987.
75. Godin JRP, Sketris IS, Belitsky P: Erythromycin-cyclosporine interaction. Drug Intell Clin Pharm 20:504–505, 1986.
76. Gonwa TA, Nghiem DD, Schulak JA, Corry RJ: Erythromycin and cyclosporine. Transplantation 41:797–799, 1986.
77. Hourmant M, LeBigot JF, Vernillet L, et al: Coadministration of erythromycin results in an increase of blood cyclosporine to toxic levels. Transplant Proc 17:2723–2727, 1985.
78. Kohan DE: Possible interaction between cyclosporine and erythromycin. N Engl J Med 314:448, 1986.
79. Martell R, Heinrichs D, Stiller CR, et al: The effect of erythromycin in patients treated with cyclosporine. Ann Intern Med 104:660–661, 1986.
80. Ptachcinski RJ, Carpenter BJ, Burckart GJ, et al: Effect of erythromycin on cyclosporine levels. N Engl J Med 313:1416–1417, 1985.

81. Vereerstraeten P, Thiry P, Kinnaert P, Toussaint C: Influence of erythromycin on cyclosporine pharmacokinetics. Transplantation 44:155–156, 1987.
82. Kreft-Jais C, Billaud EM, Gaudry C, Bedrossian J: Effect of josamycin on plasma cyclosporine levels. Eur J Clin Pharmacol 32:327–328, 1987.
83. Torregrosa JV, Campistol JM, Franco A, Andreu J: Interaction of josamycin with cyclosporin A. Nephron 65(3):476–477, 1993.
84. Gersema LM, Porter CB, Russell EH: Suspected drug interaction between cyclosporine and clarithromycin. J Heart Lung Transplant 13(2):343–345, 1994.
85. Burke MD, Omar G, Thomson AW, Whiting PH: Inhibition of the metabolism of cyclosporine by human liver microsomes by FK506. Transplantation 50:901–902, 1990.
86. Pichard L, Fabre I, Fabre G, et al: Cyclosporine A drug interactions: Screening for inducers and inhibitors of cytochrome P-450 (cyclosporine A oxidase) in primary cultures of human hepatocytes and in liver microsomes. Drug Metab Disp 18(5):595–606, 1990.
87. McNally P, Mistry N, Idle J, et al: Calcium channel blockers and cyclosporine metabolism. Transplantation 4:1071, 1989.
88. Wagner K, Philip T, Heinemeyer G, et al: Interaction of cyclosporine and calcium antagonists. Transplant Proc 21(1 Pt 2):1453–1456, 1989.
89. Brocmoller J, Neumayer HH, Wagner K, et al: Pharmacokinetic interaction between cyclosporine and diltiazem. Eur J Clin Pharmacol 38(3):237–342, 1990.
90. Grino JM, Sebate I, Castelao AM, Alsina J: Influence of diltiazem on cyclosporine clearance. Lancet 1:1387, 1986.
91. Kohlhaw K, Wonigeit K, Frei U, et al: Effect of the calcium channel blocker diltiazem on cyclosporine A blood levels and dose requirements. Transplant Proc 20:572–574, 1988.
92. Pochet JM, Pirson Y: Cyclosporine-diltiazem interaction. Lancet 1:979, 1986.
93. Renton KW: Inhibition of hepatic microsomal drug metabolism by the calcium channel blockers diltiazem and verapamil. Biochem Pharmacol 34:2549–2553, 1985.
94. Bourbigot B, Guiserix J, Airiau J, et al: Nicardipine increases cyclosporine blood levels. Lancet 1:1447, 1986.
95. Cantarovich M, Hiesse C, Lockiec F, et al: Confirmation of the interaction between cyclosporine and the calcium channel blocker nicardipine in renal transplant patients. Clin nephrol 2:190–193, 1987.
96. Kessler M, Netter P, Renoult E, et al: Influence of nicardipine on renal function and plasma cyclosporin in renal transplant patients. Eur J Clin Pharmacol 36(6):637–638, 1989.
97. Angermann CE, Spes CH, Anthuber M, et al: Verapamil increases cyclosporine-A trough levels in cardiac transplant recipients. J Am Coll Cardiol 11:206A, 1988.
98. Lindholm A, Henricsson S: Verapamil inhibits cyclosporine metabolism. Lancet 1:1262–1263, 1987.
99. Maggio TG, Bartels DW: Increased cyclosporine blood concentrations due to verapamil administration. Drug Intell Clin Pharm 22:705–707, 1988.
100. Peterson JC, Brannigan J, Pickard T, et al: Cyclosporine-verapamil interaction. Kidney Int 33:449, 1988.
101. Sabate I, Grino J, Castelao AM, Ortola J: Evaluation of cyclosporine-verapamil interaction with observations on parent cyclosporine and metabolites. Clin Chem 34:2151, 1988.
102. Henricsson S, Lindholm A: Inhibition of cyclosporine metabolism by other drugs in vitro. Transplant Proc 20:569–571, 1988.
103. Propper DJ, Whiting PH, Power DA, et al: The effect of nifedipine on graft function in renal allograft recipients treated with cyclosporine A. Clin Nephrol 32:62–67, 1989.
104. Vernillet L, Bourbigot B, Codet JP, et al: Lack of effect of isradipine on cyclosporine pharmacokinetics. Fundament Clin Pharmacol 63:367–374, 1992.
105. Grezard O, Sharobeem R, Al Najjar A, et al: Effect of amlodipine on cyclosporin pharmacokinetics. Am J Hypertens 6(5)Part 2:92A, 1993.
106. Copur MS, Tasdemir I, Turgan C, et al: Effects of nitrendipine on blood pressure and blood cyclosporine A level in patients with post-transplant hypertension. Nephron 52:227–230, 1989.
107. Butman SM, Wild JC, Nolan PE, et al: Prospective study of the safety and financial benefit of ketoconazole as adjunctive therapy to cyclosporine after heart transplantation. J Heart Lung Transplant 10(3):351–358, 1991.
108. First MR, Schroeder TJ, Michael A, et al: Cyclosporine-ketoconazole interaction: Long-term follow-up and preliminary results of a randomized trial. Transplantation 55:1000–1004, 1993.
109. Deray G, LeHoang P, Cacoub P, et al: Oral contraceptive interaction with cyclosporine. Lancet 1:158–159, 1987.
110. Ross WB, Roberts D, Griffin PJA, Salaman JR: Cyclosporine interaction with danazol and norethisterone. Lancet 1:330, 1986.
111. Watkins PB: The role of cytochrome P450 in cyclosporine metabolism. J Am Acad Dermatol 23:1301–1311, 1990.

112. Albengres E, Tillement JP: Cyclosporin and ketoconazole, drug interaction or therapeutic association? Int J Clin Pharmacol Ther Toxicol 30(12):555–570, 1992.
113. Gueco IP, Tan-Torres T, Baniga U, Alano F: Ketoconazole in posttransplant triple therapy: Comparison of costs and outcomes. Transplant Proc 24(5):1709–1714, 1992.
114. Bourge RC, Kirklin JK, Naftel DC, et al: Diltiazem-cyclosporine interaction in cardiac transplant recipients: Impact on cyclosporine dose and medication costs. Am J Med 90(3):402–494, 1991.
115. Neumayer HH, Wagner K: Diltiazem and economic use of cyclosporine. Lancet 2:523, 1986.
116. Valantine H, Keogh A, McIntosh N, et al: Cost containment: Coadministration of Diltiazem with cyclosporine after heart transplantation. J Heart Lung Transplant 11:1–8, 1992.
117. Patton PR, Brunson ME, Pfaff WW, et al: A preliminary report of diltiazem and ketoconazole. Transplantation 57:889–892, 1994.
118. Randall T: Cyclosporine-ketoconazole combination offers promise in reducing antirejection therapy costs. JAMA 264(4):430–431, 1990.
119. Becerra E, Torres H, Gonzalez R, et al: Two-year follow-up of a heart transplant patient being treated with cyclosporine and ketoconazole. J Heart Lung Transplant 12(2):338, 1993.
120. Girardet RE, Melo JC, Fox MS, et al: Concomitant administration of cyclosporine and ketoconazole for three and a half years in one heart transplant recipient. Transplantation 48(5):887–890, 1989.
121. Karlix JL, Cheng MA, Brunson ME: Decreased cyclosporine concentrations with the addition of an H_2-receptor antagonist in a patient on ketoconazole. Transplant 56(6):1554–1555, 1993.
122. Van Der Meer JW, Keuning JJ, Scheijgrong HW, et al: The influence of gastric acidity on the bioavailability of ketoconazole. J Antimicrob Chemother 6:552–554, 1993.
123. Freeman DJ, Laupacis A, Keown PA, et al: Evaluation of cyclosporine-phenytoin interaction with observations on cyclosporine metabolites. Br J Clin Pharmacol 18:887–893, 1984.
124. Keown P, Stiller CR, Laupacis AL, et al: The effects and side effects of cyclosporine A relationship to drug pharmacokinetics. Transplant Proc 14(4):659–661, 1982.
125. Keown PA, Laupacis A, Carruthers G, et al: Interaction between phenytoin and cyclosporine following organ transplantation. Transplantation 38(3):304–306, 1984.
126. Carstensen H, Jacobsen N, Dieperink H: Interaction between cyclosporine A and phenobarbitone. Br J Clin Pharmacol 21:550–551, 1986.
127. Wideman CA: Pharmacokinetic monitoring of cyclosporine. Transplant Proc 15:3168–3175, 1983.
128. Hillebrand G, Castro LA, van Scheidt W, et al: Valproate for epilepsy in renal transplant recipients receiving cyclosporine. Transplantation 43(6):915–916, 1987.
129. Lele P, Peterson P, Yang S, et al: Cyclosporine and Tegretol—Another drug interaction. Kidney Int 27:344, 1985.
130. Klintmalm G, Sawe J, Ringden O, et al: Cyclosporine plasma levels in renal transplant patients. Transplantation 39:132–137, 1985.
131. Allen RD, Hunnisett AG, Morris PJ: Cyclosporine and rifampicin in renal transplantation. Lancet 1:980, 1985.
132. Cassidy MJD, Van Zyl-Smit R, Pascoe MD, et al: Effects of rifampicin on cyclosporine A blood levels in a renal transplant recipient. Nephron 41:207–208, 1985.
133. Coward RA, Raftery AT, Brown CB: Cyclosporine and antituberculous therapy. Lancet 1:1342–1343, 1985.
134. Howard P, Bixler TJ, Gill B: Cyclosporine-rifampicin drug interaction. Drug Intell Clin Pharm 19:763–764, 1985.
135. Langhoff E, Madsen S: Rapid metabolism of cyclosporine and prednisone in kidney transplant patient receiving tuberculostatic treatment. lancet 2:1303, 1983.
136. Jones DK, Hakim M, Wallwork J, et al: Serious interaction between cyclosporine A and sulphadimidine. Br Med J 292:728–729, 1986.
137. Wallwork J, McGreggor CG, Wells FC, et al: Cyclosporine and intravenous sulphadimidine and trimethoprim therapy. Lancet 1:366–367, 1983.
138. Veremis SA, Maddux MS, Pollak R, Mozes MF: Subtherapeutic cyclosporine concentrations during nafcillin therapy. Transplantation 43:913–915, 1987.
139. Tobert JA: To the editor. N Engl J Med 318:48, 1988.
140. Ballantyne CM, Radovancevic B, Farmer JA, et al: Hyperlipidemia after heart transplantation: Report of a 6-year experience, with treatment recommendations. J Am Coll Cardiol 19(6):1315–1321, 1992.
141. Reaven P, Witztum JL: Lovastatin, nicotinic acid, and rhabdomyolysis. Ann Intern Med 109:597–598, 1988.
142. Ayanian JZ, Fuchs CS, Stone RM: Lovastatin and rhabdomyolysis. Ann Intern Med 109:682–683, 1988.
143. Corpier CL, Jones PH, Suki WN, et al: Rhabdomyolysis and renal injury with lovastatin use; report of two cases in cardiac recipients. JAMA 260:239–241, 1988.'
144. de Alava E, Sola JJ, Lozano MD, Pardo-Mindan FJ: Rhabdomyolysis and acute renal failure in a heart transplant recipient treated with hypolipemiants. Nephron 66(2):242–243, 1994.

145. East C, Alivizatos PA, Grundy SM, et al: Rhabdomyolysis in patients receiving lovastatin after cardiac transplantation. N Engl J Med 318(1):47–48, 1988.
146. Norman DJ, Illingworth DR, Munson J, Hosenpud J: Myolysis and acute renal failure in a heart-transplant recipient receiving lovastatin. N Engl J Med 318:46, 1988.
147. Marais GE, Larson KK: Rhabdomyolysis and acute renal failure induced by combination lovastatin and gemfibrozil therapy. Ann Int Med 112:228–230, 1990.
148. Pierce LR, Wysowski DK, Gross TP: Myopathy and rhabdomyolysis associated with lovastatin-gemfibrozil combination therapy. JAMA 264:71–75, 1990.
149. Wirebaugh SR, Shapiro ML, McIntyre TH, Whitney EJ: A retrospective review of the use of lipid-lowering agents in combination, specifically gemfibrozil and lovastatin. Pharmacotherapy 12(6):445–450, 1992.
150. Kuo PC, Kirshenbaum JM, Gordon J, et al: Lovastatin therapy for hypercholesterolemia in cardiac transplant recipients. Am J Cardiol 64:631–536, 1989.
151. Kobashigawa JA, Murphy FL, Stevenson LW, et al: Low-dose lovastatin safely lowers cholesterol after cardiac transplantation. Circulation 82:281–283, 1990.
152. Cheung AK, DeVault GA Jr, Gregory MC: A prospective study on treatment of hypercholesterolemia with lovastatin in renal transplant patients receiving cyclosporine. J Am Soc Nephrol 3(12):1884–1891, 1993.
153. Barbir M, Rose M, Kushwaha S, et al: Low-dose simvastatin for the treatment of hypercholesterolemia in recipients of cardiac transplantation. Int J Cardiology 33:241–246, 1991.
154. Castelao AM, Grino JM, Andres E, et al: HMGCoA reductase inhibitors lovastatin and simvastatin in the treatment of hypercholesterolemia after renal transplantation. Transplant Proc 25(1 Pt 2):1043–1046, 1993.
155. Wiklund O, Angelin B, Bergman M, et al: Pravastatin and gemfibrozil alone and in combination for the treatment of hypercholesterolemia. Am J Med 94:13–20, 1993.
156. Arnadottir M, Eriksson LO, Thysell H, Karkas JD: Plasma concentration profiles of simvastatin 3-hydroxy-3-methyl-glutaryl-coenzyme A reductase inhibitory activity in kidney transplant recipients with and without cyclosporin. Nephron 65(3):410–413, 1993.
157. Regazzi MB, Iacona I, Campana C, et al: Altered disposition of pravastatin following concomitant drug therapy with cyclosporin A in transplant recipients. Transplant Proc 25(4):2732-2733, 1993.
158. Blaison G, Weber JC, Sachs D, et al: Rhabdomyolysis caused by simvastatin in a patient following heart transplantation and cyclosporine therapy. Rev Med Interne 13(1):61–63, 1992.
159. Vanhaecke J, Cleemput JV, Lierde JV, et al: Safety and efficacy of low dose simvastatin in cardiac transplant recipients treated with cyclosporine. Transplantation 58:42–45, 1994.
160. Bennett WM, Pulliam JP: Cyclosporine nephrotoxicity. Ann Intern Med 99:851–854, 1983.
161. Greenberg A, Thompson ME, Griffith BJ, et al: Cyclosporine nephrotoxicity in cardiac allograft patients—a seven-year follow-up. Transplantation 50:589–593, 1990.
162. Hows JM, Chipping PM, Fairhead S, et al: Nephrotoxicity in bone marrow transplant recipients treated with cyclosporin A. Br J Haematol 54:69–78, 1983.
163. Whiting PH, Simpson JG, Thomson AW: Nephrotoxicity of cyclosporine in combination with aminoglycoside and cephalosporin antibiotics. Transplant Proc 15:2702–2705, 1983.
164. Whiting PH, Simpson JG, Davidson RJ, Thomson AW: The toxic effects of combined administration of cyclosporine A and gentamicin. Br J Exp Pathol 63:554–561, 1982.
165. Kennedy MS, Deeg MJ, Siegel M, et al: Acute renal toxicity with combined use of amphotericin B and cyclosporine after marrow transplantation. Transplantation 35(3):211–215, 1983.
166. Erice A, Jordan MC, Chace BA, et al: Ganciclovir treatment of cytomegalovirus disease in transplant recipients and other immunocompromised hosts. JAMA 257(22):P3082–3087, 1989.
167. Deray G, LeHoang P, Aupetit B, et al: Enhancement of cyclosporine A nephrotoxicity by diclofenac. Clin Nephrol 27(4):213–214, 1987.
168. Johnson AG, Seidemann P, Day RO: NSAID-related adverse drug interactions with clinical relevance. Int J Clin Pharmacol Ther 32(10):509–532, 1994.
169. Sesin GP, O'Keefe E, Roberto P: Sulindac-induced elevation of serum cyclosporine concentration. Clin Pharm 8:445, 1989.
170. Whiting PH, Burke MD, Thomson AW: Drug interactions with cyclosporine: Implications from animal studies. Transplant Proc 18:56–70, 1986.
171. Dale BM, Sage RE, Norman JE, et al: Bone marrow transplantation following treatment with high-dose melphalan. Transplant Proc 17:1711–1713, 1985.
172. Brunner FP, Hermle M, Mihatsch MJ, Thiel G: Mannitol potentiates cyclosporine nephrotoxicity. Clin Nephrol 25:S130–S136, 1986.
173. Christensen P, Leski M: Nephrotoxic drug interaction between metolazone and cyclosporine. Br Med J 294:578, 1987.
174. Pachon J, Lorber MI, Bia MJ: Effects of H_2-receptor antagonists on renal function in cyclosporine-treated renal transplant patients. Transplantation 47:254–259, 1989.

175. Whiting PH, Cunningham C, Thomson AW, Simpson JG: Enhancement of high dose cyclosporine A toxicity by furosemide. Biochem Pharmacol 33(7):1075–1079, 1984.
176. McNally PG, Feehally J: Pathophysiology of cyclosporin A nephrotoxicity: Experimental and clinical observations. Nephrol Dial Transplant 7(8):791–804, 1992.
177. Myers BD, Sibley R, Newton L, et al: The long-term course of cyclosporine-associated chronic nephropathy. Kidney Int 33:590–600, 1988.
178. Nagineni CD, Misra BC, Lee DB, Yanagawa N: Cyclosporine A—calcium channels interaction: A possible mechanism for nephrotoxicity. Transplant Proc 19:1358–1362, 1987.
179. Sturrock ND, Struthers AD: Hormonal and other mechanisms involved in the pathogenesis of cyclosporin-induced nephrotoxicity and hypertension in man. Clin Sci 86(1):1–9, 1994.
180. Curtis JJ, Laskow D, Jones P, et al: Captopril-induced fall in glomerular filtration rate in cyclosporine-treated hypertensive patients. J Am Soc Nephrol 9(3):1570–1574, 1993.
181. Adams MB, the Enisoprost Renal Transplant Study Group: Enisoprost in renal transplantation. Transplantation 53(2):338–345, 1992.
182. Curtis LD, Anwar N, Briggs JD, et al: Misoprostol in renal transplantation. Transplant Proc 25(1):603, 1993.
183. Makowka L, Lopatin W, Gilas T, et al: Prevention of cyclosporine nephrotoxicity by synthetic prostaglandins. Clin Nephrol 25:S89–S94, 1986.
184. Moran M, Mozes MF, Maddux MS, et al.: Prevention of acute graft rejection by the prostaglandin E_1 analogue misoprostol in renal-transplant recipients treated with cyclosporine and prednisone. N Engl J Med 322(17):1183–1188, 1990.
185. Bennett WM, Elzinga LW, Porter GA, Rosen S: The effects of pentoxifylline on experimental chronic cyclosporine nephrotoxicity. Transplantation 54(6):1118–1120, 1992.
186. Markewitz A, Hammer C, Pfeiffer M, et al: Reduction of cyclosporine-induced nephrotoxicity by cilastatin following clinical heart transplantation. Transplantation 57(6):865–870, 1994.
187. Mraz W, Sido B, Knedel M, Hammer C: Concomitant immunosuppressive and antibiotic therapy— Reduction of cyclosporine A blood levels due to treatment with imipenem/cilastatin. Transplant Proc 19:4017–4020, 1987.
188. Hummel M, Hetzer R, et al: Urodilatin, a new therapy to prevent kidney failure after heart transplantation. J Heart Transplant 12:209–218, 1993.
189. Driscoll DF, Pinson CW, Jenkins RL, Bistrian BR: Potential protective effects of furosemide against early cyclosporine-induced renal injury in hepatic transplant recipients. Transplant Proc 21:3549–3550, 1989.
190. Menta R, Rossi E, Guariglia A, et al: Reversible acute cyclosporine nephrotoxicity induced by colchicine administration. Nephrol Dial Transplant 2:380-381, 1987.
191. Murray BM, Paller MS: Beneficial effects of renal denervation and prazosin on GFR and renal blood flow after cyclosporine in rats. Clin Nephrol 25:S37–S39, 1986.
192. Petric R, Freeman D, Wallace C, et al: Amelioration of experimental cyclosporine nephrotoxicity by calcium channel inhibition. Transplantation 54(6):1103–1106, 1992.
193. Rodicio JL, Morales JM, Ruilope LM: Lipophilic dihydropyridines provide renal protection from cyclosporin toxicity. J Hypertens 11(Suppl 6):S21–S25, 1993.
194. Dawidson I, Rooth P, Fry WR, et al: Prevention of acute cyclosporine-induced renal blood flow inhibition and improved immunosuppression with verapamil. Transplantation 48(4):575–580, 1989.
195. Dawidson I, Rooth P, Alway C: Verapamil prevents posttransplant delayed function and cyclosporine A nephrotoxicity. Transplant Proc 22(4):1379–1380, 1990.
196. Chrysostomou A, Walker R, Graeme R, et al: Diltiazem in renal allograft recipients receiving cyclosporine. Transplantation 55(2):300–304, 1993.
197. Frei U, Margreiter A, Harms A, et al: Preoperative graft reperfusion with a calcium antagonist improves initial function: Preliminary results of a prospective randomized trial in 110 kidney recipients. Transplant Proc 19(5):3539–3541, 1987.
198. Morales JM, Andres A, Alvarez C, et al: Calcium channel blockers and early cyclosporine nephrotoxicity after renal transplantation: A prospective randomized study. Transplant Proc 22(4):1733–1735, 1990.
199. Oppenheimer R, Alcaraz M, Manalich A, et al: Influence of the calcium blocker diltiazem on the prevention of acute renal failure after renal transplantation. Transplant Proc 24(1):50–51, 1992.
200. Pedersen EB, Sorensen SS, Eiskjaer H, et al: Interaction between cyclosporine and felodipine in renal transplant recipients. Kidney Int 36:S82–S86, 1992.
201. Morales JM, Andres A, Rodriguez P: Calcium antagonist therapy prevents chronic cyclosporine nephrotoxicity after renal transplantation: A prospective study. Transplant proc 24(1):89–91, 1992.
202. Berg KJ, Holdaas H, Endresen L, et al: Effects of isradipine on renal function in cyclosporin-treated renal transplanted patients. Nephrol Dial Transplant 6:725–730, 1991.
203. McCrea J, Francos G, Burke J, et al: The beneficial effects of isradipine on renal hemodynamics in cyclosporine-treated renal transplant recipients. Transplantation 55(3):672–674, 1993.

204. Watschinger B, Ulrich W, Vychytil A, et al: Cyclosporine A toxicity is associated with reduced endothelin immunoreactivity in renal endothelium. Transplant Proc 24(6):2618–2619, 1992.
205. Epstein M: Calcium antagonists and the kidney. Implications for renal protection. Am J Hypertens 6(7 Pt2):251S–59S, 1993.
206. Berglund F, Killander J, Pompeius R: Effect of trimethoprim-sulfamethoxazole on the renal excretion of creatinine in man. J Urol 114:802–808, 1975.
207. Myre SA, McCann J, First MR, Cluxton RJ: Effect of trimethoprim on serum creatinine in healthy and chronic renal failure volunteers. Ther Drug Monit 9:161, 1987.
208. Thompson JF, Chalmers DH, Hunnisett AG, et al: Nephrotoxicity of trimethoprim and cotrimoxazole in renal allograft recipients treated with cyclosporine. Transplantation 36:204–206, 1983.
209. Nanni G, Magalini SC, Serino F, Castagneto M: Effect of disopyramide in a cyclosporine-treated patient. Transplantation 45:257, 1988.
210. Zazgornik J, Schindler J, Gremmel F, et al: Ranitidine does not influence cyclosporine levels in renal transplant patients. Kidney Int 28:401, 1985.
211. June CH, Thompson CB, Kennedy MS, et al: Correlation of hypomagnesemia with the onset of cyclosporine associated with hypertension in marrow transplant patients. Transplantation 41:477–451, 1986.
212. Miller LW: Long-term complications of cardiac transplantation. Prog Cardiovasc Dis 33(4):229–282, 1991.
213. Lake KD: Management of post-transplant obesity and hyperlipidemia. In Emery RW, Miller LW: Handbook of Cardiac Transplantation. Philadelphia, Hanley & Belfus, 1995.
214. Butler RT, Kalkwarf KL, Kaldahl WB: Drug induced gingival hyperplasia: Phenytoin, cyclosporine and nifedipine. J Am Dent Assoc 114:56–60, 1987.
215. King GN, Gullinfaw R, Higgins TJ, et al: Gingival hyperplasia in renal allograft recipients receiving cyclosporin-A and calcium antagonists. J Clin Periodontol 20(4):213–214, 1992.
216. Tam IM, Wandres DL: Calcium-channel blockers and gingival hyperplasia. Ann Pharmacother 26(2):213–214, 1992.
217. MacCarthy D, Claffey N: Fibrous hyperplasia of the gingiva in organ transplant patients. J Ir Dent Assoc 37(1):3–5, 1991.
218. Seymour RA, Jacobs DJ: Cyclosporin and the gingival tissues. J Clin Periodont 19(1):1–11, 1992.
219. Barclay S, Thomason JM, Idle JR, Seymour RA: The incidence and severity of nifedipine-induced gingival overgrowth. J Clin Periodontol 19(5):311–314, 1992.
220. Brown RS, Sein P, Corio R, Bottomley WK: Nitrendipine-induced gingival hyperplasia. Oral Surg Oral Med Oral Path 70(5):593–596, 1990.
221. Fattore L, Stablein M, Bredfeldt G, et al: Gingival hyperplasia: A side effect of nifedipine and diltiazem. Special Care Dentistry 11(3):107–109, 1991.
222. Lombardi T, Fiore-Donno G, Belser U, DiFelice R: Felodipine-induced gingival hyperplasia: A clinical and histologic study. J Oral Pathol Med 20(2):89–92, 1991.
223. Miller CS, Damm DD: Incidence of verapamil-induced gingival hyperplasia in a dental population. J Periodontol 63(5):453–456, 1992.
224. DeCamargo PM: Cyclosporin- and nifedipine-induced gingival enlargement: An overview. J West Soc Periodontol—Periodontal Abstr 37(2):57–64, 1989.
225. Slavin J, Taylor J: Cyclosporine, nifedipine, and gingival hyperplasia. Lancet 2:739, 1987.
226. Thomason JM, Seymour RA, Rice N: The prevalence and severity of cyclosporin and nifedipine-induced gingival overgrowth. J Clin Periodontal 20(1):37–40, 1993.
227. Modeer T, Wondimu B, Larsson E, Jonzon B: Levels of cyclosporin-A (CsA) in saliva in children after oral administration of the drug in mixture or in capsule form. Scand J Dent Res 100(6):366–370, 1992.
228. Wong W, Hodge MG, Lewis A, et al: Resolution of cyclosporin-induced gingival hypertrophy with metronidazole. Lancet 343(8903):986, 1994.
229. Peters DH, Fitton A, Plosker GL, Faulds D: Tacrolimus—A review of its pharmacology, and therapeutic potential in hepatic and renal transplantation. Drugs 46(4):746–794, 1993.
230. Christians U, Guengerich FP, Schmidt G, Sewing KF: In-vitro metabolism of FK506, cytochrome P450 and drug interactions. Ther Drug Monit 15(2):145, 1993.
231. Christians U, Braun F, Sattler M, et al: Interactions of FK506 and cyclosporine metabolism. Transplant Proc 23(6):2794–2796, 1991.
232. Pichard L, Fabre I, Domergue H, et al: Effect of FK506 on human hepatic cytochromes P-450: Interaction with CyA. Transplant Proc 23(6):2791–2793, 1991.
233. Sattler M, Guengerich FP, Yun CH, et al: Cytochrome P-450 3A enzymes are responsible for biotransformation of FK 506 and rapamycin in man and rat. Drug Metab Disp 20(5):753–761, 1992.
234. Shah AI, Whiting PH, Omar G, et al: Effects of FK506 on human hepatic microsomal cytochrome P450-dependent drug metabolism in vitro. Transplant Proc 23:2783–2785, 1991.
235. Stiff DD, Venkataramanan R, Prasad TN: Metabolism of FK 506 in differentially induced rat liver microsomes. Res Com Chem Pathol Pharmacol 78(1):121–124, 1992.

236. Vincent SH, Karanam BV, Painter SK, Chiu SHL: In vitro metabolism of FK-506 in rat, rabbit, and human liver microsomes; identification of a major metabolite and of cytochrome P450 3A as the major enzymes responsible for its metabolism. Arch Biochem Biophys 294:454–460, 1992.

237. Shaeffer MS, Collier D, Sorrell MF: Interaction between FK506 and erythromycin. Ann Pharmacother 28:280–281, 1994.

238. Manez R, Martin M, Venkataramanan R, et al: Fluconazole therapy in transplant recipients receiving FK506. Transplantation 47(10):1521–1523, 1994.

239. Venkataramanan R, Jain A, Warty VS, et al: Pharmacokinetics of FK506 in transplant patients. Transplant Proc 23(6):2736–2740, 1991.

240. Mieles L, Venkataramanan R, Yokoyama I, et al: Interaction between FK506 and clotrimazole in a liver transplant recipient. Transplantation 52(6):1086–1087, 1991.

241. Shapiro R, Venkataramanan R, Warty VS, et al: FK506 interaction with danazol. Lancet 341(8856):1344–1345, 1993.

242. Zeevi A, Eiras G, Burckart G, et al: Bioassay of plasma specimens from liver transplant patients on FK506 immunosuppression. Transplant Proc 22(1):60–63, 1990.

243. Jain AB, Venkataramanan R, Fung J, et al: Pharmacokinetics of cyclosporine and nephrotoxicity in orthotopic liver transplant patients rescued with FK506. Transplant Proc 23(6):2777–2779, 1991.

244. Steeves M, Abdallah HY, Venkataramanan R, et al: In-vitro interaction of a novel immunosuppressant, FK506, and antacids. J Pharm Pharmacol 43(8):574–577, 1991.

245. McDiarmid SV, Colonna JO, Shaked A, et al: Differences in oral FK506 dose requirements between adult and pediatric liver transplant patients. Transplantation 556):1328–1332, 1993.

246. Venkataramanan R, Warty VS: Pharmacokinetics and monitoring of FK506 (tacrolimus). In Thomson AW, Starzl TE (eds): Immunosuppressive Drugs: Developments in Anti-Rejection Therapy. Boston, Little, Brown, 1994, pp 83–94.

247. Rui X, Flowers J, Warty VS, Venkataramanan R: Drug interactions with FK506. Pharm Res 9:314, 1992.

248. Iwasaki K, Matsuda H, Nagase K, et al: Effects of twenty-three drugs on the metabolism of FK506 by human liver microsomes. Res Commun Chem Pathol Pharmacol 82(2):209–216, 1993.

249. Venkataramanan R, Jain A, Cadoff E, et al: Pharmacokinetics of FK506: Preclinical and clinical studies. Transplant Proc 22:52–56, 1990.

250. Starzl TE, Todo S, Fung J, et al: FK506 for liver, kidney, and pancreas transplantation. Lancet 2(8670):1000–1004, 1989.

251. Wu YM, Venkataramanan R, Suzuki M, et al: Interaction between FK506 and cyclosporine in dogs. Transplant Proc 23(6):2797–2799, 1991.

252. Zeevi A., Duquesnoy R, Eiras G, et al: Immunosuppressive effect of FK-506 on in vitro lymphocyte alloactivation: Synergism with cyclosporine A. Transplant Proc 19(5 Suppl 6):40–44, 1987.

253. McCauley J: The nephrotoxicity of FK506 as compared with cyclosporine. Nephrol Hypertension 2:662–669, 1993.

254. Honig PK, Woosley RL, Zamani K, et al: Changes in the pharmacokinetics and electrocardiographic pharmacodynamics of terfenadine with concomitant administration of erythromycin. Clin Pharmacol Ther 52(3):231–238, 1992.

255. Ludden TM: Pharmacokinetic interactions of the macrolide antibiotics. Clin Pharmacokinet 10(1):63–79, 1985.

256. Henry DA, MacDonald IA, Kitchingman G, et al: Cimetidine and ranitidine: Comparison of effects on hepatic drug metabolism. Br Med J 281:775, 1980.

257. Sorkin EM, Darvey DL: A review of cimetidine drug interactions. Drug Intell Clin Pharm 17:110–120, 1983.

258. Martin MF: Nephrotoxic effects of immunosuppression. Mayo Clin Proc 69:191–192, 1994.

259. Porayko MK, Textor SC, Krom RA, et al: Nephrotoxic effects of primary immunosuppression with FK-506 and cyclosporine regimens after liver transplantation. Mayo Clin Proc 69(2):105–111, 1994.

260. Sheiner PA, Mor E, Chodoff L, et al: Acute renal failure associated with the use of ibuprofen in two liver transplant recipients on FK506. Transplantation 57:1132–1133, 1994.

261. McCauley J, Takaya S, Fung J, et al: The question of FK506 nephrotoxicity after liver transplantation. Transplant Proc 23(1 Pt 2):1444–1447, 1991.

252. Jain AB, Fung JJ, Venkataramanan R, et al: FK506 dosage in human organ transplantation. Transplant Proc 22(1, Suppl 1):23–24, 1990.

263. Brooks RJ, Dorr RT, Durie BGM: Interaction of allopurinol with 6-mercaptopurine and azathioprine. Biomedicine 36:217–222, 1983.

264. Venkat Raman G, Sharman VL, Lee HA: Azathioprine and allopurinol: A potentially dangerous combination. J Int Med 228:69, 1990.

265. Chan GL, Canafax DM, Johnson CA: The therapeutic use of azathioprine in renal transplantation. Pharmacotherapy 7(5):165, 1987.

266. Ding TL, Gamberatoglio JG, Amend WJC, et al: Azathioprine (AZA) bioavailability and pharmacokinetics in kidney transplant patients. Clin Pharmacol Ther 27(2):250, 1980.
267. Boekenoogen SJ, Szefler SJ, Jusko WJ: Prednisolone disposition and protein binding in oral contraceptive users. J Clin Endocrinol Metab 56:702, 1983.
268. Kozower M, Veatch L, Kaplan MM: Decreased clearance of prednisolone, a factor in the development of corticosteroid side effects. J Clin Endocrinol Metab 38:407, 1974.
269. Jubiz W, Meikle AW: Alterations of glucocorticoid actions by other drugs and disease states. Drugs 12:113, 1979.
270. Langhoff E, Madsen S, Flachs H, et al: Inhibition of prednisolone metabolism by cyclosporine in kidney transplanted patients. Transplantation 39(1):107–109, 1985.
271. Ost L: Impairment of prednisolone metabolism by cyclosporine treatment in renal graft recipients. Transplantation 44:533–535, 1987.
272. Ost L: Effects of cyclosporine on prednisolone metabolism. Lancet 1:451, 1984.
273. Kandrotas RJ, Slaughter RL, Brass C, Jusko WJ: Ketoconazole effects on methylprednisolone disposition and their joint suppression of endogenous cortisol. Clin Pharmacol Ther 42(4):465–470, 1987.
274. Glynn AM, Slaughter RL, Brass C, et al: Effects of ketoconazole on methylprednisolone pharmacokinetics and cortisol secretion. Clin Pharmacol Ther 39:645, 1989.
275. Yamashita SK, Ludwig EA, Middleton E, Jusko WJ: Lack of pharmacokinetic and pharmacodynamic interactions between ketoconazole and prednisolone. Clin Pharmacol Ther 49:55, 1991.
276. Zurcher RM, Frey BM, Frey FJ: Impact of ketoconazole on the metabolism of prednisolone. Clin Pharmacol Ther 45:366, 1989.
277. Buffington GA, Dominguez JH, Piering WF, et al: Interaction of rifampin and glucocorticoids—Adverse effect on renal allograft function. JAMA 236(17):1958–1960, 1976.
278. McAllister WAC, Thompson MJ, Al-Habet SM, Rogers HJ: Rifampicin reduces effectiveness and bioavailability of prednisolone. Br Med J 286(6369):923–925, 1983.
279. Eradiri O, Jamili F, Thomson A: Interaction of metronidazole with phenobarbital, cimetidine, prednisone and sulfasalazine in Crohn's disease. Biopharm Drug Disp 9:219, 1988.
280. Graham GG, Champion GD, Day RO, Paull PD: Patterns of plasma concentrations and urinary excretion of salicylate in rheumatoid arthritis. Clin Pharmacol Ther 22(4):410–420, 1977.
281. Laflin MJ: Interaction of pancuronium and corticosteroids. Anesthesiology 47:471, 1977.
282. Vetten KB: Immunosuppressive therapy and anesthesia. S Afr Med J 47:767, 1973.
283. Dretchen KL, Morgenroth III VH, Standaert FG, Walts LF: Azathioprine: Effects on neuromuscular transmission. Anesthesiology 45(6):604–609, 1976.
284. Spiers ASD, Mibashan PS: Increased warfarin requirement during mercaptopurine therapy: A new drug interaction. Lancet 2:221, 1974.
285. Amacher DE, Schomaker SJ, Retsema JA: Comparison of the effects of the new azalide antibiotic, azithromycin, and erythromycin estolate on rat liver cytochrome P-450. Antimicrob Agents Chemother 35(6):1186–1190, 1991.
286. Guillemain R, Billaud E, Dreyfus G, et al: The effects of spiramycin on plasma cyclosporine A concentrations in heart transplant patients. Eur J Clin Pharmacol 36:97–98, 1989.
287. Kessler M, Netter P, Zerrouki M, et al: Spiramycin does not increase plasma cyclosporine concentrations in renal transplant patients. Eur J Clin Pharmacol 35:331–332, 1988.
288. Vernillet L, Bertault-Peres P, Bertand Y, et al: Lack of effect of spiramycin on cyclosporine pharmacokinetics. Br J Clin Pharmacol 27:789–794, 1989.
289. Baciewicz AM, Baciewicz FA: Ketoconazole and fluconazole drug interactions. Arch Intern Med 153:1970–1976, 1993.
290. Back DJ, Tjia JF: Inhibition of tolbutamide metabolism by substituted imidazole drugs in vivo. Br J Pharmacol 85:121–126, 1985.
291. Carver PL, Berardi RR, Knapp MJ, et al: In vivo interaction of ketoconazole and sucralfate in healthy volunteers. Antimicrob Agents Chemother 38(2):326–329, 1994.
292. Blum RA, D'Andrea DT, Florentino BM, et al: Increased gastric pH and the bioavailability of fluconazole and ketoconazole. Ann Intern Med 114(9):755–757, 1991.
293. Piscitelli SC, Goss TF, Wilton JH, et al: Effects of ranitidine and sucralfate on ketoconazole bioavailability. Antimicrob Agents Chemother 35(9):1765–1771, 1991.
294. Smith AG: Potentiation of oral anticoagulants by ketoconazole. Br Med J 28(6412):188–189, 1984.
295. Daneshmend TK, Warnock DW, Ene MD, et al: The influence of food on the pharmacokinetics of ketoconazole. Antimicrob Agents Chemother 25:1–3, 1984.
296. Daneshmend TK: Disease and drugs but not food decreases ketoconazole "bioavailability." Br J Pharm 29:783–784, 1990.
297. Mannisto PT, et al: Impaired effects of food on ketoconazole absorption. Antimicrob Agents Chemother 21:730–733, 1982.
298. Craven PC: Interaction of ketoconazole with rifampin and isoniazid. N Engl J Med 312:1061, 1983.

299. Englehard D, Stutman HR, Marks MI: Interaction of ketoconazole with rifampin and isoniazid. N Engl J Med 311:1681–1683, 1984.
300. McNulty RM, Lazor JA, Sketch M: Transient increases in plasma quinidine concentrations during ketoconazole-quinidine therapy. Clin Pharm 8(3):222–225, 1989.
301. Heusner JJ, Dukes GE, Rollins DE, et al: Effects of chronically administered ketoconazole on the elimination of theophylline in man. Drug Intell Clin Pharm 21(6):514–517, 1987.
302. Hoey LL, Lake KD: Does ciprofloxacin interact with cyclosporine? Ann Pharmacother 28(1):93–96, 1994.
303. Lang J, de Villaine JF, Garraffo R, Touraine JL: Cyclosporine (cyclosporine A) pharmacokinetics of renal transplant patients receiving ciprofloxacin. Am J Med (Suppl 5A):82S–85S, 1989.
304. Tan KC, Trull AK, Shawket S: Co-administration of ciprofloxacin and cyclosporine: Lack of evidence for a pharmacokinetic interaction. Br J Clin Pharmacol 28:185–187, 1989.
305. Robinson JA, Venezio FR, Costanzo-Nordin MR, et al: Patients receiving quinolones and cyclosporine after heart transplantation. J Heart Transplant 9:30–31, 1990.
306. Zazgornik J, Schein W, Heimberger K, et al: Potentiation of neurotoxic side effects by coadministration of imipenem to cyclosporine therapy in kidney transplant recipient—Synergism of side effects or drug interaction. Clin Nephrol 26:265–266, 1986.
307. Anderson JE, Blaschke TF: Ketoconazole inhibits cyclosporine metabolism in vivo in mice. J Pharmacol Exp Ther 236:671–674, 1986.
308. Thomson DJ, Menkis AG, McKenzie FN: Norfloxacin-cyclosporine interaction. Transplantation 46:312–313, 1988.
309. Kahan BD: Individualization of cyclosporine therapy using pharmacokinetic and pharmacodynamic parameters. Transplantation 40:457–476, 1985.
310. Piepho RW, Bloedow DC, Lacz JP, et al: Pharmacokinetics of diltiazem in selected animal species and human beings. Am J Cardiol 49:525–528, 1982.
311. Birx DL, Berger M, Fleisher TE: The interference of T cell activation by calcium channel blocking agents. J Immunol 133:2904–2909, 1984.
312. McMillen M, Tesi RJ, Baumgarten WB, et al: Potentiation of cyclosporine immunosuppression by verapamil in vitro. Transplantation 40:444–445, 1985.
313. Tesi RJ, Hong J, Butt KM, et al: In vivo potentiations of cyclosporine immunosuppression by calcium antagonists. Eleventh International Congress on Transplantation. Helsinki, 27,2, 1986.
314. Snyder DS: Interaction between cyclosporine and warfarin. Ann Intern Med 108:311, 1988.
315. Cockburn I: Cyclosporine A: A clinical evaluation of drug interactions. Transplant Proc 18:50–55, 1986.
316. Jadoul M, Hene RJ: Ranitidine and the cyclosporine-treated recipient. Transplantation 48, 359, 1989
317. Jarowenko MW, Buren CTV, Kramer WG, et al: Ranitidine, cimetidine and the cyclosporine-treated recipient. Transplantation 42:311–312, 1986.
318. Humphries TJ: Famotidine T: A notable lack of drug interactions. Scand J Gastroenterol 124:55, 1987.
319. Moller BB, Ekelund B: Toxicity of cyclosporine during treatment with androgens. N Engl J Med 312:416, 1985.
320. Maurer G: Metabolism of cyclosporine. Transplant Proc 17(4, Suppl 1):19–26, 1985.
321. Klintmalm G, Sawe J: High dose methylprednisolone increases plasma cyclosporine levels in renal transplant patients. Lancet 1:731, 1984.
322. Ptachcinski RJ, Venkataramanan R, Burckart GJ, et al: Cyclosporine—high dose steroid interaction in renal transplant recipients: Assessment by HPLC. Transplant Proc 19:1728–1729, 1987.
323. Boobaerts MA, Zachee P, Verwilghen RL: Cyclosporine, methylprednisolone, and convulsions. Lancet 2:1216–1217, 1982.
324. Durrant S, Chipping PM, Palmer S, Gordon-Smith EC: Cyclosporine A, methylprednisolone, and convulsions. Lancet 2:829, 1982.
325. Paul MD, Parfrey PS, Smart M, Gault H: The effect of ethanol on serum cyclosporine A levels in renal transplant recipients. Am J Kidney Dis 10:133–135, 1987.
326. Gramstad L, Gjerlow JA, Hysing ES, Rugstad HE: Interaction of cyclosporine and its solvent, cremophor, with atracurium and vecuronium. Studies in the cat. Br J Anaesth 58:1149–1155, 1986.
327. Kloke O, Osieka R: Interaction of cyclosporine A with antineoplastic agents. Klin Wöxhwnaxhe 52:1081–1082, 1985.
328. Cirella VN, Pantuck CB, Lee YJ, Pantuck EJ: Effects of cyclosporine on anesthetic action. Anesth Analg 66:703–706, 1987.

Chapter 19

Long-Term Complications of Transplantation

Peter R. Rickenbacher, MD
Sharon A. Hunt, MD

Many of the chronic complications seen in heart transplant patients occur as a consequence of immunosuppression or result from side effects of immunosuppressive agents. The most important of these conditions contributing to posttransplant morbidity and mortality are listed in Table 1.

The causes of death after cardiac transplantation are related to duration posttransplant[1] as shown in Figure 1. The majority of deaths during the immediate postoperative period are caused by technical or primary cardiac complications (e.g., donor preservation failure, acute right heart failure, hemorrhage). Subsequently, during the first few months after transplantation, infections and rejection are the most frequent causes of death. In recipients surviving longer than 6 months posttransplant, the risk of fatal infections or acute rejection episodes declines. Transplant coronary artery disease (sometimes referred to as chronic rejection) remains the leading cause of death after the first year posttransplant.[2-4] In addition, malignancy, most commonly lymphoproliferative disorders, accounts for about 10% of long-term mortality. The other side effects of immunosuppression listed in Table 1 contribute to significant long-term morbidity, impairment of quality of life, and disability posttransplant.

This chapter deals with prevalence, diagnosis, management, and prevention of infections, arterial hypertension, renal dysfunction, and osteoporosis as major manifestations of immunosuppression-related complications after cardiac transplantation. Furthermore, psychosocial issues, quality of life, and rehabilitation after cardiac transplantation are discussed. Transplant coronary artery disease, malignancy, hyperlipidemia, and obesity are discussed elsewhere in this book and therefore are not further evaluated.

TABLE 1.   Major Chronic Complications after Cardiac Transplantation

Related to chronic immunosuppression	Related to chronic immunosuppression *(cont.)*
General	Steroids
Infections	Osteoporosis
Malignancy	Hypertension
Cyclosporine	Obesity
Arterial hypertension	Hyperlipidemia
Renal dysfunction	Glucose intolerance
Hyperlipidemia	Sodium retention
Gingival hypertrophy	Myopathy
Hypertrichosis	Skin changes
Neurologic: tremor, headache	Cholelithiasis
Azathioprine	Not directly related to immunosuppression
Neutropenia	Rejection
Hepatic dysfunction	Transplant coronary artery disease
Pancreatitis	Nonspecific graft failure
	Tricuspid regurgitation

INFECTIONS

As a result of chronic immunosuppression with relatively nonspecific agents, infections involving a wide range of organisms are a major problem after transplantation. Although the overall incidence of infections is lower since the introduction of cyclosporine[5–7] and more sophisticated diagnostic methods, and more powerful antimicrobial agents have also become available in recent years, infections still remain the leading cause of morbidity and mortality after cardiac transplantation.[1,8] In a recent multicenter review from the Cardiac Transplant Research Database Group,[8] which included 814 patients, the incidence of serious infections was 0.5/patient during a mean follow-up period of 8.2 months posttransplant. Bacteria accounted for 47%, viruses for 41%, and fungi and protozoa for 12% of these infections. Overall mortality was 13% per infection and was highest with fungal infections (36%). An early peak of infections is generally noted during the first month posttransplant.[8–10] Nosocomial, often catheter-related, bacterial infections with staphylococci and gram-negative organisms dominate during this period. The peak hazard for fungal infections also falls within the first month. The following months are characterized by a second peak of infections caused by a variety of opportunistic organisms, the most important being cytomegalovirus, *Pneumocystis carinii, Toxoplasma gondii* and various fungi.[8,11,12] During long-term

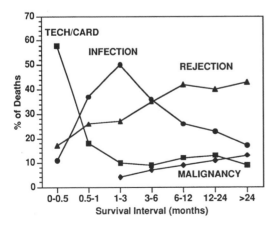

FIGURE 1.   Relationship between cause of death and survival interval in heart transplant recipients (Adapted from Kriett JM, Kaye MP, The Registry of the International Society for Heart and Lung Transplantation: Eighth official report—1991. J Heart Lung Transplant 10:491–498, 1991.)

follow-up, community-acquired bacterial infections predominate.[12] Independent of time posttransplantation, recipients are most susceptible to infectious complications after periods of augmented immunosuppression given for allograft rejection.[13] Table 2 lists some of the most common infections in transplant patients. Institutional immunosuppressive strategy and geographic local infection trends may contribute to the variable patterns of infection seen at different institutions.

Viral

Cytomegalovirus is the single most common pathogen seen after heart transplantation.[8] Infections occur by three mechanisms: primary exposure of a seronegative recipient to a seropositive allograft or blood products, reactivation of a latent virus, or reinfection with a different viral strain. Clinical presentation of cytomegalovirus infection is highly variable and can range from an asymptomatic rise in antibody titer or a mononucleosis-type febrile syndrome to life-threatening multisystem organ disease. Primary cytomegalovirus infections usually exhibit a more severe course than endogenous reactivations.[14] Laboratory methods for diagnosis of cytomegalovirus infections are currently in evolution. Rapid viral isolation, antigenemia assays, polymerase chain reaction, immunohistology, and in situ hybridization[14–17] hold great promise for complementing serology and conventional culture techniques and making rapid diagnosis possible. If cytomegalovirus infection is suspected, an aggressive diagnostic approach, including tissue biopsies when clinically indicated is mandatory to allow early institution of pharmacologic therapy. Ganciclovir has been shown to be highly effective as treatment for cytomegalovirus infections,[18–20] and, in a recent multicenter survey, the overall mortality rate from cytomegalovirus infections was only 7%.[21] The duration of ganciclovir therapy is somewhat empiric and is usually determined by clinical response and surveillance laboratory studies. In the presence of organ manifestations or life-threatening disease, administration of cytomegalovirus-specific hyperimmune globulin or pooled immunoglobulins may further enhance efficacy of antiviral therapy.[22,23] Cytomegalovirus infection predisposes to superinfection in immunosuppressed patients[24] and, therefore, the presence of concomitant infections, especially pneumocystis, must be carefully investigated in the CMV-infected patient.

TABLE 2.   Peak Incidence of Common Infections after Cardiac Transplantation

Organism	Source
Month 1 Posttransplant	
Staphylococci	Lung, wound, urine, blood
Gram-negative bacteria	Lung, wound, urine, blood
Herpes simplex virus	Mucocutaneous
Candida	Mucocutaneous
Aspergillus	Lung
Months 2 to 5 Posttransplant	
Cytomegalovirus	Lung, gastrointesinal tract, heart, eye
Herpes zoster virus	Dermatomes
Pneumocystis carinii	Lung
Toxoplasmosis gondii	Central nervous system, lung, heart
Listeria monocytogenes	Central nervous system
Legionella pneumophila	Lung
Nocardia asteroides	Lung, soft tissues
Later than 6 Months Posttransplant	
Community-acquired bacteria	Variable

Reactivation of herpes simplex virus or herpes zoster virus after transplantation are not unusual, although these infections, in most instances, either require no therapy or respond well to oral or intravenous treatment with acyclovir.

Bacterial

Bacterial infections, primarily of the lungs and urinary tract, include a wide range of organisms including *Legionella, Listeria, Nocardia*, and atypical mycobacteria, which are uncommon in immunocompetent subjects. Aggressive culturing followed by empiric antibiotic therapy and more specific treatment after the pathogen has been identified is essential in the care of these patients.

Fungal

Mucocutaneous candida infections are common posttransplant and usually can be controlled with topical nystatin or systemically with ketoconazole or fluconazole. In contrast, aspergillus infections carry a grave prognosis and outcome in patients with central nervous system involvement or disseminated disease is almost uniformly fatal.[8,25–27] Patients are at higher risk of contracting aspergillus during periods of augmented immunosuppression or treatment with antibiotics, in the presence of metabolic disorders, and if the fungal spore concentration in the air is high, such as during construction work.[28] Investigative procedures for suspected aspergillosis, mostly in the presence of localized infiltrates on the chest radiograph, include prompt bronchoalveolar lavage, or transbronchial biopsy. Standard treatment, including high daily doses (up to 0.5 mg/kg/day) of intravenous amphotericin B for prolonged periods,[26] is often limited by renal toxicity. A liposome-encapsulated form of amphotericin B seems to be less toxic,[29] and promising results have been reported with itraconazole administered orally as treatment for aspergillus infections.[30]

Protozoal

Pneumocystis carinii and *Toxoplasma gondii* are the most common protozoal infections seen after cardiac transplantation. *Pneumocystis carinii* almost exclusively infects the lung and usually presents with fever, dry cough, dyspnea, hypoxemia, and diffuse pulmonary infiltrates on chest radiograph.[31] Diagnosis can usually be established by bronchoalveolar lavage or transbronchial biopsy. Specific treatment for *Pneumocystis carinii* pneumonia (PCP) consists of high-dose trimethoprim/sulfamethoxazole[32,33] or pentamidine[34] in patients who experience side effects with, or intolerance to, sulfa drugs.

Toxoplasmosis, in most cases in transplant recipients transmitted by the donor, fortunately is rare but carries a very poor prognosis. Presentations of primary infection can include pneumonia, myocarditis, and necrotizing encephalitis. Long-term treatment with sulfonamides and pyrimethamine has been effective.[35]

Diagnostic Approaches

Expectant surveillance for infections plays a major role in the postoperative care of heart transplant recipients and an aggressive diagnostic approach is of paramount importance to ensure early treatment of potentially life-threatening infectious complications. Availability of, and close cooperation with, pulmonary and infectious disease specialists who are experienced in management of immunocompromised patients and the availability of skilled microbiology and pathology laboratories are prerequisites for successful diagnosis and management of infections. Obviously, the diagnostic approach varies with type of infection and organ system involved. The lung is the most common site of infectious complications in heart transplant recipients[5,7]; therefore, it is important to obtain routine screening chest radiographs at regular intervals posttransplant, even in asymptomatic patients. If new pulmonary pathology is observed on chest radiographs or if symptoms suggestive of pulmonary infection are present, additional diagnostic studies are warranted. Fiberoptic bronchoscopy with bronchoalveolar lavage and transbronchial biopsy, CT-guided transthoracic needle aspiration, and, ultimately, lung biopsy when other diagnostic approaches have failed are safe and accurate techniques in experienced hands.[31–33] Fever without obvious source is another common clinical problem facing transplant physicians. Further investigations are based on history, physical examination, chest radiography and routine laboratory results. They should include taking cultures of blood, urine, and sputum where appropriate. The source of infection rarely remains occult for any extended period.

Infection Prophylaxis

Because of the considerable morbidity and mortality associated with infections in transplant patients, various preventive strategies have been studied. Unfortunately, effective prophylaxis regimens exist for only a minority of the common pathogens.

Trimethoprim/sulfamethoxazole on a 3 day/week basis has been shown to be highly effective in preventing PCP;[34] this regimen is generally recommended in immunosuppressed patients. Aerosolized pentamidine is used as an alternative when trimethoprim/sulfamethoxazole is contraindicated or not tolerated.[35,37–40] Cytomegalovirus and *Toxoplasma gondii* are the most important organisms known to have a potential for transmission from donor to recipient.[35,37–40] Pretransplant serologic screening of donors and recipients is routinely performed to identify recipients at risk. Although desirable, donors seronegative for cytomegalovirus are fairly rare and matching of recipients seronegative for cytomegalovirus or *Toxoplasma* with seronegative donors is not always possible. Pyrimethamine is of proven efficacy for prophylaxis of toxoplasmosis if the donor is found to be IgM positive.[41] Prophylactic cytomegalovirus immunoglobulin[42] and high-dose oral acyclovir[43] have been used successfully in renal transplant recipients to reduce the perioperative risk of cytomegalovirus infection, but no randomized studies have been performed in heart transplant patients using these agents. In a recent prospective randomized placebo-controlled trial, prophylactic ganciclovir significantly decreased the incidence of cytomegalovirus reinfection but not of primary infection after heart transplantation.[44] Oral low-dose acyclovir has been shown to prevent reactivation of herpes simplex and herpes zoster in renal transplant recipients,[45] and clotrimazole or nystatin are used to prevent mucocutaneous candidiasis posttransplant.[46] The role of nebulized amphotericin B, oral itraconazole, or any other modality for prevention of aspergillosis in transplant recipients remains to be proved. Effective prophylaxis against aspergillus infections would be a major advance in transplant medicine.

Although infective endocarditis is rarely reported after heart transplantation, standard endocarditis prophylaxis is recommended in these patients. Recommendations for infection prophylaxis posttransplantation are summarized in Table 3.

Sound vaccination protocols for solid organ transplant recipients have yet to be established. Concerns in immunocompromised patients include risk of infection with live virus vaccines and potential triggering of rejection because of stimulation of the immune system. A consensus of opinion exists that live virus vaccines should be avoided in transplant patients. According to recent recommendations,[47] transplant candidates should be evaluated for immunity to hepatitis B, measles, mumps, rubella, poliomyelitis, and

TABLE 3. Regimens for Infection Prophylaxis

Organism	Regimen	Patients
Pneumocystis carinii	(1) TMP/SMX	All
	(2) Pentamidine	Intolerance to (1)
Cytomegalovirus	Ganciclovir	Seropositive donor (?)
Toxoplasma gondii	Pyrimethamine	Donor IgM positive
Herpes simplex/zoster	Acyclovir	Recurrence
Mucocutaneous candidiasis	Nystatin or clotrimazole	All
Aspergillus	Itraconazole or amphotericin B	Questioned, unproved efficacy
Endocarditis	Routine prophylaxis	All

TMP/SMX = trimethoprim/sulfamethoxazole.

varicella; those lacking immunity should be vaccinated, ideally avoiding live virus vaccinations within 3 months of transplantation. In addition, transplant candidates should receive pneumococcal vaccine once and a tetanus-diphtheria booster every 10 years. In the posttransplant period, pneumococcal vaccine boosters should be repeated every 5 or 6 years and tetanus boosters every 10 years (Table 4). Treatment with immunoglobulins should be considered when exposure of nonimmunized transplant patients to tetanus, measles, varicella, or hepatitis B virus occurs. A known exposure to influenza A can be treated with rimantidine or amantadine; patients developing an exanthem after exposure to varicella should be started on high dose acyclovir.[47] Use of annual influenza immunization in heart transplant recipients remains somewhat controversial because influenza does not pose a major source of morbidity in these patients.

ARTERIAL HYPERTENSION

Hypertension is a very common complication after heart transplantation, occurring in 50 to 90% of recipients on cyclosporine[48-51] Although corticosteroids clearly may contribute to the development of hypertension,[52,53] this complication is usually attributed to use of cyclosporine.[54] Several important differences exist between essential hypertension and cyclosporine-related hypertension. First, demographic characteristics associated with essential hypertension, for example, age, race, gender, body weight, and family history, do not seem to influence cyclosporine-related hypertension. Second, cyclosporine-related hypertension develops in the first weeks or months after starting cyclosporine therapy. Third, in contrast to the pattern in essential hypertension, blood pressure does not decrease during the night and the highest values in transplant patients are usually

TABLE 4. Vaccination Recommendations

Vaccine	Patients
Pretransplant	
Measles, mumps, rubella, varicella, polio, hepatitis B	No immunity
Pneumococcus	All not previously immunized
Tetanus/diphtheria	All not previously immunized
	Booster every 10 years
Influenza	Questioned, yearly
Posttransplant	
Pneumococcus	Booster every 5 to 6 years
Tetanus/diphtheria	Booster every 10 years
Influenza	Questioned, yearly (controversial)

measured in the morning. Fourth, cyclosporine-related hypertension is frequently diffi-cult to control and it often becomes necessary to combine several antihypertensive agents.[48,49,55–59] The pathogenesis of cyclosporine-related hypertension remains incom-pletely understood. Several mechanisms have been proposed, including increased sym-pathetic tone, volume expansion, elevated endothelin levels, activation of the renin-angiotensin system, elevation of vasoconstrictor prostaglandins and renal vaso-constriction.[60–75] Treatment of cyclosporine-related hypertension remains empiric be-cause no single agent or class of agents has been found to be effective. Calcium channel blockers, angiotensin-converting enzyme inhibitors, beta blockers, alpha blockers, di-uretics, and direct-acting vasodilators have all been used with varying success alone or in combination. Diltiazem deserves special attention because it not only acts as an anti-hypertensive but also substantially decreases cyclosporine requirements by increasing levels[76] and seems to reduce progression of transplant coronary artery disease.[77] Finally, a recent report suggests that blood pressure after cardiac transplantation is sensitive to reduced dietary sodium intake, which always should be considered an adjunctive non-pharmacologic approach in the management of hypertension in these patients.[78]

RENAL DYSFUNCTION

Renal dysfunction in cardiac transplant recipients is attributed to cyclosporine-re-lated nephrotoxicity.[56,71,79–83] Despite extensive investigations of the pathophysiology of cyclosporine nephropathy, specific mechanisms of renal injury are not fully understood. Chronic administration of cyclosporine leads to renal vasoconstriction, primarily of the afferent arterioles, with subsequent increase in renal vascular resistance, decrease in renal plasma flow and glomerular filtration rate and chronic ischemia resulting in irre-versible renal fibrosis.[71,84–87] Prostaglandins, angiotensin, adrenergic tone, endothelin, and catecholamines may modulate the severity of vasoconstriction.[63,72,73,88] Direct tubu-lar toxicity of cyclosporine is a second, probably less important, mechanism in the de-velopment of cyclosporine-related nephrotoxicity.[82,83,89]

Renal function declines most rapidly during the first 6 months of cyclosporine therapy.[90] Thereafter, serum creatinine levels increase more gradually and eventually stabilize,[59,90,91] presumably as a result of reduced cyclosporine doses in the long-term course.[92] The clinical picture of chronic cyclosporine nephropathy is characterized by elevation of serum creatinine levels, reduced creatinine clearance, disproportionate azotemia, hyperkalemia, elevated serum uric acid levels, proteinuria, decreased sodium excretion, hypertension, and fluid retention.[82,87,89]

Close monitoring of cyclosporine levels and adjustment of cyclosporine doses to maintain levels within the therapeutic and nontoxic range is important to limit progres-sive renal dysfunction.[92] Many drugs alter cyclosporine levels and/or exert additive nephrotoxic effects.[93] Important examples of such agents include aminoglycosides, am-photericin, trimethoprim/sulfamethoxazole, erythromycin, cimetidine, ketoconazole, and nonsteroidal antiinflammatory drugs (see chapter 18). Therefore, cyclosporine levels should be frequently checked and the cyclosporine dose adjusted after initiation or withdrawal of any of these drugs. In the presence of chronic cyclosporine-related nephropathy, improvement in renal function has been demonstrated with reduction of cyclosporine dosage,[90,.94–96] but the risks of dosage with subtherapeutic levels must be evaluated on an individual basis.

Following these guidelines and with the dosages of cyclosporine currently used, progression of cyclosporine-related nephropathy to end-stage renal disease seems to be uncommon after heart transplantation. Incidence of end-stage renal disease in heart transplant patients has been reported to be 3.8 to 10%[71,81] and may be lower with currently used lower cyclosporine dosages. At Stanford, 14 of 430 (3.3%) cardiac transplant recipients on cyclosporine-based immunosuppression therapy commenced in 1980 have developed end-stage renal disease requiring dialysis or renal transplantation an average of 82 ± 42 months posttransplant. Nine of these 14 patients underwent renal transplantation. Patient and allograft survival was 89% at both 1 and 3 years after renal transplant and serum creatinine was measured at 1.3 ± 0.6 mg/dl and 1.6 ± 0.8 mg/dl respectively.[97] According to these results, renal transplantation is a safe and effective treatment for selected patients who develop end-stage renal disease after cardiac transplantation.

OSTEOPOROSIS

Osteoporosis contributes significantly to morbidity after cardiac transplantation and may limit rehabilitation and significantly impair quality of life. The prevalence of osteoporosis has not been assessed in a consecutive series of heart transplant recipients. Up to 35% of patients develop vertebral fractures posttransplant,[98-101] whereas avascular necrosis of weight-bearing joints seems to occur less frequently.[99] Clinically, chronic and sometimes debilitating back pain due to vertebral compression fractures is the predominant manifestation. Conventional radiographic studies allow diagnosis of fractures, but more sophisticated methods are required to measure bone mass, mineral content, and density.[102-104] Bone density has been shown to correlate with risk of fractures in other patient populations[103] and has therefore been used in most studies in heart transplant patients for assessment of osteoporosis.[98,99,105-107]

The pathogenesis of osteoporosis after cardiac transplantation is clearly multifactorial. Pretransplant mean vertebral bone mineral density was 20% lower than normal in heart failure patients awaiting cardiac transplantation in a study by Muchmore and colleagues.[101] This has been attributed to therapy with loop diuretics and heparin, inactivity, cachexia, and cigarette smoking.[106,108,109] After transplant, bone density is further reduced.[101] This is thought to be primarily a consequence of steroid therapy, which is well known to cause osteoporotic fractures.[110-114] Corticosteroids affect both bone resorption and bone formation.[115-117] Direct effects of cyclosporine on bone metabolism resulting in severe osteopenia have been observed in rat models,[118] and clinical evidence exists that cyclosporine also contributes to reduced bone mineral density in heart transplant recipients.[105,110] Other contributing factors include advanced age,[100,101] postmenopausal status in female recipients[119] and renal dysfunction.

Therapeutically, withdrawal of corticosteroids or using lower steroid doses in transplant patients obviously has a major impact on slowing progression of osteoporosis. This strategy, however, is not always possible. Regular exercise, oral calcium supplementation, calcitonin injections, testosterone, estrogen, vitamin D, fluoride, anabolic steroids, and biphosphonates have been used successfully to prevent osteoporosis in different patient populations,[100,116,120-125] but no randomized studies of any of these has been performed in heart transplant patients.

QUALITY OF LIFE AND REHABILITATION AFTER TRANSPLANTATION

The stated goal of cardiac transplantation is to prolong patients' lives and restore them to an improved quality of life and enable them to resume family life and occupational pursuits.

Quality-of-life judgments are frequently subjective and the goals to be achieved are much less amenable to easy quantitation than goals such as survival. Several different tests have been employed to assess quality of life in a number of studies. These differences in methodology make direct comparisons between reports difficult.

In the first two studies addressing quality of life and rehabilitation after heart transplantation in 1973 and 1976, 16 of 25 (64%)[126] and 51 of 69 (74%)[127] patients returned to their previous occupation or activity; an additional 4 of 25 (15%) and 11 of 69 (16%) were in functional class I cardiac status but voluntarily retired. Morbidity secondary to complications of immunosuppression was the primary factor limiting more complete rehabilitation of these patients.[126] A later study from the same institution assessed quality of cardiac function and lifestyle of 25 long-term survivors of transplantation.[128] Defining rehabilitation as ability to perform tasks of interest, to work, and to have an overall sense of well being, these patients qualified as rehabilitated during 86% of their follow-up time. In a questionnaire for patients who were under age 30 at the time of transplant, 87% were moderately or very satisfied with their lives after transplantation.[129] The two largest series assessing quality of life after cardiac transplantation, the National Transplantation Study including information from 85% of all transplant programs in the United States[130] and the United Kingdom Heart Transplant Study[131,132] deserve special attention. In the former study,[130] 80 to 85% of surviving transplant recipients were physically active, but only 32% were actually employed. Although almost 90% of patients analyzed felt well and perceived themselves as healthy, 66% stated they were limited in some way from doing something they desired. Subjective quality of life in a number of areas was similar among heart transplant recipients and other solid organ transplant recipients and not significantly different from the general population. In the United Kingdom Heart Transplantation Study,[131,132] quality of life, job problems, difficulties with housework, and sexual problems significantly improved post- as compared to pretransplant. Using the Nottingham Health profile Survey,[132] scores for physical mobility, pain, energy, social isolation, and emotional reactions were similar at 1 and 2 years posttransplant compared with nontransplant controls. Transplant patients reported more difficulties sleeping than did controls. These favorable results in terms of quality of life and rehabilitation after cardiac transplantation have been confirmed by a number of studies.[133–139] Results from the United Kingdom Heart Transplantation Study[135] comparing pre- and posttransplant qualify of life in heart transplant recipients and from Evans and associates[133] comparing quality of life of heart transplant with kidney transplant recipients and the general population are shown in Tables 5 and 6.

Thus, review of the existing published data suggests that the majority of recipients of heart transplants are in fact fully functional and "well" in both subjective and objective

TABLE 5. Comparison of Quality of Life Pre- and Postcardiac Transplantation Using the Nottingham Health Profile Survey*

Dimension	No. of Ties†	Pretransplant Mean Rank Score	Posttransplant Mean Rank Score	2-Tailed p-Value
Energy	10	27.21	18.00	< 0.01
Pain	17	24.65	12.25	< 0.01
Emotional reactions	4	31.22	5.90	< 0.01
Sleep	9	30.71	11.05	< 0.01
Social isolation	19	23.86	3.88	< 0.01
Physical mobility	2	32.29	5.50	< 0.01

* Paired comparisons of most recent pretransplant and 3-month posttransplant profiles of 62 patients. Range of values 0.0 to 100.0, where lower scores indicate better health status.
† Ties represent situations in which the rank of the score did not change.
(Modified from O'Brien BJ, Buxton MJ, Ferguson BA: Measuring the effectiveness of heart transplant programmes: Quality of life data and their relationship to survival analysis. J Chron Dis 40(Suppl 1):137–153, 1987.)

TABLE 6.   Comparison of Quality of Life of Heart Transplant Recipients with Renal Transplant Recipients and the General Population

Patient Group	Objective Indicators of Quality of Life			Subjective Indicators of Quality of Life		
	Functional Impairment	Ability to Work[†]	Health Status[‡]	Well-being[§]	Psychological Affect[//]	Life Satisfaction[#]
Heart transplant patients	1.47	57.88	9.60	11.11	5.49	5.11
Kidney transplant patients	1.96	74.13	5.52	11.83	5.62	5.66
Dialysis patients	2.88	44.68	12.16	10.94	5.27	5.16
General population	N/A	N/A	N/A	11.77	5.68	5.54

* Based on the Karnofsky Index, range of values 1.0 to 10.0, where 1.0 = absence of dysfunction and 10 = maximal dysfunction (death).
† Ability to work, range of values 0.0 to 100.0, where 0.0 = patients unable and 100.00 = patients able.
‡ Total Sickness Impact Profile score, range of values 0.0 to 100.0. Lower scores indicate better health status.
§ Range of values 2.1 to 14.7, where high score = positive well-being.
// Range of values 1.0 to 7.0, where 7.0 = positive affect.
Range of values 1.0 to 7.0, where 7.0 = positive satisfaction.
(Modified from Evans RW, Manninen DL, Maier A, et al: The quality of life in kidney and heart transplant recipients. Transplant Proc 17:1579–1582, 1985.)

senses. Disability, when it exits, is not commonly due to cardiac causes but usually relates to sequelae of the immunosuppressive regimen, such as opportunistic infections or steroid side effects. Interestingly, although heart transplant recipients in general achieve reasonable functional capacity and are able to perform most desired physical activities,[129,136,140] they have a reduced maximal exercise tolerance compared with normal subjects.[141–143] The mechanisms responsible for this exercise intolerance are not entirely understood. Blunted increase of heart rate and contractility early during exercise because of loss of autonomic innervation,[142,144,145] diastolic dysfunction,[146,147] and loss of muscle strength, which occurs as a consequence of deconditioning and steroid myopathy,[148] all contribute to reduced maximal oxygen consumption[141–143] and cardiac output,[149–151] as well as rapid increase of intracardiac pressures[150,151] during exercise.

Increasingly, important and related issues in these patients frequently have a great impact on their postoperative quality of life. These issues are the patient's employability, insurability, and financial situation. Employment and job satisfaction as well as a stable financial situation have been shown to be significantly correlated with quality of life in heart transplant patients.[134,137,139] In view of the high rehabilitation rates posttransplant, previously published return-to-work rates after transplantation are surprisingly low, ranging from 32 to 86%.[129,130,137,152–159] Rates exceeding 50% have been reported from Australia and Europe, and range from 32 to 57% in the United States. Shorter periods of pretransplantation disability and/or unemployment, greater control over working conditions, extensive previous work history, age from 35 to 50 years, a longer period of time after transplantation, retention of health insurance, a professional job, expectation of returning to work, education level above 12 years, and no loss of disability income have been shown to be the factors associated with a patient's return to work.[129,163–159]

Unless a patient is self-employed or on medical leave from a job being held open for him or her, finding a job after heart transplantation can be quite difficult in the United States. Many employers do not want to hire a person with what they view as serious health problems, and the potential for unpredictable and possibly lengthy hospitalizations or time off the job. Also, health insurance, if not continued from the preoperative period, is virtually unavailable through any but the largest employers in the current U.S. health care system. These factors, which are clearly societal rather than medical, can make what would otherwise be an excellent quality of life, most difficult socioeconomically for many patients. They are issues that need to be addressed more actively in our society over the coming years as increasing numbers of transplant recipients each year return to a functional life and seek to exercise that function in society.

REFERENCES

1. Kriett JM, Kaye M: The Registry of the International Society for Heart and Lung Transplantation: Eighth official report—1991. J Heart Lung Transplant 10:491–498, 1991.
2. Bieber CP, Hunt SA, Schwinn DA, et al: Complications in long-term survivors of cardiac transplantation. Transplant Proc 8:207–322, 1981.
3. Cooper DKC, Novitsky D, Hassoulas J, et al: Heart transplantation: The South African experience. J Heart Transplant 2:78–84, 1982.
4. Jamieson SW, Oyer PE, Baldwin J, et al: Heart transplantation for end-stage ischemic heart disease: The Stanford experience. Heart Transplant 3:224–227, 1984.
5. Dummer JS, Bahnson HT, Griffith BP, et al: Infections in patients on cyclosporine and prednisone following cardiac transplantation. Transplant Proc 15:2779–2781, 1983.
6. Dresdale AR, Drusin RE, Lamb J, et al: Reduced infection in cardiac transplant recipients. Circulation 72:(Suppl II):237–240, 1985.
7. Hofflin JM, Potasman J, Baldwin JC, et al: Infectious complications in heart transplant recipients receiving cyclosporine and corticosteroids. Ann Intern Med 106:209–216, 1987.
8. Miller LW, Naftel DC, Bourge RC, et al: Infection after heart transplantation: A multiinstitutional study. J Heart Lung Transplant 13:381–393, 1994.
9. Dummer SJ, Hardy A, Poorsattar A, Ho M: Early infections in kidney, heart, and liver transplant recipients on cyclosporine. Transplantation 36:259–267, 1984.
10. Dresdale A, Diehl J: Early postoperative care. Prog Cardiovasc Dis 33:1–9, 1990.
11. Hosenpud D, Hershberger RE, Pantely GA, et al: Late infection in cardiac allograft recipients: Profiles, incidence and outcome. J Heart Transplant 10:39–80–86, 1987.
12. Dummer SJ: Infectious complications of transplantation. Cardiovasc Clin 20:163–178, 1990.
13. Mason JW, Stinson EB, Hunt SA: Infections after cardiac transplantation: Relation to rejection therapy. Ann Intern Med 85:69–72, 1976.
14. Dummer SJ, White LT, Ho M, et al: Morbidity of cytomegalovirus infection in recipients of heart or heart-lung transplants who received cyclosporine. J Infect dis 152:1182–1191, 1985.
15. Spector SA: Diagnosis of cytomegalovirus infection. Semin Hematol 27(Suppl):11–16, 1990.
16. Chou S: Newer methods for diagnosis of cytomegalovirus infection. Rev Infect Dis 12(Suppl 7):727–736, 1990.
17. The TH, van den Berg AP, van Son WJ, et al: Monitoring for cytomegalovirus after organ transplantation: A clinical perspective. Transplant Proc 25(Suppl 4):5–9, 1993.
18. Keay S, Peterson E, Icenogle T, et al: Ganciclovir treatment of serious cytomegalovirus infection in heart-lung transplant recipients. Rev Infect Dis 10(Suppl):563–572, 1988.
19. Watson FS, O'Connell JB, Amber IJ, et al: Treatment of cytomegalovirus pneumonia in heart transplant recipients with 9(1,3-dihydroxy-2-proproxymethyl)-guanine (DHPG). J Heart Transplant 7:102–105, 1988.
20. Cooper DKC, Novitzky D, Schlegel V, et al: Successful management of symptomatic cytomegalovirus disease with ganciclovir after heart transplantation. J Heart Lung Transplant 10:656–666, 1991.
21. Kirklin JK, Naftel DC, Levine TB, et al: Cytomegalovirus after heart transplantation. risk factors for infection and death: A multiinstitutional study. J Heart Lung Transplant 13:394–404, 1994.
22. Emanuel D, Cunningham I, Jules-Elysee K, et al: Cytomegalovirus pneumonia after bone marrow transplantation successfully treated with the combination of ganciclovir and high-dose intravenous immune globulin. Ann Intern Med 109–777–782, 1988.
23. Reed EC, Bowden RA, Dandliker PS, et al: Treatment of cytomegalovirus pneumonia with ganciclovir and intravenous cytomegalovirus immunoglobulin in patients with bone marrow transplants. Ann Intern Med 109:783–788, 1988.
24. Rand KH, Pollard RB, Merigan TC: Increased pulmonary superinfections in cardiac transplant patients undergoing primary cytomegalovirus infection. N Engl J Med 298:951–953, 1978.
25. Gurwith MJ, Stinson EB, Remington JS: Aspergillus infection complicating cardiac transplantation. Arch Intern Med 128:541–545, 1971.
26. Denning DW, Stevens DA: Antifungal and surgical treatment of invasive aspergillosis: Review of 2,121 published cases. Rev Infect Dis 12:1147–1201, 1990.

27. Hummel M, Thalmann U, Jautzke G, et al: Fungal infections following heart transplantation. Mycoses 35:23–34, 1992.
28. Opal SM, Asp AA, Cannady PB, et al: Efficacy of infection control measures during a nosocomial outbreak of disseminated aspergillosis associated with hospital construction. J Infect Dis 153:634–637, 1986.
29. Wiebe VJ, DeGregorio MW: Liposome-encapsulated amphotericin B: A promising new treatment for disseminated fungal infections. Rev Infect Dis 10:1097–1101, 1988.
30. Denning DW, Tucker RM, Hanson LH, Stevens DA: Treatment of invasive aspergillosis with itraconazole. Am J Med 86:791–800, 1989.
31. Hedemark LL, Kronenberg RS, Rasp FL, et al: The value of bronchoscopy in establishing the etiology of pneumonia in renal transplant recipients. Am Rev Respir Dis 126:981–985, 1982.
32. Young JA, Hopkins JM, Cuthbertson WP: Pulmonary infiltrates in immunocompromised patients: Diagnosis by cytological examination of bronchoalveolar lavage fluid. J Clin Pathol 37:390–394, 1985.
33. Bandt PD, Blank N, Castellino RA: Needle diagnosis of pneumonitis: Value in high risk patients. JAMA 220:1578–1580, 1972.
34. Hughes WT, Rivera GK, Schell MJ, et al: Successful intermittent chemoprophylaxis for Pneumocystis carinii pneumonitis. N Engl J Med 316:1627–1632, 1987.
35. Ryning FW, McLeod R, Maddox JC, et al: Probable transmission of Toxoplasma gondii by organ transplantation. Ann Intern Med 90:27–31, 1983.
36. Golden JA, Chernoff D, Hollander H, et al: Prevention of Pneumocystis carinii pneumonia by inhaled pentamidine. Lancet 1:654–657, 1989.
37. Siegel SE, Lunde MN, Gelderman AH, et al: Transmission of toxoplasmosis by leukocyte transfusion. Blood 37:388–394, 1971.
38. Luft BJ, Naot Y, Araujo FG, et al: Primary and reactivated toxoplasma infection in patients with cardiac transplantation. Ann Intern Med 99;27–31, 1983.
39. Prince AM, Szmuness W, Millian SJ, David DS: A serologic study of cytomegalovirus infections associated with blood transfusions. N Engl J Med 284:1125–1131, 1971.
40. Ho M, Suwannsirikul S, Dowling JN, et al: The transplanted kidney as a source of cytomegalovirus infection. N Engl J Med 293:1109–1112, 1975.
41. Holliman RE, Johnson JD, Adams S, et al: Toxoplasmosis and heart transplantation. J Heart Transplant 10:608–610, 1991.
42. Snydman DR, Werner BG, Heinze-Lacey B, et al: Use of cytomegalovirus immune globulin to prevent cytomegalovirus disease in renal transplant recipients. n Engl J Med 317:1049–1054, 1987.
43. Balfour HH, Chace BA, Stapleton JT, et al: A randomized, placebo-controlled trial of oral acyclovir for the prevention of cytomegalovirus disease in recipients of renal allografts. N Engl J Med 320:1381–1387, 1989.
44. Merigan TC, Renlund DG, Keay S, et al: A controlled trial of gancyclovir to prevent cytomegalovirus disease after heart transplantation. N Engl J Med 326:1182–1186, 1992.
45. Seale L, Jones CJ, Kathpalia S, et al: Prevention of herpesvirus infections in renal allograft recipients by low-dose oral acyclovir. JAMA 254:3435–3438, 1985.
46. Gombert ME, duBouchet L, Aulcino TM, Butt KM: A comparative trial of clotrimazole troches and oral nystatin suspension in recipients of renal transplants. Use in prophylaxis of oropharyngeal candidiasis. JAMA 258:2553–2555, 1987.
47. Houston SH, Glossa JS, Fisher A, et al: Immunization of solid organ transplant candidates and recipients. Infect Dis Newsletter 12:86–87, 1993.
48. Thompson ME, Shapiro AP, Johnson AM, et al: New onset of hypertension following cardiac transplantation: A preliminary report and analysis. Transplant Proc 15(Suppl 1):2573–2577, 1983.
49. Thompson ME, Shapiro AP, Johnson AMN, et al: The contrasting effects of cyclosporine A and azathioprine on arterial pressure and renal function following cardiac transplantation. Int J Cardiol 11:219–229, 1986.
50. Greenberg ML, Uretsky BF, Reddy PS, et al: Long-term hemodynamic follow-up of cardiac transplant patients treated with cyclosporine and prednisone. Circulation 71:487–494, 1985.
51. Olivari MT, Kubo SH, Braunlin EA, et al: Five-year experience with triple-drug immunosuppressive therapy in cardiac transplantation. Circulation 83(Suppl 4):276–280, 1990.
52. Moore CK, Renlund DG, Rasmussen LG, O'Connell JB: Long-term morbidity of cyclosporine with corticosteroid-free maintenance immunosuppression in cardiac transplantation. Transplant Proc 22(Suppl 1):25–29, 1990.
53. Renlund DG, O'Connell JB, Gilbert EM, et al: Feasibility of discontinuation of corticosteroid maintenance therapy in heart transplantation. J Heart Transplant 6:71–78, 1987.
54. Starling RC, Cody RJ: Cardiac transplant hypertension. Am J Cardiol 65:106–111, 1990.
55. Rodney RA, Johnson LL: Myocardial perfusion scintigraphy to assess heart transplant vasculopathy. J Heart Lung Transplant 11:S74-S78, 1992.

56. Miller LW, Pennington DG, McBride LR: Long-term effects of cyclosporine in cardiac transplantation. Transplant Proc 22(Suppl 1):15–20, 1990.
57. Olivari MT, Antolick A, Ring WS: Arterial hypertension in heart transplant recipients treated with three-drug immunosuppressive therapy. J Heart Transplant 8:34–39, 1989.
58. Reeves RA, Shapiro AP, Thompson ME, et al: Loss of nocturnal decline in blood pressure after cardiac transplantation. Circulation 73:401–408, 1986.
59. Wenting GJ, Van den Meiracker AH, van Eck HJ, et al: Lack of circadian variation of blood pressure after heart transplantation. J Hypertens 4 (Suppl 6):78–80, 1986.
60. Scherrer U, Vissing SF, Morgan BJ, et al: Cyclosporine-induced sympathetic activation and hypertension after heart transplantation. N Engl J Med 323:693–699, 1990.
61. Porter GA, Bennett WM, Sheps SG: Cyclosporine associated hypertension. Arch Intern Med 150:280–283, 1990.
62. Mark AL: Cyclosporine, sympathetic activity, and hypertension. N Engl J Med 323:748–750, 1990.
63. Perico N, Dadan J, Remuzzi G: Endothelin mediates the renal vasoconstriction induced by cyclosporine in the rat. J Am Soc Nephrol 1:76–83, 1990.
64. Curtis JJ, Luke RG, Jones P, et al: Hypertension in cyclosporine-treated renal transplant recipients is sodium dependent. Am J Med 85:134–138, 1988.
65. Meyer-Lehnert H, Schrier RW: Potential mechanisms of cyclosporine A induced vascular smooth muscle contraction. Hypertension 13:352–360, 1989.
66. Lustig S, Stern N, Eggena P, et al: Effect of cyclosporine on blood pressure and renin aldosterone axis in rats. Am J Physiol 253:H1596–H1600, 1987.
67. Bellet M, Carol C, Sassano P, et al: Systemic hypertension after cardiac transplantation: Effect of cyclosporine on the renin-angiotensin system. Am J Cardiol 56:927–931, 1985.
68. Garr MD, Paller MS: Cyclosporine augments renal but not systemic vascular reactivity. Am J Physiol 258:F211–F217, 1990.
69. Bantee JP, Nath KA, Sutherland DE, et al: Effects of cyclosporine on the renin-angiotensin system and potassium excretion in renal transplant patients. Arch Intern Med 145:505–508, 1985.
70. Bantle JP, Boudreau RJ, Ferris TF: Suppression of plasma renin activity by cyclosporine. Am J Med 83:59–64, 1987.
71. Myers BD, Sibley R, Newton L, et al: The long-term course of cyclosporine-associated chronic nephropathy. Kidney Int 33:590–600, 1988.
72. Neild GH, Rocchi G, Imberti L, et al: Effect of cyclosporine on prostacyclin synthesis by vascular tissue in rabbits. Transplant Proc 15(Suppl 1):2398–2400, 1983.
73. Coffman IM, Carr DR, Yarger WF, et al: Evidence that renal prostaglandins and thromboxane production is stimulated in chronic cyclosporine nephrotoxicity. Transplantation 43:282–285, 1987.
74. Morgan BJ, Lyson T, Scherrer U, Victor RG: Cyclosporine causes sympathetically mediated elevations in arterial pressure in rats. Hypertension 18:458–466, 1991.
75. Kaye D, Thompson J, Jennings G, Esler M: Cyclosporine therapy after cardiac transplantation causes hypertension and renal vasoconstriction without sympathetic activation. Circulation 88:1101–1109, 1993.
76. Bourge RC, Kirklin JK, Figg WD, et al: Diltiazem-cyclosporine interaction in cardiac transplant patients: Impact on cyclosporine dose and medication costs. Am J Med 90:402–404, 1991.
77. Schroeder JS, Gao S, Alderman EL, et al: A preliminary study of diltiazem in the prevention of coronary artery disease in heart-transplant recipients. N Engl J Med 328:164–170, 1993.
78. Singer DRJ, Markandu ND, Buckley MG, et al: Blood pressure and endocrine responses to changes in dietary sodium intake in cardiac transplant recipients. Circulation 89:1153–1159, 1994.
79. Hunt SA, Gamberg P, Stinson EB, et al: The Stanford Experience: Survival and renal function in the pre-sandimmune era compared to the sandimmune era. Transplant Proc 22(Suppl 1):1–5, 1990.
80. Constanzo-Nordin MR, Grady KL, Johnson MR, et al: Long-term effects of cyclosporine-based immunosuppression in cardiac transplantation: The Loyola experience. Transplant Proc 22(Suppl 1):6–11, 1990.
81. Greenberg A, Thompson ME, Griffith BJ, et al: Cyclosporine nephrotoxicity in cardiac allograft patients—a seven year follow-up. Transplantation 50:589–593, 1990.
82. Myers BD: Cyclosporine nephrotoxicity. N Engl J Med 30:964–974, 1986.
83. Mihatsch MJ, Thiel G, Ryfel B: Cyclosporine nephrotoxicity. Adv Nephrol 17:303–320, 1988.
84. Bennett WM, Pulliam JB: Cyclosporine nephrotoxicity. Ann Intern Med 99:851–854, 1983.
85. Kahan BD: Cyclosporine nephrotoxicity: Pathogenesis, prophylaxis, therapy and prognosis. Am J Kidney Dis 8:323–331, 986.
86. Myers BD, Newton L: Cyclosporine-induced chronic nephropathy: An obliterative microvascular renal injury. J Am Soc Nephrol 2(Suppl 1):S45–S52, 1991.
87. Lorber MI: Cyclosporine: Lessons learned—Future strategies. Clin Transplant 5:505–516, 1991.
88. Barros EJG, Boim MA, Ajyen H, et al: Glomerular hemodynamics and hormonal participation on cyclosporine nephrotoxicity. Kidney Int 32:19–25, 1987.

89. Kahan BD: Cyclosporine. N Engl J Med 321:1725–1738, 1989.
90. Lewis RM, Van Buren CT, Radovancevic B, et al: Impact of long-term cyclosporine immunosuppressive therapy on native kidneys versus renal allografts: Serial renal function in heart and kidney transplant recipients. J Heart Lung Transplant 10:63–70, 1991.
91. McKenzie N, Keown P, Stiller C, et al: Effects of cyclosporine on renal function following orthotopic heart transplantation. Heart Transplant 4:400–403, 1985.
92. Moyer TP, Post GR, Sterioff S, et al: Cyclosporine nephrotoxicity is minimized by adjusting dosage on the basis of drug concentration in blood. Mayo Clin Proc 63:241–247, 1988.
93. Lake KD: Cyclosporine drug interactions: A review. Cardiac Surgery: State of the Art Reviews 2:617–630, 1988.
94. Spratt P, Esmore D, Bzron D, et al: Effectiveness of minimal dosage cyclosporine in limiting toxicity and rejection. J Heart Transplant 5:8–12, 1986.
95. Imoto EM, Glanville AR, Baldwin JC, et al: Kidney function in heart lung transplant recipients: The effect of low-dose cyclosporine therapy. J Heart Transplant 6:204–213, 1987.
96. Sibley RK, Rynasiewicz J, Ferguson RM, et al: Morphology of cyclosporine nephrotoxicity and acute rejection in patients immunosuppressed with cyclosporine and prednisone. Surgery 94:255–234, 1983.
97. Kuo PC, Luikart H, Busse-Henry S, et al: Clinical outcome in interval cadaveric renal transplantation in cardiac allograft recipients. Clin Transplant (in press).
98. Shane K, Rivas MDC, Silverberg SJ, et al: Osteoporosis after cardiac transplantation. Am J Med 94:257–264, 1993.
99. Sambrook PN, Kelly PJ, Keogh AM, et al: Bone loss after heart transplantation: A prospective study. J Heart Lung Transplant 13:116–121, 1994.
100. Olivari MT, Antolick A, Kaye MP, et al: Heart transplantation in elderly patients. J Heart Transplant 7:258–264, 1988.
101. Muchmore JS, Cooper DKC, Ye Y, et al: Loss of vertebral bone density in heart transplant patients. Transplant Proc 23:1184–1185, 1991.
102. Krolner B, Nielsen SP: Bone mineral content of the lumbar spine in normal and osteoporotic women: Cross-sectional and longitudinal studies. Clin Sci 62:329–336, 1982.
103. Hui SL, Slemenda CW, Johnson CC: Baseline measurement of bone mass predicts fracture in white women. Ann Intern Med 111:355–361, 1989.
104. Pocock NA, Eberl S, Eisman JA, et al: Dual-photon bone densitometry in normal Australian women: A cross-sectional study. Med J Aust 146:293–297, 1987.
105. Rich GM, Mudge GH, Laffel GL, LeBoff MS: Cyclosporine A and prednisone-associated osteoporosis in heart transplant recipients. J Heart Lung Transplant 11:950–958, 1992.
106. Lee AH, Mull RL, Keenan GF, et al: Osteoporosis and bone morbidity in cardiac transplant recipients. Am J Med 96:35–41, 1994.
107. Muchmore JS, Cooper DKC, Ye Y, et al: Prevention of loss of vertebral bone density in heart transplant patients. J Heart Lung Transplant 11:959–964, 1992.
108. Heidrich FE, Stergachis A, Gross KM: Diuretic drug use and the risk of hip fracture. Ann Intern Med 115:1–6, 1991.
109. Krolner B, Toft B: Vertebral bone loss: An unheeded side effect of therapeutic bed rest. Clin Sci 64:537–540, 1983.
110. Katz IA, epstein S: Posttransplantation bone disease. J Bone Miner Res 7:123–126, 1992.
111. Lukert BP, Raisz LG: Glucocorticoid-induced osteoporosis: pathogenesis and management. Ann Intern Med 112:352–164, 1990.
112. Seeman E, Wahner HW, Offord KP, et al: Differential effects of endocrine dysfunction on the axial and the appendicular skeleton. J Clin Invest 69:1302–1309, 1982.
113. Adinoff AD, Hollister JR: Steroid-induced fractures and bone loss in patients with asthma. N Engl J Med 309:265–268, 1983.
114. Baylink DJ: Glucocorticoid-induced osteoporosis. N Engl J Med 309:306–308, 1983.
115. Jowsey J, Riggs BL: Bone formation in hypercortisonism. Acta Endocrinol 63:61–68, 1970.
116. Jowell PS, Epstein S, Fallon MD, et al: 1,25-Dihydroxy-vitamin D3 modulates glucocorticoid induced alteration in serum bone gla protein and bone histomorphometry. Endocrinology 120:531–536, 1987.
117. Dempster PW: Perspectives: Bone histomorphometry in glucocorticoid-induced osteoporosis. J Bone Miner Res 4:237–241, 1989.
118. Schlosberg M, Movsowitz C, Epstein S, et al: The effect of cyclosporine A administration and its withdrawal on bone mineral metabolism in the rat. Endocrinology 124:2179–2184, 1989.
119. Kossoy LR, herbert CM, Wentz AC: Management of heart transplant recipients: Guidelines for the obstetrician-gynecologist. Am J Obstet Gynecol 159:490–499, 1988.
120. Pocock NA, Eisman JA, Yeates MG, et al: Physical fitness is a major determinant of femoral neck and lumbar spine bone mineral density. J Clin Invest 78:618–621, 1986.

121. Krolner B, Toft B, Port Nielson S: Physical exercise as prophylaxis against involutional vertebral bone loss: A controlled trial. Clin Sci 64:541–545, 1983.
122. Adami S, Fossaluzza V, Rossini M, et al: The prevention of corticosteroid-induced osteoporosis with nandrolone decanoate. Bone Miner 15:72–81, 1991.
123. Stein B, Takizawa M, Katz I, et al: Salmon calcitonin prevents cyclosporin A induced high turnover bone loss. Endocrinology 129:92–96, 1991.
124. Klein RG, Arnaud SB, Gallagher JC, et al: Intestinal calcium absorption in exogenous hypercortisolism, role of 25-hydroxy-vitamin D and corticosteroid use. J Clin invest 60:253–259, 1977.
125. Reid IR, King AR, Alexander CJ, Ibbertson HK: Prevention of steroid-induced osteoporosis with (3-amino-1-hydroxypropylidene)-1,1-biphosphonate (APD). Lancet 1:143–146, 1988.
126. Graham AF, Schroeder JS, Griepp RB, et al: Does cardiac transplantation significantly prolong life and improve its quality? Circulation 47-48(Suppl III):116–119, 1973.
127. Hunt SA, Rider AK, Stinson EB, et al: Does cardiac transplantation prolong life and improve its quality? An updated report. Circulation 54(Suppl III):56–60, 1976.
128. Gaudiani VA, Stinson EB, Alderman E, et al: Long-term survival and function after cardiac transplantation. Ann Surg 194:381–385, 1981.
129. Samuellson RG, Hunt SA, Schroeder JS: Functional and social rehabilitation of heart transplant recipients under age thirty. Scand J Thor Cardiovasc Surg 18:97–103, 1984.
130. Evans RW: Executive summary: The National cooperative Transplantation Study: BHARC-100-91-020. Seattle, Battelle-seattle Research Center, 1991.
131. Buxton MJ, Acheson R, Caine N, et al: Costs and benefits of the heart transplant programmes at Harefield and Papworth Hospitals. DHSS Research Report No. 12. London: Her Majesty's Stationer's Office, 1985.
132. Caine N, O'Brien B: Quality of life and psychological aspects of heart transplantation. In Wallwork J (ed): Heart and Heart-Lung Transplantation. Philadelphia: W.B. Saunders, 1989, pp 389–422.
133. Evans RW, Manninen DL, Maier A, et al: The quality of life in kidney and heart transplant recipients. transplant Proc 17:1579–1582, 1985.
134. Lough ME, Lindsey Am, Shinn JA, Stotts NA: Impact of symptom frequency and symptom distress on self-reported quality of life in heart transplant recipients. Heart and lung 16:193–200, 1987.
135. O'Brien BJ, Buxton MJ, Ferguson BA: Measuring the effectiveness of heart transplant programmes: Quality of life data and their relationship to survival analysis. J Chron Dis 40(Suppl 1):137–153, 1987.
136. Bunzel B, Grundböck A, Laczkovics A, et al: Quality of life after orthotopic heart transplantation. J Heart Lung Transplant 10:455–459, 1991.
137. Angerman CE, Bullinger M, Spes CH, et al: Quality of life in long-term survivors of orthotopic heart transplantation. Z Kardiol 81:411–417, 1992.
138. Riether AM, Smith SL, Lewison BJ, et al: Quality-of-life changes and psychiatric and neurocognitive outcome after heart and liver transplantation. Transplantation 54:444–450, 1992.
139. Rosenblum DS, Rosen ML, Pine ZM, et al: Health status and quality of life following cardiac transplantation. Arch Phys Med Rehabil 74:490–493, 1993.
140. Christopherson LK, Griepp RB, Stinson EB: Rehabilitation after cardiac transplantation. JAMA 236:2082–2084, 1976.
141. Degre SG, Niset GL, DeSmet JM, et al: Cardiorespiratory response to early exercise testing after orthotopic cardiac transplantation. Am J Cardiol 60:926–928, 1987.
142. Kavanagh T, Yacoub MH, Mertens DJ, et al: Cardiorespiratory responses to exercise training after orthotopic cardiac transplantation. Circulation 77:162–171, 1988.
143. Savin WM, Haskell WL, Schroeder JS, Stinson EB: Cardiorespiratory responses of cardiac transplant patients to graded, symptom-limited exercise. Circulation 62:55–60, 1980.
144. Pope SE, Stinson EB, Daughters GT, et al: Exercise response of the denervated heart in long-term cardiac transplant recipients. Am J Cardiol 46:214–218, 1980.
145. Uretsky BF: Physiology of the transplanted heart. Cardiovascular Clin 20:23–56, 1990.
146. Young JB, Leon CA, Short HD, et al: Evolution of hemodynamics after orthotopic heart and heart/lung transplantation: Early restrictive patterns persisting in occult fashion. J Heart Transplant 6:34–43, 1987.
147. Tischler MD, Lee RT, Plappert T, et al: Serial assessment of left ventricular function and mass after orthotopic heart transplantation: A four-year longitudinal study. J Am Coll Cardiol 19:60–66, 1992.
148. Drexler H: Skeletal muscle failure in heart failure. Circulation 85:1621–1622, 1992.
149. McLaughlin PR, Kleiman JH, Martin RP, et al: The effect of exercise and atrial pacing on left ventricular volume and contractility in patients with innervated and denervated hearts. Circulation 58:576–583, 1978.
150. Verani MS, George SE, Leon CA, et al: Systolic and diastolic ventricular performance at rest and during exercise in heart transplant recipients. J Heart Transplant 7:145–151, 1988.
151. Pflugfelder PW, Purves PD, McKenzie FN, Costuk WJ: Systolic and diastolic ventricular performance at rest and during exercise in heart transplant recipients. J Am Coll Cardiol 10:336–341, 1987.

152. Jones BM, Chang VP, Esmore D, et al: Psychological adjustments after cardiac transplantation. Med J Aust 149:118–122, 1988.
153. Harvison A, Jones BM, McBride M, et al: Rehabilitation after heart transplantation: The Australian experience. J Heart Transplant 7;337–341, 1988.
154. Niset G, Coustry-Degre C, Degre S: Psychosocial and physical rehabilitation after heart transplantation: 1-year follow-up. Cardiology 75:311-317, 1988.
155. Evans RW: The economics of heart transplantation. Circulation 75:63–76, 1987.
156. Shapiro PA: Life after heart transplantation. Prog Cardiovasc Dis 32:405–418, 1990.
157. Meister ND, McAleer MJ, Meister JS, et al: Returning to work after heart transplantation. J Heart Transplant 5:154–161, 1986.
158. Wallwork J, Caine N: A comparison of the quality of life of cardiac transplant patients before and after surgery. Qual Life Cardiovasc Care 2:317–331, 1985.
159. Paris W, Woodbury A, Thompson S, et al: Returning to work after heart transplantation. J Heart Lung Transplant 12:46–54, 1993.

Chapter 20

Photopheresis in Transplantation: Evolution of a Novel Immunotherapy

Mark L. Barr, MD

Current immunosuppressive protocols with cyclosporine, azathioprine, and corticosteroids, with or without induction protocols utilizing monoclonal or polyclonal antibodies such as OKT3 or ATG, have resulted in dramatically increased survival of transplanted organs. However, in addition to suppressing the immune response to the allograft, they impair immune function in a nonspecific and often toxic fashion, leaving the host susceptible to increased risk of opportunistic infections, malignancy, and the direct side effects of these drugs. Moreover, there remains significant morbidity and mortality from both acute and chronic forms of organ rejection, as seen with the development of transplant coronary artery disease. Thus, despite the toxic effects of current immunosuppressive protocols, a significant number of patients continue to die from organ-specific underimmunosuppression. Although percentages may vary, these problems continue to plague all varieties of solid organ transplantation. The inability to discriminate between individual clones of pathogenic and benign T cells and the persistent problem with ongoing chronic B-cell-related humoral immunity has led to the use of novel therapies.

Photopheresis is a technique in which peripheral-blood mononuclear cells of patients previously given a photoactivatable substance, such as 8-methoxypsoralen (8-MOP), are exposed extracorporeally to ultraviolet-A light (UVA). After the patient has taken an oral dose of psoralen, blood is removed through a peripheral intravenous line. Using a cell separator, the leukocyte-depleted blood is returned to the patient while the leukocyte-enriched plasma containing the systemically absorbed psoralen is exposed to ultraviolet light in the 320 to

400 nm range. The photoexposed white blood cells are then returned to the patient. Theoretically, photoactivated 8-MOP binds covalently to DNA pyrimidine bases, cell surface molecules, and cytoplasmic components in the exposed white blood cells.[1] The altered lymphocytes are then reinfused to produce a suppressor response that targets unirradiated T cells of similar clones in a mechanism that is not yet elucidated.

The first disease successfully treated with photopheresis in humans was cutaneous T-cell lymphoma, a disease characterized by massive expansion of a single clone of T cells.[2] Based on work with this disease, photopheresis received FDA approval for this indication. Additional disease states in which there have been laboratory and/or clinical work[3] include scleroderma (on which a major trial is ongoing in the United States), pemphigus vulgaris, rheumatoid arthritis, systemic lupus erythematosus, multiple sclerosis, and solid organ and bone marrow transplantation. All of these disease states are in part potentially mediated by expanded populations of unregulated effector T cells.

Based on prior experimental work done with 8-MOP and UVA treatment in rat autoimmune encephalitis[4] and murine lupus models,[5] a study was performed in which CBA/j mouse donor skin was grafted onto Balb/c mice to introduce histoincompatible tissue with disparity in the H2 locus.[6] Upon skin graft rejection, the spleen from the transplanted mouse was removed, splenic lymphocytes were cultured, and then treated with 8-MOP and UVA. These photoinactivated recipient splenic lymphocytes were then reinfused into a naive Balb/c mouse. These immunized Balb/c mice were tested for specific T-cell immunoresponsiveness to CBA/j alloantigens through the use of mixed lymphocyte cultures (MLC) and cytotoxicity assays. The ability to mount a delayed type hypersensitivity reaction and reject a CBA/j skin allograft was also tested. Compared with controls, Balb/c mice treated with the photoinactivated CBA/j spleen cells demonstrated decreased MLC proliferation and cytotoxic activity to CBA/j antigens. In vivo, the treated mice had significantly longer survival of CBA/j skin allografts yet retained the ability to respond to other third party skin grafts. This series of experiments represented a major finding because donor-specific immunosuppression, rather than panimmunosuppression, was seen.

With a goal of applying photopheresis to human cardiac transplantation, studies on primate cardiac xenografting were performed.[7] Using a heterotopic cynomolgous monkey-to-baboon model, a maintenance cyclosporine and steroid-based regimen was used. The experimental group in addition was started on prophylactic photopheresis beginning 3 days posttransplant and then weekly thereafter. Similar to the mouse skin graft model, the photopheresis group had an increased donor-specific immunosuppression, as shown by inhibited mixed lymphocyte culture responses compared with controls and decreased formation of lymphocytotoxic antibodies to the donor, with prolonged xenograft survival. In addition, resolution of an acute rejection episode was seen in one animal following photopheresis therapy without the need for augmented conventional immunosuppression.

Based on experimental murine and primate work and the clinical experience and safety as seen in cutaneous T-cell lymphoma, human cardiac transplantation trials were begun. In one study, high-risk patients with elevated levels of non–donor-specific anti-HLA antibody (PRA) were treated with adjuvant photopheresis.[8] Three of four patients were multiparous women and two of four were retransplants. Oral 8-MOP and the Therakos UVAR system were used in a treatment schedule of 2 days sequentially every 3 to 4 weeks for the first postoperative year and every 6 to 8 weeks during the second year. Although there was no control group and this study was purely observational, an early decrease in PRA was seen and there was a relatively low incidence of rejection.

In another study, a single photopheresis treatment was compared with 3 days of high-dose steroids in the treatment of hemodynamically stable cardiac rejection.[9]

Photopheresis alone was capable of reversing acute cellular rejection, although the success and time to complete resolution of the episode was inferior to corticosteroids. Of additional importance, the photopheresis treatment group had a trend toward less postrejection treatment infections.

Atherosclerosis in cardiac allografts is regarded as a manifestation of chronic vascular (humoral) rejection. Earlier work has shown an association between the production of non–donor-specific panel reactive anti-HLA antibody and the development of transplant atherosclerosis.[10] Based on these observations and earlier animal and human work, a phase II pilot clinical study under FDA monitoring was performed to determine whether the addition of monthly photopheresis to standard triple-drug therapy with cyclosporine, azathioprine, and corticosteroids is safe and results in lower levels of panel-reactive antibodies and transplant atherosclerosis.[11] Photopheresis was begun within 1 month of transplantation and was performed on two successive days every four weeks. Oral 8-MOP and the Therakos UVAR photopheresis system were used in this study. Patients were randomized to either adjunctive photopheresis (n = 10) or only standard triple-drug therapy (n = 13). Mean follow-up was 19 months. Both groups were comparable in terms of the following demographics: age, sex, race, pretransplant heart disease, graft ischemic time, HLA mismatch, and donor–recipient CMV status. During the follow-up period, cyclosporine level, azathioprine dose, and cumulative steroid dose were similar between the two groups. No difference in average white blood cell counts, cholesterol levels, or infection rates was seen. Rejection incidence and grades of rejection were also not significantly different. Non–donor-specific panel-reactive anti-HLA antibody levels were significantly reduced in the photopheresis group compared with the control group by postoperative months 3 or 4 ($p < 0.03$) and remained significantly lower through postoperative month 6 ($p < 0.05$). Of patients surviving at least 1 year follow-up, 2 of 10 patients in the photopheresis group had transplant atherosclerosis on coronary angiography compared with 4 of 11 in the control group ($p = $ ns). If the patient did not have obvious transplant atherosclerosis at the time of the angiogram, intravascular ultrasound testing was performed to determine coronary artery intimal thickness. Intimal thickness at one year was 0.23 mm (± 0.09) in the photopheresis group vs. 0.49 mm (± 0.20) in the control group ($p < 0.04$). At 2 year follow-up, intimal thickness was 0.28 (± 0.08) in the photopheresis group vs. 0.46 mm (± 0.07) in the control group ($p < 0.02$). No difference existed at 2 years in the incidence of death in the two groups—2 of 10 in the photopheresis group vs. 3 of 13 in the control group. Photopheresis was safe, well-tolerated, and did not increase morbidity of triple-drug immunosuppression in cardiac transplant patients. Treated patients showed early reduction in non–donor-specific panel-reactive anti-HLA antibody levels. Of greater clinical importance was the finding of a significantly decreased coronary artery intimal thickness at up to 2 year follow-up—the first immunotherapy that has resulted in this finding in humans.[12]

In a subsequent European study[13] using an earlier, and more frequent, treatment schedule, and using liquid 8-MOP (which is more reliable than the oral form) added directly to the extracorporeal buffy coat, rejection and infection rates were reduced compared with the control group. Based on these earlier studies, an international, multicenter, randomized clinical trial utilizing liquid 8-MOP and the Therakos UVAR system is in progress to investigate the impact of prophylactic therapy on the incidence of acute cellular rejection and infection in cardiac transplant patients. Potential mechanisms of photopheresis may involve generation of CD8 positive clonotypic T cells; increased expression and/or recognition of immunogenic peptides in Class I HLA clefts; inhibition of second signal transmission from antigen presenting cells; and production of cytokines by irradiated leukocytes. Further research must establish the optimal and minimal treatment frequency and duration and potential synergy with other new immunoregulatory agents. Characterization of the host response needs to define the mechanism of action and may lead to future new drug development. Finally, effects on the development of microchimerism need to be investigated. Future transplant studies will involve other solid organs as well as effects on graft vs. host disease in bone marrow transplantation. Increasing anecdotal clinical experience with photopheresis for resistant rejection in cardiac, pulmonary, and renal transplant patients has led to development of "rescue" protocols. This may prove of great importance in the areas of lung and small bowel transplantation in which current clinical results with conventional immunosuppressive agents have been disappointing. These current studies and future experimental and clinical trials will help define the role of this novel, safe, and nontoxic immunomodulating technology in the field of transplantation.

REFERENCES

1. Gasparro F, Dall'Amico R, et al: Molecular aspects of extracorporeal photochemotherapy. Yale J Biol Med 62:579–594, 1989.
2. Edelson R, Berger C, Gasparro F, et al: Treatment of cutaneous T-cell lymphoma by extracorporeal photochemotherapy—Preliminary results. N Engl J Med 316:297–303, 1987.
3. Rook A, Cohen J, et al: Therapeutic applications of photopheresis. Dermatol Clin 11:339–347, 1993.
4. Lider O, Reshef T, Beraud E, et al: Anti-idiotypic network induce by T-cell vaccination against experimental autoimmune encephalomyelitis. Science 239:181–183, 1988.
5. Berger C, Perez M, Laroche L, Edelson R: Inhibition of autoimmune disease in a murine model of systemic lupus erythematosus induced by exposure to syngeneic photoinactivated lymphocytes. J Invest Dermatol 94:52–57, 1990.
6. Perez M, Edelson R, Laroche L, Berger C: Specific suppression of anti-allograft immunity by immunization with syngeneic photoinactivated effector lymphocytes. J Invest Dermatol 92:669–676, 1989.
7. Pepino P, Berger C, et al: Primate cardiac allo and xeno transplantation: Modulation of the immune response with photochemotherapy. Eur Surg Res 21:105–113, 1989.
8. Rose E, Barr M, et al: Photochemotherapy in human heart transplant recipients at high risk for fatal rejection. J Heart Lung Transplant 11:746–750, 1992.
9. Costanzo-Nordin M, Hubbell E, et al: Photopheresis versus corticosteroids in the therapy of heart transplant rejection. Circulation 86(II):242–250, 1992.
10. Rose E, Pepino P, Barr M, et al: Relation of HLA antibodies and graft atherosclerosis in human cardiac allograft recipients. J Heart Lung Transplant 11:S120–S123, 1992.
11. Barr M, Berger C, et al: Photochemotherapy for the prevention of graft atherosclerosis in cardiac transplantation. J Heart Lung Transplant 12:S85, 1993.
12. Barr M, McLaughlin S, Murphy M, et al: Prophylactic photopheresis and effect on graft atherosclerosis in cardiac transplantation. Transplant Proc 27:1993–1994, 1995.
13. Meiser B, Kur F, Reichenspurner H, et al: Reduction of the incidence of rejection by adjunct immunosuppression with photochemotherapy after heart transplantation. Transplantation 57:563–568, 1994.

Chapter **21**

New Diagnostic Modalities in the Assessment of Transplant Coronary Disease

Todd J. Anderson, MD
Ian T. Meredith, MBBS, PhD
Stacy F. Davis, MD
Gilbert H. Mudge, MD
Andrew P. Selwyn, MD
Peter Ganz, MD
Alan C. Yeung, MD

Allograft cardiac transplantation is now an accepted treatment option for patients with many forms of end-stage heart disease. Survival rate exceeds 85% at 1 year and 70% at 5 years. Despite this, long-term survival is threatened by the development of transplant coronary disease.[1] Angiographic studies identify abnormalities of the coronary arteries in as many as 50% of patients at the 5-year evaluation.[2] Significant progression of disease with ischemic manifestations often develops at this stage and treatment is difficult.[3] Coronary angiography provides a *lumenogram* and can underestimate the burden of disease particularly when the intimal thickening is smooth and diffuse as is the case in transplant coronary disease. Extensive evidence now suggests that early intimal thickening is common and can be identified by using intravascular ultrasound (IVUS) long before angiographic evidence of atherosclerosis exists.[4] This technique provides a sensitive method of quantitating the burden of atherosclerosis, following patients longitudinally, and identifying risk factors leading to transplant coronary disease.

The etiology of transplant coronary disease has not been clearly elucidated, but is likely a form of chronic rejection in the setting of traditional cardiac risk factors. Immunologic and ischemic endothelial injury have been implicated in this process.[5] Endothelium-derived nitric oxide has important anti-atherogenic properties including vasodilation, inhibition of platelet aggregation and smooth muscle cell proliferation, and leukocyte-endothelial cell adhesion.[6] Clinical studies that assess coronary vasomotion in response to infused endothelium-dependent agonists (such as acetylcholine) have demonstrated endothelial dysfunction in the setting of both native and transplantation atherosclerosis.[7,8] Endothelial dysfunction is known to precede structurally significant atherosclerosis and is likely important in its pathogenesis.[9] Abnormal vasomotor responses may thus serve as a marker in patients at increased risk of atherosclerosis progression.

This review discusses our current understanding of the use of intravascular ultrasound and endothelial function testing in the diagnosis and follow-up of patients after cardiac transplantation.

INTRAVASCULAR ULTRASOUND

High frequency (20 to 30 Mhz) ultrasound systems have been developed to image intravascular structures. Both mechanical and phase-array techniques have been successfully employed to create real-time cross-sectional images of the coronary arteries.[10] Early studies established that a reasonable correlation by IVUS with angiographic measurement of cross-sectional area could be obtained in relatively nondiseased arteries.[11] If the image is taken at a site of an eccentric stenosis, or if the IVUS catheter is aligned obliquely across the vessel, correlation with angiographic areas can be poor. In vitro studies have also demonstrated that IVUS is able to identify thickened intima, with a typical three-layer appearance.[12] In a normal coronary artery, the single layer intima cannot be visualized. After the intima thickens beyond 150 µm, however, it can be identified by IVUS. The echogenic intima is separated from the media by the internal elastic lamina, creating a boundary between intima and media. Tobis and colleagues reported in nontransplant patients that intimal thickening could be prominently seen when the angiogram appeared completely normal.[13] This has been subsequently confirmed by other studies, suggesting that angiography is not sensitive in detecting early coronary atherosclerosis.

IVUS in Transplantation

St. Goar and colleagues at Stanford were among the first to report on the use of intravascular ultrasound in transplant patients.[14] Using a 30-MHz mechanical system (CVIS, Sunnyvale, CA), they compared coronary diameters with IVUS and quantitative angiography. They confirmed that ultrasound tended to overestimate the diameter, and that the correlation between the two was improved when the ultrasound catheter was positioned parallel to the long axis of the vessel. Subsequent to this, the same investigators reported on vessel wall morphology in 80 patients posttransplantation.[4] They developed a grading system based on the overall thickness and circumferential extent of disease (Table 1). They noted that some degree of atherosclerosis was present in all 60 patients studied at least 1 or more years posttransplantation. The majority of these patients had angiographically normal coronary arteries. They could not identify any patient or donor demographic factors associated with intimal thickening. The utility of intravascular ultrasound in detecting "angiographically silent" atherosclerosis has been confirmed by other studies as well.[15] The consistent finding among these studies is that intimal thickening is common within a year posttransplantation and increases in proportion and magnitude with increasing time posttransplantation. A report from the Brigham and Women's Hospital was only able to demonstrate intimal thickening in

TABLE I.   Stanford Ultrasound Classification of Coronary Artery Disease after Cardiac Transplantation

Classification	Normal	I	II	III	IV
Severity	None	Minimal	Mild	Moderate	Severe
Intimal thickness	None	< 0.3 mm	> 0.3 mm	0.3 to 0.5 mm or	> 1.0 mm or
		< 180°	> 180°	> 0.5 mm < 180°	> 0.5 mm > 180°

Angle = extent of circumferential intimal thickening.
From St. Goar, et al: Intracoronary ultrasound in cardiac transplant recipients: in vivo evidence of "angiographically silent" intimal thickening. Circulation 85:979–987, 1992, with permission.

about a third of patients studied 1 year posttransplantation.[15] A similar incidence has been demonstrated by other investigators.[16] However, by 5 or more years posttransplantation, all patients have intimal thickening by ultrasound.[15] The only factor that predicted the degree of thickening in this study was the time posttransplantation and a history of hypercholesterolemia before transplant.

St. Goar and colleagues studied 25 patients within 1 month of transplantation for whom the mean age of the donor was 28 years.[17] Of these, 14 subjects had intimal thickening and 5 patients with cardiac risk factors had discrete stenoses. This study confirmed previous pathologic studies that demonstrated that young subjects with angiographically normal vessels have a range of coronary intimal thickening. Studies from our own laboratory at Brigham and Women's have demonstrated moderate to severe intimal thickening in transplanted hearts from older donors, particularly if there was a history of cigarette smoking.

From the cross-sectional studies done to date, certain IVUS features of transplantation atherosclerosis appear (Table 2). The process starts soon after transplantation and is often patchy and eccentric. Not all segments studied will be affected, and a thin eccentric-to-concentric rim of intimal thickening is often the first manifestation. In patients studied further out after transplantation, the proportion of segments with intimal thickening increases, and more concentric lesions are present. Calcification, which is common in native vessel atherosclerosis, is distinctly uncommon in the first 10 years posttransplantation (Fig. 1). Longitudinal studies are ongoing to confirm what has been suggested by cross-sectional studies. Preliminary work by the Stanford group has shown that about 30% of lesions progress over a 1-year period. Risk factors for progression are not clear at this time.

Safety

Although IVUS provides very useful information about the pathology of the intima, its safety in patients undergoing repeated studies has been questioned. All patients are

TABLE 2.   Intravascular Ultrasound Features of Transplantation Atherosclerosis

Onset	Progression
Occurs within first year	$^1/_3$ segments will progress over 1 year
Begins as eccentric rim	Becomes concentric, or eccentric with greater thickness
Often patchy, involving only a portion of vessel	Involves a greater proportion of segments
Calcification not seen	Calcification is rare in first 5 years

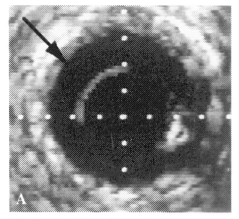

FIGURE 1.   A, Normal intravascular ultrasound image. Black arrow shows lumen-media border with no thickened intima. B, Mild eccentric thickening as shown by the black arrow. Thickening extends from 9 o'clock to 6 o'clock. C, Moderate concentric thickening. D, Concentric thickening which is more severe on the right side of the image (black arrow). E, Severe concentric thickening, more severe on the right side of the image.

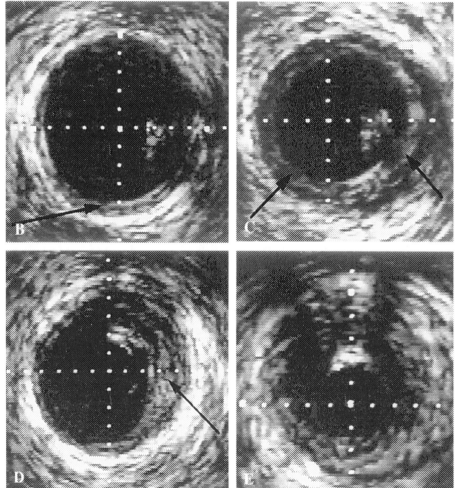

treated with systemic anticoagulation therapy and sublingual nitroglycerin before study. Arteries less than 2.0 mm are avoided, because risk probably increases in these patients. In patients in whom the device is used to assess coronary interventions, the incidence of complications is very low. Coronary spasm requiring termination of the study occurs in about 3 to 4% of cases. No serious or lasting complications resulted from this spasm.[18] Serious complications, including arterial dissection or myocardial infarction, are distinctly uncommon. Using quantitative angiography, Pinto and colleagues also assessed imaged and nonimaged vessels and demonstrated no difference in vessel diameter changes over a 1-year period. This suggests that IVUS does not accelerate progression of transplantation atherosclerosis and can be used safely.[18]

Future Directions

The potential advantage of intravascular ultrasound is its ability to detect intimal thickening long before it can be seen by angiography. This will provide an opportunity to follow the progression of atherosclerosis in a longitudinal fashion. It is hoped that risk factors for the progression of disease will be identified, thus allowing a better understanding of its pathogenesis.

A multicenter IVUS transplant group, headed by researchers from Stanford, has been gathering data on patients in the first 2 years posttransplantation. Preliminary data on 300 patients were presented at the American Heart Association in November 1994. Longitudinal data available in 1995 should provide insights into potential risk factors for transplant atherosclerosis (Yeung and associates, personal communication). Because of the relatively small number of patients receiving transplants at individual centers, multicenter studies will have much better power to answer these difficult questions.

In the next several years, improvements in catheter design will allow interrogation of more of the coronary vasculature. Three-dimensional reconstruction with detail plaque burden quantification may also become routinely used.

ENDOTHELIAL FUNCTION TESTING

In 1980 Furchgott and Zawadski made the simple yet important discovery that the endothelium was required to mediate vasodilation to acetylcholine.[19] They speculated that an endothelium-derived relaxing factor (EDRF) was responsible for this action. Subsequent work has confirmed that EDRF is likely nitric oxide, which is synthesized from the guanidino nitrogen atom of L-arginine by the endothelium-constitutive nitric oxide synthase (Fig. 2).[20] Endothelial-derived nitric oxide is an important mediator of vasodilation in health. It also, however, inhibits platelet aggregation and adhesion, smooth muscle cell proliferation, and leukocyte adhesion. All of these actions can be viewed as antiatherogenic. Nitric oxide is released from vascular endothelium in response to a number of pharmacologic agonists including acetylcholine, and physiologic stimuli including shear stress. Ludmer and coworkers were among the first to infuse acetylcholine into the coronary arteries of patients in the catheterization laboratory.[7] They observed in healthy subjects without cardiac risk factors that acetylcholine with final estimated coronary concentration of 10^{-8} to 10^{-6} M, resulted in coronary vasodilation. In patients with luminal irregularities or coronary stenoses, however, acetylcholine results in vasoconstriction. In vivo, the observed effect of acetylcholine is a balance of its direct vasoconstricting effects through smooth muscle muscarinic receptors and its dilating effect through the release of endothelium-derived nitric oxide. In health, the balance favors dilation, whereas vasoconstriction is observed when the activity of nitric oxide is diminished. This so-called endothelial dysfunction is observed in

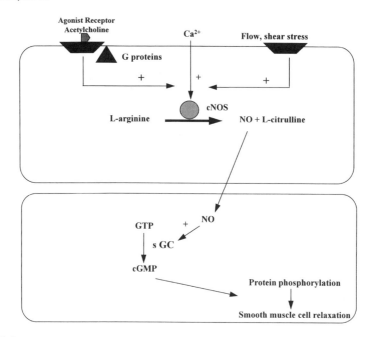

FIGURE 2.   The L-arginine nitric oxide pathway. Acetylcholine or shear stress, for example, interacts with receptors leading to stimulating of cNOS, a Ca++-dependent process. L-arginine is converted to nitric oxide, which then interacts with soluble guanylate cyclase, leading to an increase in cGMP; cGMP leads to protein phosphorylation and subsequent smooth muscle cell relaxation. cNOS = constitutive nitric oxide synthase; NO = nitric oxide; Ca++ = calcium; sGC = soluble guanylate cyclasel; GTP = guanosine triphosphate; cGMP = cyclic guanosine monophosphate.

patients with atherosclerosis, or risk factors for atherosclerosis, and a variety of other conditions (Table 3). Intravascular ultrasound studies have confirmed that abnormal vasoconstrictor responses precede intimal thickening and may be an early marker of endothelial dysfunction and subsequent progression of atherosclerosis.

Endothelial Function Testing Post-Cardiac Transplantation

Conduit Vessel Responses

Fish and colleagues were the first to describe acetylcholine testing in patients posttransplantation.[8] In 12 patients 1 or 2 years posttransplant, they observed vasoconstriction in all segments with angiographic evidence of luminal irregularities. However, they also observed vasoconstriction in the majority of coronary segments with smooth coronary angiograms. They concluded that impaired responses to acetylcholine were common and may be important in the development of atherosclerosis. A study by Nellessen and colleagues assessed acetylcholine responses in 10 heart transplant patients with normal coronary angiograms.[21] They observed vasoconstriction in all patients, but at doses of 10^{-5} M, which has subsequently been shown to induce nonspecific vasoconstriction.

Other groups have suggested that substance P, an endothelium-dependent vasodilator, may also be an appropriate agent for testing endothelial function. Kushwaha and coworkers used substance P to demonstrate that vasodilation was maintained in 12 patients posttransplant with normal coronary arteries.[22] They have also presented

TABLE 3.   Conditions Associated with Endothelial Dysfunction

Atherosclerosis	Syndrome X
Hypercholesterolemia	Variant angina
Hypertension	Cocaine use
Diabetes mellitus	Dilated cardiomyopathy
Cigarette smoking	Chagas' disease
Transplantation atherosclerosis	

preliminary data showing a shift in the dose-response curve in patients with and without angiographic coronary artery disease. However, response to the maximum dose of substance P was not different between the two groups. Mügge and coworkers were able to demonstrate a trend for a difference in the conduit vessel dilator response to substance P in patients with normal coronary arteries compared to those with angiographic atherosclerosis (11% vs. 5% dilation; 0 = 0.06).[23] They also observed that flow-mediated vasodilation to the distal infusion of papaverine was impaired in patients with transplant vasculopathy. This has been confirmed in a recently published study.[24] Response to the smooth muscle dilator nitroglycerin is preserved in patients with transplant atherosclerosis, suggesting the defect in dilator responses is at the level of the endothelium.

These studies have suggested that abnormal vasodilator responses are commonly seen by 1 year posttransplant. Ultrasound studies have also confirmed that intimal thickening is common by the 1 year exam as well.[4] We postulated that immunologic and ischemic injury to the endothelium in the perioperative period may be important in the pathogenesis of atherosclerosis. As such, we evaluated the acetylcholine response in 35 patients within the first month posttransplantation.[25] We observed vasoconstriction to acetylcholine in two out of three of these patients. No donor or recipient characteristics predicted the Ach response. The long-term significance of this early impairment of dilator responses must await longitudinal studies.

Resistance Vessel Responses

Coronary blood flow is mainly determined at the resistance vessel level (< 100 μm), and as such, the blood flow flow response to infused agonists is a measure of resistance vessel function. Treasure and colleagues studied patients 1 to 3 years posttransplantation with acetylcholine and adenosine.[26] Blood flow was measured using a Miller Doppler catheter. There was no difference in the flow response to the endothelium-independent agonist adenosine, but patients 3 years posttransplantation had decreased responses to acetylcholine and a decrease in the acetylcholine/adenosine flow ratio, compared with patients 1 or 2 years following transplantation. Mügge and coworkers studied the blood flow responses to a bolus infusion of substance P.[23] The peak blood flow response was decreased in patients with angiographic evidence of atherosclerosis. both of these studies suggest that impaired dilator responses to endothelium-dependent agonists also occur in the coronary microvasculature.

Structure-Function Correlation

A recent study from our laboratory assessed the relationship between conduit vessel dilator responses to acetylcholine and the intravascular ultrasound appearance of the vessel.[15] Forty patients from 1 to 8 years posttransplant were studied. The relationship between acetylcholine response and intimal thickening is complex and time dependent. The majority of coronary segments studied in patients 1 year posttransplant had no evidence of intimal thickening, but had endothelial dysfunction. This confirmed that endothelial dysfunction could precede structural atherosclerosis, which has been shown in nontransplant patients as well. Interestingly, in patients more than 5 years posttransplantation who were healthy clinically, preserved endothelial function was observed in segments with moderate intimal thickening. The variable nature between intimal pathology and endothelial function is likely a result of an episodic nature of immune injury.

Treatment of Endothelial Dysfunction

Studies in animals and humans involving nontransplanted patients have demonstrated that endothelial dysfunction can be improved by a variety of methods including lowering cholesterol and L-arginine infusion.

Drexler and associates have recently administered L-arginine to 18 patients post-cardiac transplantation.[27] L-arginine alone did not change conduit vessel diameter nor coronary blood flow. It did, however, attenuate acetylcholine-induced vasoconstriction (−6.8% before vs. −2.8% after L-arginine). The acetylcholine-induced increase in blood flow was significantly enhanced with L-arginine as well (+121% vs. +176%). A subgroup of patients also had intravascular ultrasound studies; data suggested that reversibility of epicardial endothelial dysfunction was more likely to occur in arteries with a normal vessel wall morphology. The effect of chronic supplementation of L-arginine on endothelial function has not been studied.

Fleischhauer and partners administered omega-3 fatty acids (fish oil) to 7 transplant patients for 3 weeks and then measured acetylcholine responses, comparing them with 7 patients not treated with fish oil.[28] The patients treated with omega-3 fatty acid had better vasodilator response than the control patients, suggesting that fish oil alters endothelium-dependent coronary vasodilation. Clearly studies must be done in which responses are measured before and after an intervention. However, improvement in endothelium-dependent vasodilation to acetylcholine has been shown in nontransplanted patients treated for 6 months as well with omega-3 fatty acids.[29] No other studies have aimed to improve endothelial function in patients after cardiac transplantation.

Endothelial Function as a Predictor of Atherosclerosis Development

Ergonovine does not test the release of endothelium-dependent nitric oxide but is known to cause vasoconstriction in areas of intimal thickening in patients with variant angina. Kushwaha and colleagues administered ergonovine to a small series of patients after transplantation.[30] Patients who demonstrated a marked vasoconstrictor response to ergonovine were more likely to demonstrate angiographic evidence of atherosclerosis than those who did not constrict. Matsuguchi and colleagues, from our laboratory, evaluated patients who were clinically well 5 or more years posttransplantation and those who had died of graft atherosclerosis.[31] The patients who were clinically well had minimal loss of coronary diameter with serial quantitative angiographic studies and had normal vasodilator responses to acetylcholine. Patients who died of graft atherosclerosis had normal vasodilator responses to acetylcholine. Patients who died of graft atherosclerosis had a greater loss of coronary diameter over the same period and an abnormal response to acetylcholine. This small retrospective study of highly selected patients suggested that constriction to acetylcholine 1 year posttransplantation may be associated with development of graft atherosclerosis.

We sought to address the discriminative ability of the acetylcholine vasodilator response to predict the development of atherosclerosis in a more rigorous fashion.[32] We identified 38 patients who had acetylcholine testing 1 year posttransplantation and had at least 4 years of follow-up. Of these, 21 had endothelial dysfunction and 17 had preserved endothelial function. Patients were evaluated for death caused by atherosclerosis, myocardial infarction, ischemic left ventricular dysfunction, and angiographic evidence of coronary stenoses. The change in coronary diameter by serial quantitative angiographic studies, over a mean 3-year period, was also assessed. No significant difference existed in the number of atherosclerotic events in the dysfunction and normal function group (8 vs. 5). There was also no difference in the number of patients with angiographic evidence of atherosclerosis (8 vs. 5). A weak trend showed a greater loss of coronary caliber (0.11 mm/year vs. 0.07 mm/year) in patients with endothelial dysfunction, but this did not reach significance. We were thus unable to demonstrate in this limited study that a vasoconstrictor response to acetylcholine 1 year posttransplant was associated with a higher angiographic incidence of atherosclerosis or ischemic complications.

We recently completed a study in which we assessed the acetylcholine response immediately posttransplantation and performed serial intravascular ultrasound studies over the next year. We hypothesized that vasoconstriction early after transplantation is a result of ischemic and immunologic injury and would predispose patients to development of accelerated atherosclerosis. We chose intravascular ultrasound as a more sensitive end-point than clinical events and demonstrated that patients with an early constrictor response to acetylcholine developed more intimal thickening in the first year than those with normal endothelial function.[33]

CONCLUSIONS

Coronary angiography has been the gold standard for assessing coronary anatomy after cardiac transplantation. However, studies have shown that it is not sensitive for the early detection and follow-up of these patients. Intravascular ultrasound allows much more detailed interrogation of the thickened intima, which has been shown to occur early after transplantation. Endothelial dysfunction manifested as as an abnormal vasomotor response to acetylcholine also occurs early after transplantation and may serve as a marker of accelerated atherosclerosis. If this proves true, then endothelial function testing will allow identification of patients who would have the most to gain from prospective multicenter studies aimed at decreasing the progression of atherosclerosis. Much needs to be learned about the complex interaction between standard cardiac risk factors, immunologic and ischemic factors, and their impact on endothelial function and transplantation coronary disease. Studies which address the functional aspects of coronary atherosclerosis provide information about the biology of the endothelium above and beyond that which can be obtained with angiography. A combination of functional and structural assessments with acetylcholine and intravascular ultrasound at yearly intervals may allow a better insight into the accelerated atherosclerosis that threatens long-term survival in these patients.

Acknowledgment.   This work was supported by a Clinical Fellowship of the Alberta Heritage Foundation for Medical Research (TJA); a National Heart Foundation of Australia Ralph Reader Overseas Research Fellowship (ITM); NHLBI Research Career Development Award 1 K04 HL-02566 (PG); NHLBI R01 HL-38780-05 (APS); NHLBI Clinician-Investigator Development Award 1 K08 HL-02787 (ACY).

REFERENCES

1. Gao SZ, Schroeder JS, Alderman EL, et al: Clinical and laboratory correlations of accelerated coronary artery disease in the cardiac transplant patient. Circulation 76:V:56–61, 1987.
2. Gao SZ, Alderman EL, Schroeder JS, et al: Accelerated coronary vascular disease in the heart transplant patient: Coronary arteriographic findings. J Am Coll Cardiol 12:334–340, 1988.
3. Miller LW: Long-term complications of cardiac transplantation. Prog Cardiovasc Dis 33:229–282, 1991.

4. St. Goar FG, Pinto FJ, Alderman EL, et al: Intracoronary ultrasound in cardiac transplant recipients—in vivo evidence of "angiographically silent" intimal thickening. Circulation 85:979–987, 1992.
5. Salomon RN, Hughs CW, Schoen FJ, et al: Human coronary transplantation-associated evidence for chronic immune reaction to activated graft endothelial cells. Am J Pathol 138:791–798, 1991.
6. Moncada S, Higgs A: The L-arginine-nitric oxide pathway. N Engl J Med 329:2002–2012, 1993.
7. Ludmer PL, Selwyn AP, Shook, et al: Paradoxical vasoconstriction induced by acetylcholine in atherosclerotic coronary arteries. N Engl J Med 315:1046–1051, 1986.
8. Fish RD, Nabel EG, Selwyn AP, et al: Responses of coronary arteries of cardiac transplant patients to acetylcholine. J Clin Invest 8–21, 1988.
9. Reddy KG, Nair RN, Sheehan HM, Hodgson JMcB: Evidence that selective endothelial dysfunction may occur in the absence of angiographic or ultrasound atherosclerosis in patients with risk factors for atherosclerosis. J Am Coll Cardiol 23:833–843, 1994.
10. Yock PG, Johnson EL, Linker DT: Intravascular ultrasound: Development and clinical potential. Int J Card Imag 2:185–193, 1988.
11. Nissen SE, Gurely JC, Grines CL, et al: Intravascular ultrasound assessment of lumen size and wall morphology in normal subjects and patients with coronary artery disease. Circulation 84:1087–1099, 1991.
12. Fitzgerald PJ, St. Goar FG, Connolly AJ, et al: Intravascular ultrasound imaging of coronary arteries: Is three layers the norm? Circulation 86:154–158, 1992.
13. Tobis JM, Mallery J, Mahon D, et al: Intravascular ultrasound imaging of human coronary arteries in vivo. Circulation 83:L913–L926, 1991.
14. St. Goar FG, Pinto FJ, Alderman EL, et al: Intravascular ultrasound imaging of angiographically normal coronary arteries: an in vivo comparison with quantitative angiography. J Am Coll Cardiol 18:952–958, 1991.
15. Anderson TJ, Meredith IT, Uehata A, et al: Functional significance of intimal thickening as detected by intravascular ultrasound early and late after cardiac transplantation. Circulation 88:1093–1100, 1993.
16. Ventura HO, Ramee SR, Ashit J, et al: Coronary artery imaging with intravascular ultrasound in patients following cardiac transplantation. Transplantation 53:216–219, 1992.
17. St Goar FG, Pinto FJ, Alderman EL, et al: Detection of coronary atherosclerosis in young adult hearts using intravascular ultrasound. Circulation 86:756–763, 1992.
18. Pinto FJ, St. Goar FG, Gao SZ, et al: Immediate and one-year safety of intracoronary ultrasonic imaging: Evaluation with serial quantitative angiography. Circulation 88;1709–1714, 1993.
19. Furchgott RF, Zawadski JV: The obligatory role of endothelial cells in the relaxation of arterial smooth muscle by acetylcholine. Nature 28:373–376, 1980.
20. Palmer RMJ, Ashton D, Moncada S: Vascular endothelial cells synthesize nitric oxide from L-arginine. Nature 333:664–666, 1988.
21. Nellessen U, Lee TC, Fischell TA, et al: Effects of acetylcholine on epicardial coronary arteries after cardiac transplantation without angiographic evidence of fixed graft narrowing. Am J Cardiol 62:1093–1097, 988.
22. Kushwaha SS, Crossman DC, Bustami M, et al: Substance P for evaluation of coronary endothelial function after cardiac transplantation. J Am Coll Cardiol 17:1537–1544, 1991.
23. Mügge A, Heublein B, Kuhn M, et al: Impaired coronary dilator responses to substance P and impaired flow-dependent dilator responses in heart transplant patients with graft vasculopathy. J Am Coll Cardiol 21:163–170, 1993.
24. Heroux AL, Silverman P, Costanzo MR, et al: Intracoronary ultrasound assessment of morphological and functional abnormalities associated with cardiac allograft vasculopathy. Circulation 89:272–277, 1994.
25. Meredith IT, Anderson TJ, Uehata A, et al: Early dysfunction of the coronary endothelium after cardiac transplantation [abstract]. Aust N Z J Med 22(4 Suppl):45, 1992.
26. Treasure CB, Vita JA, Ganz P, et al: Loss of the coronary microvascular response to acetylcholine in cardiac transplant patients. Circulation 86:1156–1164, 1992.
27. Drexler H, Fischell TA, Pinto FJ, et al: Effect of L-arginine on coronary endothelial function in cardiac transplant recipients: Relation to vessel wall morphology. Circulation 89:1615–1623, 1994.
28. Fleischhauer FJ, Yan W-D, Fischell TA: Fish oil improves endothelium-dependent coronary vasodilation in heart transplant recipients. J Am Coll Cardiol 21:982–989, 1993.
29. Vekshtein VI, yeung AC, Vita JA, et al: Fish oil improves endothelium-dependent relaxation in patients with coronary artery disease [abstract]. Circulation 80:II-434A, 1989.
30. Kushwaha S, Lythall D, Maseri A, et al: Coronary reactivity to ergonovine—Possible relationship to accelerated coronary arterial disease in cardiac transplant recipients. Eur Heart J 12:520–525, 1991.
31. Matsuguchi T, Ryan TJ Jr, Vekshtein VI, et al: Endothelial vasomotor function in the long term follow-up of coronary disease in cardiac transplant patients. Circulation 84(Suppl II):353, 1991.
32. Anderson TJ, Meredith IT, Selwyn AP, et al: Early endothelial dysfunction does not predict the development of transplant coronary atherosclerosis [abstract]. Can J Cardiol 9(Suppl E):29E, 1993.
33. Davis SF, Yeung AC, Meredith IT, et al: Early endothelial dysfunction predicts the development of transplant coronary artery disease at one year posttransplant. Circulation (in press).

Chapter 22

Cardiac Xenotransplantation: Experimental Advances, Ethical Issues, and Clinical Potential

Robert E. Michler, MD

Jonathan M. Chen, MD

With the development of increasingly effective immunosuppressive agents, cardiac transplantation has progressed to the point at which it currently represents the best therapeutic option available to patients with end-stage heart disease. Despite this, the supply of human donor hearts remains inadequate to meet the ever-increasing demand. Evans and colleagues recently estimated that whereas approximately 17,000 people per year under the age of 55 could conceivably benefit from cardiac allotransplantation in the United States, no more than about 2,200 viable donor hearts per year are currently available.[1-3]

This national shortage of cardiac donors is reflected by the calculated 30% national mortality rate of adult patients awaiting cardiac transplantation and is further supported by our experience from the Cardiac Transplantation Service of the Columbia-Presbyterian Medical Center (CPMC) in New York. Similarly, the Pediatric Heart and Lung Transplantation Working Group of the International Society of Heart and Lung Transplantation documented that in 1993, of the 153 United Network for Organ Sharing (UNOS) Status I pediatric patients listed for transplantation, 38 (25%) died while on the waiting list; of the 72 neonates (ages 0 to 30 days) listed, 22 (31%) died awaiting transplantation, and of the 95 patients ages 0 to 6 months listed, 26 (27%) died awaiting transplantation.[4] This is further supported by our experience at CPMC where 26 (28%) of 92 pediatric patients listed for transplantation between 1988 and 1994 died awaiting cardiac transplantation.

Thus, although the 1-year survival rate of cardiac transplantation currently exceeds 80% at most centers, because of the lack of organ donors, the risk of awaiting heart transplantation is now greater than the risk of undergoing the procedure. If the field of cardiac transplantation is to overcome the current shortage of donors, alternatives to allografts for cardiac replacement must be explored.

The experimental search for a "bridge" to human heart transplantation has focused primarily on two alternatives: mechanical devices and biologic devices (xenografts). Although mechanical left-ventricular assist devices have witnessed relative success in carefully selected patients with isolated left-ventricular failure, exclusion criteria for their use eliminate patients with biventricular failure, and because of the physical size of the device, also those with a total body surface area (BSA) less than 1.5 square meters. Thus, many women, and virtually all children, are not candidates for mechanical left-ventricular assistance owing to their small size.

Biologic cardiac replacement obviates the major problems of mechanical cardiac assistance (e.g., external power supply, infection, thromboembolism), yet instead poses the immunologic problems of rejection and infection associated with transplantation. Decades of clinical experience have shown that these problems can be managed successfully in most patients who receive cardiac allografts. Although the introduction of cyclosporine as the primary immunosuppressive agent for cardiac transplant recipients resulted in excellent survival rates and significantly decreased recipient morbidity, the immunologic barrier that must be overcome in cross-species xenotransplantation is unquestionably greater than that in allotransplantation. Hence, the overall immunosuppression that must be maintained for prolonged graft survival—as well as its ill effects—is greater in the case of xenografts when compared with allografts. It is clear, however, that only by refining the methods by which we may overcome these cross-species immunologic barriers will the clinical success of xenotransplantation be realized.

This chapter discusses three topics in cardiac xenotransplantation: (1) immunologic barriers and potential immunosuppressive strategies, (2) ethical issues, and (3) the potential for clinical reality.

IMMUNOLOGIC BARRIERS

Rejection in xenotransplantation historically has been categorized according to effector mechanism: whether preformed natural antibodies against donor-tissue antigens are present (as in xenografts between distantly related species, or so-called "discordant" xenografts) or absent (as in xenografts between closely related species, or so-called "concordant" xenografts).[5] Thus, whereas rejection between distantly related species (hyperacute) commonly takes place rapidly, that between closely-related species (acute, chronic) may take substantially longer.

In any host, the distinction between self and nonself relies on the immune system for its detection and effector functions. Although discordant xenotransplantation has come to be associated primarily with humoral effectors of the immune system, and concordant xenotransplantation, like allotransplantation, primarily with cell-mediated effectors, both humoral and cell-mediated arms of the immune system are potentially active in every rejection event. Indeed, the only difference among the individual categories of rejection is the immune mechanism that predominates in the given rejection episode (e.g., humoral mechanisms predominate in hyperacute rejection; cellular mechanisms predominate in chronic rejection). In general, this predominance is also temporally related. Thus, the clinician may largely predict which arm of the immune response exerts the greatest influence on the rejection episode simply by the time interval between transplantation and rejection. However, these predominances express but one aspect of

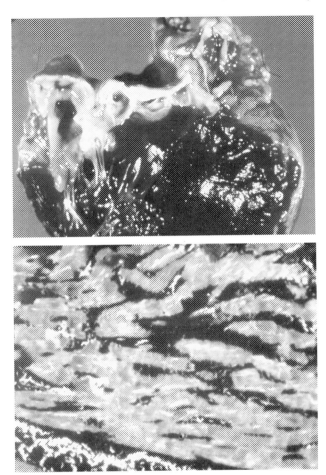

FIGURE I.   Gross specimen and microscopic examination of a pig heart following 43 minutes of implantation in an untreated baboon recipient. Extensive hemorrhage and thrombus formation, indicative of hyperacute rejection, are apparent.

the total immune response that is itself—regardless of the host and recipient or the time interval following transplantation—universal.

Hyperacute Rejection

Hyperacute rejection is the immediate barrier to successful discordant xenotransplantation (e.g., pig-to-human). Rejection between discordant species depends on the presence of preformed natural antibodies (primarily IgM) that, by binding antigen and activating the classic complement pathway, cause platelet aggregation, granule release, endothelial damage, thrombus formation, ischemia in blood vessels, and graft loss (Fig. 1).[6,7] This result is not surprising, for unlike allotransplantation in which species differ only in their transplantation antigens (present at a comparatively low density), in discordant xenotransplantation, grafts express multiple different, recognizable antigens at a higher overall density for immune detection. Platt and associates suggested that these xenoantigens (collectively termed the gp115/135 complex) are actually glycoproteins (not glycolipids or proteoglycans) associated with pig endothelial cell surfaces.[8]

Interestingly, in the guinea pig-to-rat discordant model, hyperacute rejection has also been achieved through direct activation of the alternative complement pathway by xenograft endothelial antigens without involvement of natural antibody.[9] However, this has not been demonstrated to occur in either primates or humans. Strategies to overcome the hyperacute barrier to transplantation therefore have been targeted at the main mechanisms of this process: (1) natural antibody and (2) activation of the complement cascade.

Techniques that have been developed to deplete recipient natural antibody include plasma exchange, plasmapheresis, organ adsorption, and administration of exogenous antibody binding compounds. Results using various discordant models suggest that these techniques must be performed immediately before transplantation to reduce titers of preformed natural antibody effectively.[10–12] In addition, resynthesis of natural antibody may be suppressed with the use of either cyclosporine, RS-61443, 15-deoxyspergualin (15-DSG) or splenectomy.[13] Studies in a guinea pig-to-rat model indicate that plasma exchange may, if combined with either cyclosporine or pretransplant splenectomy, yield even greater prolongation of xenograft survival when compared with grafts in untreated animals.[14] Cooper and colleagues have achieved limited success in a pig-to-baboon heart transplant model through the introduction of donor organ hemoperfusion, a process that increased graft survival from an average 3.1 hours to 4 go 5 days.[15] Similarly, Platt and coworkers extended graft survival time significantly through donor organ hemoperfusion with additional splenectomy and plasmapheresis yielding an increase in graft survival time from 3.5 days to 8 days.[16]

Studies from our Transplantation Research Laboratory have demonstrated an absence of preformed natural IgM antibodies in newborn baboon and human sera to pig lymphocytes and cultured pig aortic endothelial cells (Fig. 2).[17] We subsequently

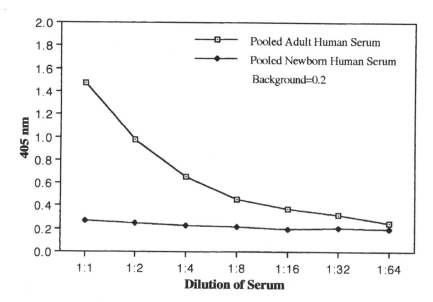

FIGURE 2.   Binding of newborn and adult human natural IgM xenoantibody to cultured pig aortic endothelial cells (background = 0.2) as measured by ELISA assay. Unlike adult human sera, newborn human sera contained very low levels of natural anti-pig IgM xenoantibodies bound to target cells.

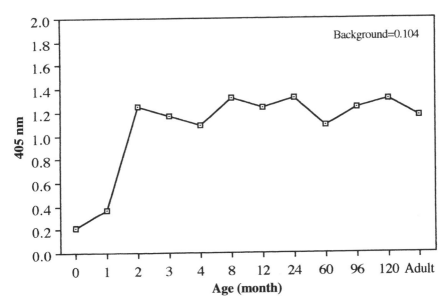

FIGURE 3. Binding, over time, of newborn human natural IgM xenoantibody to cultured pig aortic endothelial cells as measured by ELISA assay. These data demonstrate that natural xenoantibodies in the human develop over time, being initially detectable in the newborn at very low levels but by 2 months of age having achieved levels of antibody binding comparable to those of adult humans.

demonstrated that natural xenoantibodies in the human develop over time, being initially detectable at very low levels, but by 8 weeks of age, they have achieved levels of antibody binding comparable with those of adult humans (Fig. 3).[18] These findings from our in vitro studies have been correlated in vivo with the demonstration of the absence of hyperacute rejection and 3-day graft survival of newborn pig-to-baboon cardiac xenografts.[19] Finally, we also have shown a dramatic decrease in cytotoxicity of baboon and human preformed IgM xenoantibodies following therapy with dithiotreitol (DTT) and penicillamine, both of which are thiolic compounds known to cleave IgM disulfide bonds and thus to render the antibody inactive.[20] However, while the prolongations of graft survival achieved with these measures are statistically significant, the degree of prolongation is not yet clinically relevant.

Complement inhibitors have also been studied in an effort to overcome the hyperacute rejection barrier to xenotransplantation. These agents have been shown to produce the greatest prolongation of rodent discordant xenograft survival. One such agent, cobra venom factor (which acts to deplete C3), has resulted in prolongation of guinea pig-to-rat cardiac xenograft survival from 12 minutes to 3 days.[21,22] Efforts to prolong discordant xenograft survival have also been described using antibodies against B-cell growth factor receptor, blocking strategies that utilize antibody fragments, plasmapheresis combined with cytotoxic drugs, and antiidiotypic strategies.[23] Success of these therapies individually and their likely success in combination gestures toward the potential clinical application of discordant xenotransplantation.

Clinical evidence to support the notion of the potential for successful discordant xenotransplantation also comes from data collected in the setting of human kidney allotransplantation between ABO incompatible donors and recipients.[24] Here, it has been shown that depletion of preformed antibodies to blood group antigens before transplantation and the subsequent short-term maintenance of low antibody levels ultimately may lead to graft survival even in the later presence of antibody and complement.

One hypothesis to explain this observation is known as "accommodation," defined as a condition of dynamic tension between the donor and the recipient of discordant xenografts in which preformed natural antibodies with or without complement are depleted from the recipient for an unspecified time and then allowed to return to the circulation, resulting in continued graft survival despite the presence of tissue-bound antibody.[25] Potential mechanisms to explain this phenomenon include donor graft endothelial cell antigen modulation, resistance of graft endothelial cells to complement activity, and modulation of the binding capabilities of natural antibody.[25] Clearly, clinical examples of accommodation are of great interest because they strongly support the position that discordant xenotransplantation may be an achievable clinical goal.

One of the most remarkable clinical examples of xenotransplantation between distantly-related species came from Poland by Czaplicki and associates in 1991, in which hyperacute rejection was absent 24 hours following xenotransplantation of a pig heart into a human recipient.[26] The protocol used conventional immunosuppression and included the circulation of recipient blood trough two pig hearts before orthotopic transplantation of the third heart (the functional transplant). This process of serial organ hemoperfusion reportedly succeeded in allowing the functional graft to evade hyperacute reaction, presumably by adsorbing the circulating preformed natural xenoantibody before the ultimate functional heart engraftment. Data from this event, however, are incomplete, so it remains difficult to determine the exact mechanism of graft loss (Fig. 4).

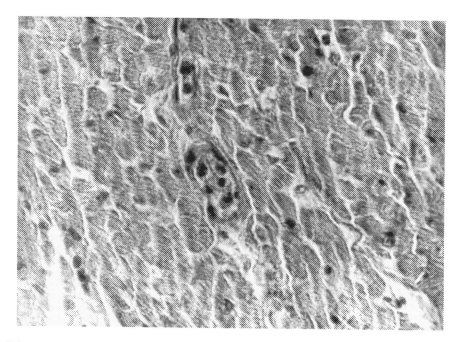

FIGURE 4. Postmortem examination of a cardiac xenograft transplanted from a pig door to a human recipient 23 hours and 42 minutes following transplantation. Isolated mononuclear cells are seen without evidence of rejection by light microscopy. (Stained with hematoxylin and eosin. Original magnification × 200.) (Courtesy of Dr. Michael Kaye.)

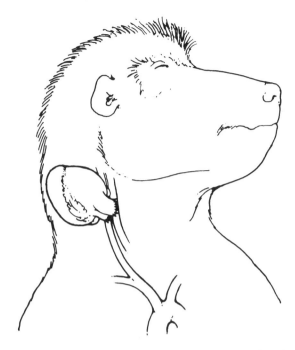

FIGURE 5.   Technique by Michler and colleagues for heterotopic transplantation of the donor heart into the recipient's neck. In this location, the graft may be readily observed without requiring recipient sedation to assess graft viability.

Acute and Chronic Rejection

Although traditionally associated with cellular mediators of the immune response, the processes of acute and chronic rejection in allotransplantation are probably controlled by *both* humoral and cell-mediated arms of the immune system. The exact mechanisms involved in acute and chronic rejection in xenotransplantation remain unclear but are likely to be composed of complex and heterogeneous phenomena. Many investigators believe these processes are predominantly T-cell mediated events, as evidenced by the inconsistent, but promising, results associated with therapy using cyclosporine, total lymphoid irradiation (TLI), or horse antithymocyte globulin (ATG).[27] In hamster-to-rat cardiac xenografts, the beneficial effects of TLI, splenectomy, cyclophosphamide and 15-deoxyspergualin (15 DSG, an inhibitor of antibody resynthesis and monocyte/macrophage interactions), however, make it difficult to deny at least some role to a B-cell mediated process.[28-34] These latter effects are thus hypothesized to result from the removal of mature, primed antibody-producing B cells that ultimately may be regenerated from hematopoietic stem cells.

Michler and colleagues established a concordant heterotopic cardiac xenograft model using cynomolgus monkey (*Macaca fascicularis*) donors in baboon (*Papio anubis*) recipients (Fig. 5).[35] They described a 10-fold increase in mean graft survival time with cyclosporine and steroids that was as effective as when other agents (e.g., azathioprine and ATG) were added.[36,37] Although hyperacute rejection was not encountered in this model, development of cytotoxic antibodies to donor lymphocytes correlated chronologically with graft loss, thus lending support to the hypothesis that the humoral arm of the immune system can be induced to produce xenogeneic antibody.[38,39]

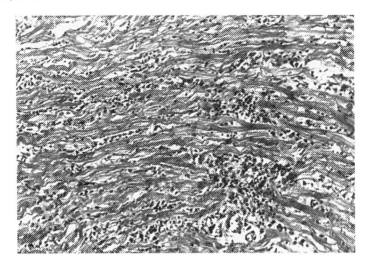

FIGURE 6. Light micrograph of a cardiac xenograft transplanted from a cynomolgus monkey (*Macaca fascicularis*) into a baboon (*Papio anubis*). Striking similarities in parenchymal pathology are noted here when compared with human allograft pathology. (Original magnification × 200.)

Histologic examination both of serial biopsies as well as of the rejected hearts in this nonhuman primate concordant cardiac xenograft model showed striking similarities between parenchymal pathology in allografts and xenografts (Fig. 6).[32,40] Thus, it is not unlikely that the mechanisms of rejection in concordant xenografts are similar to those in allografts: namely, that both humoral and cell-mediated events contribute to the process of acute and chronic rejection. Because the titer development of recipient cytotoxic antibodies to donor lymphocytes correlated chronologically with xenograft failure, and because vasculitis tends to be more prominent in xenografts than allografts, it follows that humoral mechanisms may play a more important role in rejection of xenografts than of allografts.[23,40,41]

In considering the strategies to overcome these barriers in concordant xenografts, humoral and cellular immunity are targeted. Unlike allograft immunosuppression, however, the methods of immunosuppression used to prolong concordant xenograft survival must be more potent because the barriers to graft acceptance are greater. Many of the immunosuppressive strategies investigated have been already discussed and are directed at cell-mediated rejection (cyclosporine-based immunosuppression, TLI, ATG) as well as at humorally based rejection (TLI, splenectomy, 15-DSG, RS-61443).

A relatively new therapeutic approach, photochemotherapy, has been developed that targets donor-specific suppression of the host immune system (i.e., both cell-mediated and humoral mechanisms).[42] The process is similar to phototherapy used in the treatment of psoriasis in which lymphocytes are pretreated with psoralen (8-methoxypsoralen) that intercalates into the DNA helix. The lymphocytes are then exposed extracorporeally to ultraviolet A light (UVA) that allows the psoralen-added DNA to crosslink and thus cease further cellular replication. Phototreated cells are then returned to the patient for recirculation and subsequent physiologic clearance. Photochemotherapy has also been used in other disease processes (e.g., cutaneous T-cell lymphoma) associated with (1) a high mitotic rate and (2) a situation in which selective accessibility of a population of cells to UV light exists.[23,42] The mechanism of action presumably involves the death of phototreated lymphocytes activated against specific antigens that become, upon return to the circulation, targets for immunologic attack resulting in their down regulation. Thus, the goal of photochemotherapy is to develop circulating anti-idiotypic T cells and antibodies, yielding an antigen-specific immunosuppression.

Photochemotherapy has shown promise for application as an immunosuppressant in xenotransplantation. Studies using murine models of graft tolerance (in both a histoincompatible and syngeneic system) have shown that photochemotherapy may promote suppression of the cytotoxic response to alloantigens.[23,43] Thus, it is suggested that photochemotherapy could suppress the xenorejection response specifically by down regulating the cytotoxic response without compromising the global immune response to challenge by microbial antigens.

New, more potent immunosuppressive agents, such as FK506, rapamycin, 15-DSG, and mycophenolic acid derivatives (RS-61443) may also result in significant prolongation of graft-survival after cardiac xenotransplantation, while limiting the amount of generalized immunosuppression currently required to achieve successful engraftment. FK506, like cyclosporine (CsA), selectively inhibits the transcription of cytokine and other specific genes in T cells. In contrast, unlike CsA, 15-DSG inhibits antibody formation and suppresses the monocyte system. RS-61443, a mycophenolic acid derivative and anti-B-cell immunosuppressant may similarly inhibit preformed antibody formation. These agents, in conjunction with some of the previously mentioned therapies, may well yield sufficient means to overcome the concordant xenograft immunologic barriers with fewer undesirable effects. thus rendering the potential clinical application of concordant xenotransplantation a reality.

Clinical Xenotransplantation

Clinical cross-species transplantation dates to the early twentieth century, with kidney xenografts having been performed from rabbit, pig, goat, nonhuman primate, and lamb donors (Table 1).[44] Following these early failures, the scientific literature was devoid of reports of clinical xenotransplantation for over 40 years. In 1963, Reemtsma and colleagues at Tulane University transplanted a chimpanzee kidney into a uremic human patient.[45] A total of six patients received chimpanzee kidney xenografts, with the longest survivor dying at 9 months of a presumed electrolyte imbalance. To date, no clinical results have equaled this original survival.

Since 1964, when Hardy and associates at the University of Mississippi performed the world's first cardiac xenotransplant using a chimpanzee as a donor, there have been nine documented attempts at clinical heart transplantation (Table 1). Five of these donors were nonhuman primates (2 baboons, 3 chimpanzees) and three were domesticated

TABLE I.   Clinical Cardiac Xenotransplantation World Experience

Year	Surgeon	Donor	Position	Outcome	Reference
1964	Hardy	Chimpanzee	Orthotopic	Functioned for 2 hrs	46
1968	Cooley	Sheep	Orthotopic	Immediate cessation	47
1968	Ross	Pig	Heterotopic	Immediate cessation	48
1969?	Marion	Chimpanzee	Orthotopic*	Unclear, ?functioned for several hrs	49
1977	Barnard	Baboon	Heterotopic	Functioned for 5 hrs	50
1977	Barnard	Chimpanzee	Heterotopic	Functioned for 4 days	50
1984	Bailey	Baboon	Orthotopic	Functioned for 20 days	51
1991	Czaplicki	Pig	Orthotopic	Functioned for 24 hrs	26

* Unclear from reference; presumed to be orthotopic.

farm animals (1 sheep, 2 pigs).[46–50] Most recently, the attempt of Czaplicki and colleagues in Poland to transplant a pig heart into a patient with Marfan's syndrome (discussed earlier) concluded with a poor clinical, but promising histopathologic, outcome. The patient survived for 24 hours when the pig xenograft apparently failed to provide adequate support of the patient's circulation. On postmortem examination, the pig heart xenograft was reportedly free of hyperacute rejection. In addition, the longest survival of a concordant xenograft in an ABO-incompatible host was demonstrated to be 21 days in the case of Baby Fae.[51]

Current experimental investigations offer encouraging evidence that the immunologic barriers to xenotransplantation may be overcome. Lessons learned in rodent xenotransplantation have been applied with success in larger animals such as nonhuman primates, so that primate-to-primate concordant xenografts have survived beyond 1 year in the orthotopic position.[52] The increasing sophistication with which modern immunosuppressive therapies have surmounted many of the immunologic barriers posed by experimental xenotransplantation is evidence that concordant xenotransplantation may currently be feasible.

Most recently, in 1992, Starzl and colleagues at the University of Pittsburgh transplanted baboon livers into two human recipients. In the first, a 35-year-old man suffering from irreversible hepatic damage secondary to chronic hepatitis B infection, they achieved a 70-day survival; in the second a 35-day survival was achieved. Before the first patient's death from a cerebrovascular hemorrhage, however, he reportedly suffered six infectious episodes with *Staphylococcus, Cytomegalovirus, Candida albicans, Enterococcus,* and *Aspergillus fumigatus.*[53] This case clearly delineates the point that prevention of xenotransplant rejection is currently achieved at the price of massive immunosuppression and subsequent increased risk of infection. Although some would argue that further experimental work is required before additional attempts are made to advance cardiac xenotransplantation to the clinical arena, many scientific questions regarding this issue may require the ultimate experiment (i.e., in humans) for answers to be obtained.

ETHICAL ISSUES

Concurrent with advances in cardiac xenotransplantation have been the necessary ethical debates concerning the appropriateness of this endeavor.[54] In addition, many have raised the question of whether it is ethically warranted for humans to use animals in this capacity. Kushner and Belliotti noted in their examination of the Baby Fae case that in order for unequal treatment of the two groups to be moral, it must be justified.[55] That is, the unequal treatment of being X and being Y must be justified by a morally relevant difference between X and Y. In this context, children may be relieved of many of the social responsibilities held by adults, and the use of animals (especially nonhuman primates) may be justified for xenograft research and clinical application.

Clearly, in order for this research to be justifiable, there must be made a morally relevant distinction between humans and animals, such as nonhuman primates. It is not, for example, enough to state that primates can be used for any purpose humans deem fit simply because they are members of a different species. Indeed, some have raised the issue that there are humans with diminished mental capacities who could never approach the cognitive and emotional level that some primates exhibit. Is there a difference between the species that can be emphasized as a rationale to warrant the use of nonhuman primates for experimentation? If not, the procedures discussed could not be justified because the act of doing good for the human (beneficence) would not outweigh the absence of regard (denial of maleficence) for the animal.

Kushner and Belliotti refer to the human ability to carry out complex cognitions, and Caplan has identified the capacity for complex emotional relationships between human beings as the morally significant difference between species.[55,56] However, even if one accepts the above distinctions as morally valid, what should be said about human beings with diminished mental capacities? Are they less human? Should they be used as experimental subjects or as organ donors? Proponents of research involving primates who oppose the use of anencephalic or cortically dead humans focus on the impact that the use of these individuals would have on other human beings—namely, the subject's family. As Caplan has noted, "it is in the relationships with others, both family and strangers, that the moral worth and standing of these children are grounded."[56]

If one accepts that the morally reasonable distinction between humans and non-human primates is rooted in the complex emotional relationships that humans share and nonhumans do not, then Caplan's argument appears valid. In other words, because these humans may be part of a familial or social structure that is weighted emotionally with regard to others, they should be given moral preference over nonhuman primates. If this is the case, the donation of organs by nonhuman primates for transplantation or research is acceptable.

However, even if one does accept that there is a valid moral distinction between humans and nonhuman primates, the next logical question is whether it is necessary to use primates in this manner. Ethical justification naturally does not make an action a moral imperative. Disputes regarding animal experimentation notwithstanding, such ethical issues raised regarding the advancement of xenotransplantation to the clinical arena are themselves strikingly similar to those put forth 25 years ago in reference to the (then new) field of cardiac allotransplantation. As was the case in Christian Barnard's era, so too now must one evaluate whether a sufficient level of success has been attained experimentally to warrant clinical application.

Defining Experimental Success

Can one ever hope to determine if or when the clinical application of cardiac xenotransplantation is justified? The assessment of any experimental therapy, as Fox and Swazey have suggested, should encourage the investigator to address three critical questions. Although far from a precise algorithm, the threefold inquiry that can be applied to transplantation may also allow for a systematic assessment of clinical application, namely: (1) in the laboratory, what defines success as sufficient to warrant advancement to the clinical arena; (2) under what clinical conditions should this advancement proceed; and (3) in the clinical arena, what defines success as sufficient to warrant further evaluations?[57] However, the ability to provide answers to this threefold inquiry problematically requires a reliance upon defined success, itself an appraisal of judgment that can be made confidently only in retrospect.

After discussion of experimental advances in cardiac xenotransplantation, the next logical question is whether we now have reached an appropriate stage in laboratory experimentation to justify further attempts at advancing cardiac xenotransplantation to the clinical arena. If we view the current status of experimental accomplishments in xenotransplantation with the same scrutiny as that afforded allotransplantation at the time of Barnard's endeavor, we are left with similar conclusions: first, comparable graft survival time has been achieved in animal models of xenotransplantation as present for allotransplantation before 1967. Second, with our current understanding of cardiac allotransplantation has also come a greater awareness of its limitations. Thus, conditions for the advancement of xenotransplantation arguably could be fulfilled by a patient with end-stage heart disease who is a candidate for allotransplantation but for whom a donor cannot be identified in time. Finally, the clinical success of xenotransplantation might also be considered (as was the case for allotransplantation) *any* graft survival, and the goal of xenotransplantation to strive for extended graft survival.

Under what conditions will clinical advancement of cardiac xenotransplantation proceed? For initial patients in whom clinical xenotransplantation will first be applied, clinical urgency, in the complete absence of other suitable alternatives, undoubtedly will represent the motivating factor to proceed.

Finally, in this new clinical arena, what will define success of cardiac xenotransplantation of a level sufficient to warrant its further investigation? Survival beyond the perioperative period? Survival beyond 6 months? One year? Here, as with the case of allotransplantation, it is difficult to assess predicted life expectancy following unprecedented transplantation. In 1964, for example, Shumway and colleagues achieved autograft survival in dogs beyond 2 years following transplantation. These investigations were hailed as triumphs insofar as they allowed for physiologic assessment of graft function in a controlled experiment free of immunologic rejection.[58] Undoubtedly, to have gauged the initial clinical success of allotransplantation by utilizing these laboratory findings with autotransplantation as a standard would have been imprudent and meant the certain cessation of further advancement in allotransplantation. It is now similarly unreasonable to set an arbitrary survival expectancy by which clinical xenotransplantation may be defined as successful in the absence of clinical results. Thus, we believe that clinical applications of cardiac xenotransplantation is ethically justified; we now must consider issues specific to its undertaking.

THE POTENTIAL FOR CLINICAL REALITY

In considering the selection of potential sources of organs for clinical xenotransplantation, several criteria must first be considered. The species must readily be available in large numbers, free of transmissible epizootic disease, manifest cardiac physiology similar to humans', and, in all likelihood, be ABO compatible. Nonhuman primates as organ donors have been favored by those wishing to minimize genetic disparity between donor and human recipients. Although most compatible with the above selection criteria, chimpanzees are currently unavailable as an adequate source for clinical xenotransplantation. The next logical choice is the baboon. Although a potential source of epizootic disease, it, unlike the chimpanzee, is not considered endangered. Unfortunately, the size of baboons currently limits their potential use to pediatric patients.

Furthermore, as the experience with Baby Fae would indicate, ABO blood group compatibility is mandatory before primate xenotransplantation.[51] A distribution comparable to that of the human blood groups is found in cynomolgus monkeys and baboons, with approximately one-third group A, one-third group B, and one-third group AB.[59,60] Universal donor group O is exceedingly rare and has been found only in cynomolgus monkeys (*Macaca fascicularis*) of mainland China and Guinea baboons (*Papio papio*)[60]

Although nonhuman primates represent the best alternative to human allografts for management of end-stage biventricular heart failure, ethical concerns asserted by a vocal minority in the public and the unresolvable issue of small primate size has created a renewed enthusiasm for the selection of domesticated farm animals as donors for man. The pig, in fact, fulfills all of the criteria described above: it is available in large numbers (approximately 90 million are slaughtered yearly for food for this nation), it could be bred in a controlled environment so as to eliminate epizootic disease more effectively, and it has strikingly similar cardiac anatomy and hemodynamic parameters when compared with humans. It is likely that opposition to the use of pig heart donors would be less vociferous than that to the use of nonhuman primates.

Undoubtedly other concerns will be raised about the suitability of the pig as an ideal xenogeneic organ donor for humans. For example, the status of ABO antigens on pig tissues and the significance of these antigens for xenograft survival are unknown. Results from investigations concerning the topic have been inconclusive. Thus, although the pig appears to be an intriguing and appropriate donor for man on the basis of size, availability, anatomy, and physiology, surmounting the immunologic barriers to rejection remains its primary limitation.

CLINICAL GOALS

What is the ultimate goal of the clinical application of xenotransplantation? The need for donor organs irrefutably outweighs the resources currently available. Mechanical devices and xenotransplantation have emerged as the two most promising alternatives to allograft cardiac replacement. In the immediate future, cardiac xenotransplantation will most likely first undergo clinical trials as a bridge-to-transplantation procedure before being applied as destination therapy.

Some have raised the question about whether *any* artificial device, biologic or mechanical, should be used as a bridge to allotransplantation. This argument maintains that the use of bridge transplants not only increases the morbidity of the entire endeavor, thus diminishing the overall success of the transplantation effort, but also does not address directly the lack of organ donors.[62–63] However, the experience with left ventricular assistance devices (LVADs) as a bridge-to-allotransplantation has already demonstrated an improvement in hepatic, renal, and other end-organ function during LVAD support.[16] Thus, in contrast with the previous argument, we feel that providing temporary support as a bridge-to-transplantation, biologic devices (xenotransplants)—like their mechanical counterparts (LVADs)—will allow patients to await transplantation in a more stable clinical state, making them better candidates for longer survival times after transplantation. Indeed, for the pediatric population, it is also reasonable to suggest that because of the current disparity between the size of donors most commonly available and the size of recipients most in need, bridging to allotransplantation with a xenograft may actually increase the efficacy of donor-organ usage. Further, although initial clinical experiences with a xenograft will not directly affect the donor organ shortage, they represent obligatory intermediate steps that must be undertaken before full application.

FUTURE OF XENOTRANSPLANTATION

It is our hope that more sophisticated and directed immunosuppressive therapy will be developed that is both highly specific and efficacious. The ability of the clinician to use therapies more specific to either (1) the particular arm of the immune system predominating in the rejection process or (2) the actual mechanism of rejection itself (e.g., development of antiidiotypic antibodies or cells) would allow continued more accurate treatment. These future treatment protocols, in their specificity, would not subject the patient to the same profound and generalized immunosuppression currently required, and thus would not compromise the patient's immunologic defenses against microbial infections to the same degree.

Over the past quarter century, substantial strides have been made in our understanding of the xenograft reaction. Investigations in xenotransplantation have also led to a more complete understanding of the mechanisms of allograft rejection and its modification. Ultimately, we feel that xenotransplantation will no longer be viewed as an experimental procedure. Rather, the ultimate goal of its advancement must be to have a positive impact on the current shortage of human donor organs.

The desperate shortage of human donor hearts, the limited use of left-heart mechanical assist devices for smaller individuals and those with biventricular heart failure, and the recent success in clinical and experimental trials of xenografting justify the future clinical application of cardiac transplantation. We are confident that, in the foreseeable future, clinical xenotransplantation will achieve its target of extended graft survival. Although reservations have been voiced regarding the cohort of initial recipients who undoubtedly will be patients for whom no therapeutic alternative exists or is likely to exist imminently, one must also recall, as Shimkin has suggested:

> To do nothing, or to prevent others from doing anything, is itself a type of experiment, for the prevention of experimentation is tantamount to the assumption of responsibility for an experiment different from the one proposed.[64]

REFERENCES

1. Evans RW, Orians CE, Ascher NL: The potential supply of organ donors: An assessment of the efficiency of organ procurement efforts in the United States. JAMA 267:239–246, 1992.
2. Oriens CE, Evans RW, Ascher NL: Estimates of organ-specific donor availability for the United States. Transplant Proc 25(1):1541–1542, 1993.
3. United Network for Organ Sharing (UNOS) Update 9(2):25, 1993.
4. Michler RE, McManus RP, Smith CR, et al: Prolongation of primate cardiac xenograft survival with cyclosporine. Transplantation 44:632–636, 1987.
5. Calne RY: Organ transplantation between widely disparate species. Transplant Proc 2:550, 1970.
6. Jamieson SW: Xenograft hyperacute rejection. A new model. Transplantation 17:533, 1974.
7. Cattell V, Jamieson SW: Hyperacute rejection of guinea-pig to rat cardiac xenografts. J Pathol 115:183–189, 1974.
8. Platt JL, Lindman BJ, Chen H, et al: Endothelial cell antigens recognized by xenoreactive human natural antibodies. Transplantation 50:817, 1990.
9. Johnston P, Li S, Wright L, White D: Hyperacute xenograft rejection takes place in the complete absence of antibodies but requires the presence of functional complement. Transplant Proc 23:877, 1991.
10. Van de Stadt J, Vendeville B, Weill B, et al: Discordant heart xenografts in the rat. Additional effect of plasma exchange and cyclosporine, cyclophosphamide or splenectomy in delaying hyperacute rejection. Transplantation 45:514–528, 1988.
11. Watkins JF, Edwards NM, Sanchez JA: Specific elimination of preformed antibody activity against xenogeneic antigens by use of an extracorporeal immunoadsorptive circuit. Transplant Proc 23(1):360–364, 1991.
12. Reding R, Davies HS, White DJG, et al: Effect of plasma exchange on guinea pig-to-rat heart xenografts. Transplant Proc 21:534, 1989.
13. Valdivia LA, Monden M, Gotoh M, et al: Prolonged cardiac xenograft survival by 15-deoxyspergualin combined with splenectomy. Transplant Proc 21:532–533, 1989.
14. Valdivia LA, Monden M, Gotoh M, et al: An important role of the spleen in rejection of hamster-to-rat xenografts. Transplant Proc 20:329–330, 1988.
15. Cooper DKC, Lexer G, Rose AG, et al: Effects of cyclosporine and antibody adsorption on pig cardiac xenograft survival in the baboon. J Heart Transplant 7;238, 1988.
16. Platt JL: Personal communication.
17. Xu H, Edwards NM, Kwiatkowski P, et al: Absence of anti-pig natural xenoantibodies from newborn human and baboon serum (submitted for publication).
18. Xu H, Edwards NM, Mittra A, et al: Age-related development of human anti-pig antibodies (submitted for publication).
19. Kaplon RJ, Michler RE, Xu H, et al: Absence of hyperacute rejection in newborn pig-to-baboon cardiac xenografts. Transplantation (in press).
20. Xu H, Edwards NM, Kaplon RJ, et al: Identification and functional analysis of human preformed anti-pig xenoantibodies. Transplant Proc 26(3):1365–1368, 1993.
21. Adachi JH, Rosengard BR, Hutchins GM, et al: Effects of cyclosporine, aspirin and cobra venom factor on discordant xenograft survival in rats. Transplant Proc 19:1145, 1987.
22. Miyagawa S, Hirose H, Shirakura R, et al: The mechanism of discordant xenograft rejection. Transplantation 46:825, 1988.

23. Rose EA, Pepino P, Fuzesi L, Sanchez JA: Cardiac xenotransplantation. Prog Cardiovasc Dis 33(2):105–117, 1990.
24. Chopek MW, Simmons R, Platt JL: ABO-incompatible kidney transplantation: Initial immunopathologic evaluation. Transplant Proc 19:4534-4557, 1987.
25. Platt JL, Bach FH: The barrier to xenotransplantation. Transplantation 52(6):937–937, 1991.
26. Czaplicki J, Blonska B, Religa Z: The lack of hyperacute xenogeneic heart transplant rejection in a human. J Heart Lung Transplant 11:393–397, 1992.
27. Sakakibara N, Click RE, Condie RM., Jamieson SW: Rejection/acceptance of xenografts. Transplant Proc 21:524, 1989.
28. Knechtle SJ, Haperin EC, Bollinger RR: Xenograft survival in two species combinations using total lymphoid irradiation and cyclosporine. Transplantation 43:173–175, 1987.
29. Monden M, Valdivia LA, Gotoh M, et al: A crucial effect of splenectomy on prolonging cardiac xenograft survival in combination with cyclosporine. Surgery 105:535–542, 1989.
30. Steinbruichel DA, Madsen HH, Nielsen B, et al: Graft survival in a hamster-to-rat heart transplantation model with total lymphoid irradiation, cyclosporine A, and anti-T-cell antibody. Transplantation 22:1088, 1990.
31. Valdivia LA, Monden M, Gotoh M, et al: An important role of the spleen in rejection of hamster-to-rat xenografts. Transplant Proc 20:329–330, 1988.
32. Valdivia LA, Monden M, Gotoh M, et al: Prolonged cardiac xenograft survival by 15-deoxyspergualin combined with splenectomy. Transplant Proc 231:532–533, 1989.
33. Valdivia LA, Monden M, Gotoh M, et al: Hepatic xenografts from hamster to rat. Transplant Proc 19:1158–1159, 1987.
34. Norin AJ, Roslin MS, Panza A, et al: TLI induces specific B-cell unresponsiveness and long-term monkey heart xenograft survival in cyclosporine-treated baboons. Transplant Proc 24:508–510, 1992.
35. Michler RE, McManus RP, Smith CR, et al: Technique of primate heterotopic cardiac transplantation. J Med Primatol 14:357–362, 1985.
36. Michler RE, McManus RP, Smith CR, et al: Prolongation of primate cardiac xenograft survival with cyclosporine. Transplantation 44:632–636, 1987.
37. Sadeghi AM, Robbins RC, Smith CR, et al: Cardiac xenograft survival in baboons treated with cyclosporine in combination with conventional immunosuppression. Transplant Proc 19:1149–1152, 1987.
38. Michler RE, McManus RP, Sadeghi AM, et al: Prolonged primate cardiac xenograft survival with cyclosporine. Surg Forum 36:359, 1985.
39. Sadeghi AM, Robbins RC, Smith CR, et al: Cardiac xenotransplantation in primates. J Thorac Cardiovasc Surg 93:809–817, 1987.
40. Perper RJ, Najarian JS: Experimental renal heterotransplantation I. In widely divergent species. Transplantation 4:377, 1966.
41. Rosenberg JC, Hawkins E, Rector F: Mechanisms of immunologic injury during antibody-mediated hyperacute rejection of renal heterografts. Transplantation 11(Suppl 2):151–157, 1971.
42. Edelson RL, Berger CL, Gasparro FP, et al: Treatment of cutaneous T-cell lymphoma by extracorporeal photochemotherapy. N Engl J Med 316:297–303, 1985.
43. Perez MI, Gaspas Y, O'Neil D: Inhibition of murine autoimmune disease by reinfusion of syngeneic lymphocytes inactivated with psoralen and ultraviolet A light. J Invest Dermatol 86:499, 1986.
44. Reemtsma K: Xenotransplantation—A brief history of clinical experiences: 199–1965. In Cooper DKC, Kemp E, Reemtsma K, White (eds): Xenotransplantation. New York, Springer-Verlag, 1991, pp 10–12.
45. Reemtsma K, McCracken BH, Schlegel JU, et al: Renal heterotransplantation in man. Ann Surg 160:384–410, 1964.
46. Hardy JD, Kurrus FE, Chavez CM, et al: Heart transplantation in man: Developmental studies and report of a case. JAMA 188:11342, 1964.
47. Cooley DA, Hallman GL, Bloodwell RD, et al: Human heart transplantation: Experience with 12 cases. Am J Cardiol 22:804, 1968.
48. Ross DN: In Shapiro H (ed): Experience with Human Heart Transplantation. Durban, Butterworth, 1969, p 227.
49. Marion P: Les transplantations cardiaques et les transplantations hepatiques. Lyon Med 222:585, 1969.
50. Barnard CN, Wolpowitz A, Losman JG: Heterotopic cardiac transplantation with a xenograft for assistance of the left heart in cardiogenic shock after cardiopulmonary bypass. S Afr Med J 52:1035, 1977.
51. Bailey LL, Nehlensen-Bannarella SL, Concepcion W, et al: Cardiac xenotransplantation in a neonate. JAMA 254:3321–3329, 1985.
52. Kawauchi M, Gundry SR, de Begona JA, et al: Prolonged orthotopically transplanted heart xenografts in infant baboons. J Thorac Cardiovasc Surg 106:779–786, 1993.
53. Fung J: Case report (presentation): Consortium for Clinical Xenotransplantation. N Y Acad Med, Sept. 12, 1992.

54. Chen JM, Michler RE: Heart xenotransplantation: Lessons learned and future prospects. J Heart Lung Transplant 12(5):869–875, 1993.
55. Kushner T, Bellotti R: Baby Fae: A beastly business. J Med Ethics 11:178–183, 1985.
56. Caplan AL: Is xenografting morally wrong? Transplant Proc 24(2):722–727, 1992.
57. Fox RC, Swazey JP: The experimental-therapy dilemma. In The Courage to Fail. Chicago, The University of Chicago Press, 1974, pp 60–83.
58. Dong E, Hurley EJ, Lower RR, Shumway NE: Performance of the heart two years after autotransplantation. Surgery 56:270–247, 1964.
59. Moor-Jankowski J, Socha WW: Blood groups of macaques. A comparative study. J Med Primatol 7:136, 1978.
60. Wiener AS, Moor-Jankowski J: The ABO blood groups of baboons. Am J Phys Anthropol 30:117, 1969.
61. Socha WW: Personal communication.
62. Auchincloss H: Are we ready to try clinical xenotransplantation? Xeno 1(1):2–4, 1993.
63. Levin HR, Chen JM, Oz MC, et al: Potential of left ventricular assist devices as outpatient therapy while awaiting transplantation. Ann Thorac Surg 58:1515–1520, 1994.
64. Shimkin MR: The problem of experimentation on human beings: The research worker's point of view. In Edsall G: A Positive Approach to the Problem of Human Experimentation. Daedalus 98:463–479, 1969.

SPECIAL SITUATIONS IN CARDIAC TRANSPLANTATION

Edited by Frances Hoffman, MS, RN, CCTC

Prolonged Waiting Periods for Heart Transplantation: Impact on Patients, Family, and Staff

Late Noncompliance

The Adolescent Patient: Psychosocial Considerations

Biopsy Negative Graft Dysfunction

Pregnancy after Heart Transplantation

Prolonged Waiting Periods for Heart Transplantation: Impact on Patients, Family, and Staff

Linda Ohler, MSN, RN, CCTC, CNS
Catherine Crone, MD
Sandra Cupples, DNSc, RN, CCRN

The average waiting time for a heart transplant has increased considerably over the last 5 years. As a result, many patients are becoming more critically ill and requiring hospitalization and therapy with pharmacologic or mechanical support until a suitable donor heart is available. Having a loved one become critically ill and confined to intensive care stresses family members physically, emotionally, and economically. Staff nurses and physicians are also affected, especially those who care for the patients and families in the cardiac intensive care units. It is here that most patients wait for their heart transplant, and many die waiting. It is important to explore the impact of the morbidity and mortality of this patient population on staff, family, and on the patients themselves, who experience a decline in their health status, require intensive care, and confront the reality of their own mortality.

UNITED NETWORK FOR ORGAN SHARING

The United Network for Organ Sharing (UNOS) operates a computerized national registry for patients in need of organ transplantation.[1] Heart transplant candidates are listed with UNOS as a Status 1 (urgent), 2 (nonurgent), or 7 (inactive).[2] Table 1 describes the significance of each status. Organ sharing is coordinated through UNOS with local organ procurement organizations (OPOs). Allocation of a donor heart

TABLE I.   UNOS Classification System for Heart Transplant Candidates

Status 1	Status 2
In the intensive care unit **and** On inotropic agents to maintain adequate cardiac output or On mechanical assist device (L-VAD, R-VAD) Intraaortic balloon pump Total artificial heart	All other patients awaiting heart transplantation who do not meet the Status 1 criteria Status 7 Inactive

Data from Feree DM: Cardiac organ sharing: The organ center. In Phillips M (ed): UNOS: Organ Procurement, Preservation and Distribution in Transplantation. Richmond, William Byrd Press, 1991.

is based on several factors, which include time waiting, UNOS status, blood type, and size. Hearts are distributed to local patients first and are stratified within each blood group according to severity of illness (UNOS Status) and time waiting.[2] Initially, the majority of patients who are listed for transplant are in UNOS category 2. Reports from the Cardiac Transplant Research Database (CTRD) have demonstrated that 41% of candidates awaiting transplantation in 1990 progressed to UNOS Status 1, and in 1993 48% of patients on the heart transplant waiting list progressed to Status 1 before receiving a donor heart.[3] Approximately 20 to 22% of patients waiting for a heart transplant die before a donor heart can be identified for them.[4–6]

PATIENT STRESS AND COPING

For most patients, stress levels begin to rise with the realization that they have developed a life-threatening illness. That the heart is often conceptually associated with physical and emotional well-being perhaps adds to the psychologic impact of learning that one's heart is functioning poorly. Being accepted as a candidate for heart transplantation brings the fear of dying into sharp focus for most patients.[7]

In one retrospective study, the four most common stressors identified by patients awaiting heart transplantation were the fear of death, financial burdens, deteriorating health/loss of control, and stress related directly to the paging device they carried as a means of contact when a suitable donor becomes available.[8] Some have stated that it is stressful simply to carry the pager knowing that it may be activated either by the transplant team or inadvertently. Both possibilities are stressful.

A prospective study examined the stress and coping of patients waiting for heart transplantation and identified the three most common stressors to be (1) requiring a heart transplant, (2) having terminal heart disease, and (3) causing family members to worry.[9] The three most common coping mechanisms were (1) thinking positively, (2) keeping a sense of humor, and (3) trying to keep life as normal as possible.[9] This study was done at a single point in time, usually within a month after listing for heart transplantation. A more recent, unpublished study is currently being conducted using the same tools but looking at the stress and coping over five different data collection times. The original study was completed in 1990; it was noted that waiting times were increasing. The authors subsequently decided to review stress and coping over time to determine if stress increased and coping skills decreased or changed during prolonged waiting.

In the longitudinal study, patients are reporting the greatest stressors at time one, which is within 2 weeks after being listed for transplantation, and at time four, which is usually 9 to 10 months after being listed.[10] Table 2 lists the most stressful factors identified by candidates waiting for heart transplantation. The most frequently used coping

TABLE 2.   Most Stressful Factors in Waiting for a Heart Transplant

• Being away from home	• Being away from family
• Having terminal heart disease	• Spending time in the hospital
• Needing a heart transplant	

strategies and the most effective coping strategies identified in this study are listed in Table 3. An interesting preliminary finding in this study is the change in types of coping styles being used at different data collection times. In the first data collection period, patients are using confrontive coping skills most frequently, followed by self-reliant and optimistic coping.[10] By the time of the fourth data collection, evasive coping mechanisms are being used most frequently, followed by fatalistic and supportive coping.[10] Table 4 provides examples of the various coping mechanisms being used by patients. The majority of patients completing data at time four are classified as UNOS Status 2.

Use of confrontive coping skills at first collection time may reflect the recent transplant evaluation, in which an individual has met with numerous members of the transplant team and has had education for transplantation. The need to face the unpleasant, frightening task of accepting that one needs a heart transplant may be the reason for developing confrontive coping skills. At the time of fourth collection, use of evasive coping skills, such as wishing the problem would go away, may be related to the fear that the individual may not live to receive a transplant.[10] Analysis of these data provides information about the impact of a life-threatening illness on individuals awaiting cardiac transplantation in terms of individual stress and coping skills.

FAMILY REACTIONS

There are several challenging points to the transplant process for both patients and families alike. The first is accepting the diagnosis of end-stage heart disease and that a heart transplant offers the best option for survival. The second is coping with the potentially long wait for a donor heart. This is probably one of the greatest challenges a patient and family must confront during the transplant process and perhaps during a lifetime, for it is during this waiting period that the greatest risk lies for becoming a statistic who did not survive the long wait. If the patient is at home, role changes may occur that make it difficult for the family to function in its usual style. Disruptions in family patterns begin with the transplant candidate's inability to work or function in his or her usual role, which may lead to financial problems and to lowered self-esteem.[8] Candidates for transplantation have stated that they would prefer to die rather than leave their families in financial crisis as a result of their illness. Statements such as these are examples of the development of low self-esteem as a result of severe illness.

Stress levels and coping mechanisms have also been assessed in families of candidates awaiting transplantation.[9] This study reported levels of stress and coping at a single point soon after the family member was placed on the waiting list for a donor

TABLE 3.   Most Frequently Used and Most Effective Coping Strategies

Most Frequently Used	Most Effective
• Humor	• Humor
• Thinking positively	• Thinking positively
• Trying to keep life normal	• Trying to keep life normal
• Thinking of good things in life	• Thinking of good things in life
• Trying to learn more about the problem	• Prayer

TABLE 4. Examples of Coping Strategies

Evasive Daydreaming Sleeping more than usual Convincing one's self that the problem will go away	**Supportant** Talking with family/friends Seeking counseling
Confrontive Facing the problem Developing a plan of action	**Fatalistic** Pessimistic outlook Expecting the worst outcome
Self-Reliant Preferring to work things out by oneself Keeping feelings under control Not sharing one's feelings	**Emotive** Blaming others Doing risky/impulsive things
Optimistic Positive thinking Expecting good results	**Palliative** Eating more Drinking/smoking

heart. Results showed that families used an increased number of coping skills to effectively mediate their stresses.[9] Table 5 demonstrates the most effective coping skills used by families of transplant candidates. Families generally scored lower on passive coping mechanisms, which may reflect the selection process for candidates and families.[9] Families who demonstrated passive behaviors in the evaluation phase may have been determined to be too weak to cope with the challenges of the transplant process.[9] Therefore, the selection process may have filtered out passive families and determined them incapable of coping. Further studies need to look at families' stress and coping over time in a longitudinal study designed to compare families of patients who are Status 1 and those who are Status 2.

STAFF ATTITUDES

Although a proportion of patients waiting for heart transplantation die of rhythm disturbances at home, many die in hospital cardiac intensive-care units, which can promote hopeless attitudes in staff, as well as create an environment of stress and anxiety related to a sense of personal failure.[11–12] To compensate for these feelings of failure and guilt, physicians and nurses may respond with defensive anger, avoidance, overtreatment, overattachment to the patient, and increased criticism of colleagues.[12] Because transplant candidates are often confined to the intensive care unit for weeks or months before a suitable organ donor is identified, the likelihood for attachment or overattachment becomes greater. Long-term stays in cardiac intensive-care units are relatively uncommon for most patients admitted for myocardial infarctions or severe rhythm disturbances. Staff members, including nurses and physicians, often feel a certain amount of guilt, failure, and loss following the death of a patient for whom they have cared for several weeks. There is seldom time for grieving the loss of a patient when the nurse and physician are expected to deal with the next patient being admitted to the unit.[11] Stresses such as these have been reported to lead to emotional withdrawal, social isolation, denial of professional problems, and cynicism in physicians.[13] In emotional withdrawal, health care professionals who have met with unresolved stressors retreat

TABLE 5. Most Frequently Used Coping Mechanisms for Family Members

Knowing the family has the strength to solve problems
Facing the problems head on
Seeking support from friends

from family life and may become overdedicated to their profession. These individuals may become socially isolated by becoming locked into their professional roles.[13]

Studies have been done in the areas of oncology and critical care to determine the effects of patients' deaths on staff.[14–15] Oncology nurses often choose to enter this profession to assist in prolonging life and increasing the quality of life for individuals with health-related problems. Critical care nurses choose to work in intensive care environments with the idea that they may have an impact on prolonging an individual's life.[14] Critical care nurses are often confronting issues related to death and dying, yet seldom are they given time to resolve these issues. Hospice nurses enter their profession with the knowledge that their patients will die soon. When studied, critical care nurses reported significantly more stress, experienced more death anxiety, and showed more burnout than the hospice nurses.[14] Hospice nurses demonstrated a greater sense of personal accomplishment and reported becoming emotionally involved with patients and their families.[14] Surgeons who deal with oncology and cardiac patients were studied to determine the impact of surgical failure.[15] In cases where patients did not improve following surgery, the surgeons reported shame for their inability to assist the patients. In following these patients beyond the usual postoperative period, surgeons were able to compare the vulnerability they experienced with that of their patients.[15] Perhaps this could be compared with the overinvolvement described earlier as a reaction to patients' deaths. Surgeons usually follow the patient for a short time postoperatively. This study encouraged a longer follow-up period that permitted the surgeons and patients to recognize the mutual pain and limits within each.[15]

Problems such as these were identified in the Cardiac Care Unit (CCU) at Fairfax Hospital when three patients awaiting heart transplantation died within a short period. The patients had each been confined to the CCU for 8 to 10 weeks when their deaths occurred. Nursing staff had bonded with each of the patients, one of whom was a young female with postpartum cardiomyopathy and a severely elevated panel of reactive antibodies (PRA = 95%). Two of the patients had severe right heart failure and were not candidates for the left ventricular assistance device. Following these deaths, nursing staff were stating openly that they were going to refuse to care for transplant candidates because they could not cope with losing another young patient. The transplant team psychiatrist was asked to consult with this group to identify ways in which the staff could be helped to cope with the losses. Nurses were invited to discuss their feelings with the team psychiatrist and heart transplant coordinator. The group was able to express anger over the deaths and to ask questions about why they had occurred. There were misconceptions about the criteria for use of the left ventricular assist device as well as concerns about the allocation of organs. Some staff members needed additional information about antibody titers in transplant patients. Questions were answered, and frustrations and anger were expressed.

From this meeting a questionnaire was developed and mailed to transplant coordinators and physicians at 150 transplant centers in the United States to determine how deaths of transplant candidates are dealt with in each institution. Results of this survey are still being analyzed. Individuals at 120 transplant centers in the United States responded.[15] Sample questions from the survey can be found in Table 6. Results indicate that ICU/CCU staff, transplant coordinators, social workers, and cardiologists are affected most by deaths of patients awaiting transplantation.[15] Most centers address the deaths of these patients at weekly transplant meetings or at morbidity and mortality rounds. Many centers stated that staff members attended the patient's funeral as part of addressing the issue of patient deaths. Most transplant teams include social workers and psychiatrists and/or psychologists to assist team members in dealing with patient deaths. Data from this study demonstrate that transplant staff often react with emotional

TABLE 6.   Sample Survey Questions to Staff on Patient Deaths

1. Do you have mental health professionals participate in the care of transplant patients?
2. Which mental health professionals do you use?
3. During the waiting period, how often is a patient seen in your outpatient clinic?
4. How many candidates died while waiting for a donor heart in

        Outpatient   Inpatient

  1990
  1991
  1992

5. Is there a dedicated unit for candidates awaiting transplantation in your hospital?
6. Does your center use left ventricular assist device as a bridge to transplantation?
7. From our experience, we have noticed that staff reacts to patient deaths during the waiting period in several different ways. From your observations, please indicate how often your staff have reacted to pretransplant patient deaths by:

              Never Infrequently Sometimes Frequently Always

  Depression
  Guilt/sense of failure
  Anger
  Rationalizing
  Blaming others
  Apathy/decrease in morale
  Temporary withdrawal from
    transplant patients
  Job transfer
  Changing patient selection
    criteria
  Other, please specify

8. Which team/staff members participate in dealing with deaths?

distress, which is not consistently addressed in an effective manner. Staff members who have the closest contact with transplant candidates are frequently the most strongly affected by deaths in this population.[15] Guilt, anger, and depression are commonly experienced by staff. These unresolved feelings may lead to patient avoidance, overprotective behaviors, or overtreatment.

CONCLUSION

Patients, families, and staff caring for candidates awaiting transplantation are all affected by prolonged waiting periods for donor hearts and the associated morbidity and mortality. The shortage of organs for transplantation has led many medical ethicists and health care providers to explore alternatives to current organ allocation policies, as well as alternative methods of transplantation, such as xenografts and mechanical devices. Until these alternatives are implemented as successful treatment options, patients will continue to die while awaiting heart transplantation. Research that focuses on patients, families, and staff must continue to guide us in assisting those affected by the impact of these unfortunate deaths. Learning how to recognize and address our own stress levels will be important in helping us learn to be more effective and therapeutic in intervening with patient and family stresses.

BIBLIOGRAPHY

1. Pierce E: UNOS history. In Phillips M (ed): UNOS: Organ Procurement, Preservation and Distribution in Transplantation. Richmond, William Byrd Press, 1991.

2. Feree DM: Cadaveric organ sharing: The organ center. In Phillips M (ed): UNOS: Organ Procurement, Preservation and Distribution in Transplantation. Richmond, William Byrd Press, 1991.
3. Miller LW, Merkle EJ, Jennison SH: Outpatient use of dobutamine to support patients awaiting heart transplantation. J Heart Lung Transplant 13(4):S126–S129, 1994.
4. O'Connell JB, Gunnar RM, Evans R, et al: Task force 1: Organization of heart transplantation in the U.S. J Am Coll Cardiol 22(1):8–14, 1993.
5. Stevenson LW, Miller LW: Cardiac transplantation as therapy for heart failure. Curr Prob Cardiol 16:221–305, 1991.
6. Kubo SH, Ormaza SM, Francis GS, et al: Trends in patient selection for heart transplantation. J Am Coll Cardiol 21(4):975–81, 1993.
7. Christopherson LK: Cardiac transplantation: A psychological perspective. Circulation 75(1):57-62, 1987.
8. Porter R, Bailey C, Bennett G, et al: Stress during the waiting period. Crit Care Nurse 4(1):25–31, 1991.
9. Porter RR, Krout L, Parks V, et al: Perceived stress and coping strategies among candidates for heart transplantation during the organ waiting period. J Heart Lung Transplant 13(1):102–107, 1994.
10. Cupples SA, Nolan MG, Ohler L: Perceived stress and coping among candidates for heart transplantation during the organ waiting period: A longitudinal study. (Unpublished report, ongoing research, 1994).
11. Riether AM, Boudreau MZ: Heart Transplant: Impact on CCU nurses. Am J Nursing 11:1521–1524, 1988.
12. Spikes J, Holland J: the physician's response to the dying patient. In Strin JJ, Grossman S (eds): Psychological Care of the Medically Ill. New York, Appleton-Century Crofts, 1975.
13. McCue JD: The effects of stress on physicians and their medical practice. N Engl J Med 306(8):458–463, 1982.
14. Mallet K, Price JH, Jurs SG, Slenker S: Relationship among burnout, death anxiety and social support in hospice and critical care nurses. Psychol Rep 68:1347–1359, 1991.
15. Crone C, Ohler L: The impact of heart transplant candidate deaths on healthcare providers. Unpublished report, 1994.

Chapter 24

Late Noncompliance

Frances Hoffman, MS, RN, CCTC

SCOPE OF THE PROBLEM

Noncompliance, or failure to follow medical instructions, is an important cause of posttransplant graft loss and patient mortality. A study of renal transplant recipients found medication noncompliance to be the third leading cause of graft loss.[1] In a multicenter survey of renal transplant recipients, 16% of the respondents acknowledged some form of noncompliance with immunosuppression.[2] This finding compares closely with a retrospective study of renal transplant recipients from 1971–1984 (noncompliance with medications or office visits, 18%) and a prospective survey of renal recipients transplanted from 1984–1987 (noncompliance rate, 15%).[3]

Unlike renal transplant recipients who can return to dialysis, heart recipients have no readily available long-term support for loss of allograft function, and results of noncompliance can be devastating. In an early study, Lanza and Cooper found that patient noncompliance was related to 23% of deaths or loss of graft function.[4]

Though noncompliance with medication can lead to the most devastating consequences of graft loss or death, dietary noncompliance and obesity may also have an impact on morbidity or mortality. A review of studies evaluating nonimmunologic risk factors for the development of posttransplant coronary disease identified many studies suggesting a relationship among hypercholesterolemia, hypertriglyceridemia, and obesity in the development of posttransplant coronary disease.[5] A study of luminal narrowing of the coronary tree in 15 explanted allografts found mean luminal narrowing to be significantly greater in patients with higher vs. lower mean cholesterol and triglyceride levels, and body-mass indices. The single most predictive risk factor was posttransplant body mass index.[6] Additionally, noncompliant patients have been found to have more hospital readmissions, longer lengths of stay, and increased medical costs.[7]

Compliance is considered an important criterion in transplant candidate selection. In a recent international survey of transplant program psychosocial evaluation of heart transplant candidates, most transplant programs reported considering medication and dietary noncompliance, significant obesity, AMA hospital discharge history, current cigarette smoking, heavy alcohol consumption, or addictive drug use to be either absolute or relative contraindications to heart transplantation. However, this survey also discovered wide discrepancies between programs in rates of patients excluded on psychosocial grounds.[8] Denial of transplantation for nonmedical reasons is difficult because of the subjective nature of nonmedical criteria, potential for bias, and possibility of misjudgment.[9]

Compliance behavior is difficult to measure objectively. Commonly used methods are patient self-reports, in which compliance can be overestimated, and using pill counts, which are logistically cumbersome and potentially inaccurate. Drug serum–level monitoring is most helpful for those drugs with long half-lives, because the results provide an approximation of use during the preceding week.[10] Drug levels can also be confounded, however, by patients wishing to mask noncompliance by manipulation of dosage before testing. Several authors have reported more accurate monitoring of drug-taking behavior through the use of Medication Event Monitoring System (MEMS, Aprex Corporation, Fremont, California).[10,11] A microprocessor located in the medication bottle cap records each bottle opening as a presumptive dose. Clinical outcomes have also been used as an indirect measure of compliance, with noncompliance suspected or assumed in situations such as late rejection without other explanation.

RELATED FACTORS

It is often difficult for health care providers to understand noncompliant behavior. Christensen has suggested that compliance and noncompliance should not be regarded as mutually exclusive behaviors but as opposite ends of a continuum.[12] Christensen further suggests that patient perceptions of the importance of compliance change over time, and individuals consciously or unconsciously reassess their decision to comply. Donovan has described a process of cost/benefit analysis with patients weighing costs and risks of compliance against perceived benefits, influenced by lay beliefs, and the personal and social circumstances in which they live. Patients are most compliant when they perceive the treatment as effective and possible to carry out within the constraints of their everyday lives.[13]

The Health belief Model, first proposed by Rosenstock to explain preventive heath behavior, describes health behavior as dependent on an individual's readiness to take action, assessment of benefits and costs, and a cue or stimulus to trigger action.[14] Readiness to take action is determined by perception of seriousness of disease and one's susceptibility to the disease or its sequelae. Costs can include time, inconvenience, physical, psychologic, and economic impact. Cues to action can be internal (symptoms) or external (social pressure, daily rituals).[14]

The complexity of the medical regimen has been shown to correlate with the degree of compliance. In general, the more complex the demands of treatment, the poorer the rates of adherence.[15] A study measuring compliance with epilepsy medication found a decline in rate of compliance between patients prescribed once daily dosing (compliance rate 87%) to those with twice daily dosing (81%), three times a day (77%), and four times (39%).[10] Several studies have shown relationships between medication side effects and noncompliance, with compliance diminishing as incidence and severity of side effects increases.[12]

Compliance has been shown to be negatively associated with length of treatment.[12,15] A recent study of heart transplant recipients showed progressive declines in compliance with annual diagnostic testing over the first 5 posttransplant years. Compliance with angiogram was 92% at 1 year and 77% at 5 years.[16] Compliance with medications has also been shown to decline between clinic visits. In a study using MEMS electronic monitoring of compliance with epilepsy medications, Cramer found increased compliance for a period immediately preceding and immediately following a clinic appointment, but diminished compliance 1 month later.[17] Transplant recipients generally have less frequent clinic visits with advancing posttransplant years.

Sociologic factors such as gender, socioeconomic status, education, occupation, income, or marital status do not consistently correlate with compliance. Psychiatric factors, such as major psychiatric disorders (major depression, bipolar disorders, schizophrenia, dementia, alcohol or drug dependence) may increase the likelihood of noncompliance.[18]

The adolescent population has been identified as a high-risk group for noncompliant behavior. Related developmental factors that have been described include the cognitive inability to project into the future to perceive long-term consequences, using noncompliance as a means to exert control or test limitations, the importance of body image, and the commonly used defense mechanisms of denial and acting out.[19]

Finally, quality of the health care provider-patient relationship is believed to affect patient compliance.[3,18–20] Factors enhancing compliance are good communication, patient satisfaction, and continuity of care. Table 1 lists factors correlated with noncompliance.

STRATEGIES TO INCREASE COMPLIANCE

A first step in facilitating patient compliance is to become aware of the pervasiveness of noncompliant behavior and the complexity of factors that may influence a patient's decision about whether to comply. Rather than assuming that medication schedules will be automatically followed, the transplant team should consider whether the patient has the knowledge, motivation, and ability to comply. Realizing that compliance behavior can change over time, the team should monitor the patient's level of compliance longitudinally. Rather than viewing noncompliance as a patent-controlled variable, the team should recognize their ability to create an environment that supports patients and fosters compliance.

At the core of compliance-fostering strategies is a positive health team–patient relationship.[13] Working in partnership is recommended over the didactic approach.[20]

Educational approaches, including discussion of the diagnosis and rationale for treatment, therapeutic benefits, possible adverse reactions, and the importance of

TABLE I. Correlates of Noncompliance[3,10,12–20]

Patient Factors	Treatment Factors
• Denial of illness severity/susceptibility	• Complexity of medical regimen
• Lack of perceived benefits of treatment	• Costs of therapy
• Psychiatric factors	• Treatment side effects
• Adolescent age group	• Increased length of treatment
• Lack of trust in health care providers	• Poor communication with patient
• Lack of knowledge	• Lack of continuity of care
• Lack of resources	• Complexity of health care system

follow-up, help provide the patient with information needed in the decision to comply. Sensitivity to issues of volume of information, timing, and patient readiness to learn must be addressed. Written instructions can supplement those given verbally. Allowing time for questions and assessing patient understanding are also important. Although patient knowledge is believed to be significant in treatment compliance, educational techniques should not be used as the sole intervention in fostering compliance.[18]

Simplification of the treatment regimen, especially reducing the frequency of dosage, can foster compliance.[10] The daily rituals of life such as meals and bedtime can serve as organizational cues to remind the patient to take scheduled doses.[18] The social worker or financial liaison can play an important role in securing insurance or obtaining financial assistance for the high cost of immunosuppression.

The family or other significant individuals in the patient's life may support compliance.[21] A study of spousal supportive behavior identified the significant role a spouse plays in learning the medical regimen and providing informational reinforcement, guidance, feedback, physical assistance, and material aid that supports patient compliance after discharge.[22] Effective parental involvement in adolescent's health care is predictive of increased compliance.[19]

Efforts to improve the patient's experience during clinic visits may reduce the cost associated with keeping follow-up appointments. Streamlining processes and reducing delays can reduce patient inconvenience and may improve compliance. Individualized appointment times set with a specific health care provider are recommended over block scheduling.[15] Patients who do not comply with office visits should receive immediate communication, because noncompliance with office follow-up can be related to noncompliance with medication.[3]

Patients with identified compliance difficulty can be assisted by increasing the frequency of clinic visits or drug level monitoring, arranging home visits, short hospitalizations, or involvement of family members. Utilization of MEMS electronic monitoring can identify patient individual dosing patterns more accurately than pill counts.[10] Using behavior modification techniques, such as goal-setting, behavioral contracting, and reinforcement, can assist patients in compliance with chronic medical regimens.[15]

Referral for psychiatric evaluation is recommended in cases of major affective disorders, including alcohol and drug dependence, severe anxiety disorders, psychosis, severe personality disorders, dementia, or in patients manifesting pathologic denial.[18] Chemical-dependency treatment and a monitored chemical-free period may be required before accepting the patient as a transplant candidate. Longitudinal evaluation of compliance in patients who initially were denied transplant acceptance successfully identified patients who could adhere to a complicated medical regimen, and they were subsequently accepted as candidates.[9] Table 2 outlines strategies to improve patient compliance.

TABLE 2.   Strategies to Increase Compliance[3,10–13,15,18–22]

• Facilitate clear and open communication	• Streamline clinic process
• Foster positive patient/team relationships	• Increase frequency of clinic visits or drug level monitoring
• Simplify treatment regimen	• Establish mutual goals or behavioral contracts
• Deal with side effects	• Utilize psychiatric referral
• Provide effective education	• Treat chemical dependency
• Assist with financial issues	• Follow-up after missed appointments
• Involve family/significant others	• Monitor compliance longitudinally

DISCUSSION

In 1992, we reported a retrospective review of transplant recipients selected with liberal psychosocial criteria. Recipients deemed at higher psychosocial risk were provided with aggressive psychological intervention. Medical outcomes of these high-risk recipients were similar to the control group at 1 year posttransplant.[23] Paris found similar results in a review of heart transplant recipients (mean follow-up at 18 months). Psychosocial factors that existed before transplant did not adversely affect medical outcome, with the exception of a higher rate of infection. However, Paris also found the presence of psychosocial factors and noncompliance associated with increased hospital readmissions after the first year.[7]

In a study that compared posttransplant survival between heart recipients with a history of substance abuse and those without such a history, Hanrahan found equal survival at 1 year (88%). However, long-term survival tended to be lower, and deaths directly related to noncompliance were significantly higher in patients with a substance abuse history.[24]

There is clearly a subset of patients who have difficulty maintaining compliance after transplantation. Positive early posttransplant outcomes described in the above studies indicate it is possible for high psychosocial risk candidates to do well after transplantation, at least in the short term. However, in a recent review of our patient data, we found that 33% of all mortality after one year could be related to noncompliance.

Further study is needed to determine factors related to late noncompliance, and methods which promote continued compliance after transplantation, not only for those patients identified at risk, but all recipients.

CONCLUSION

Compliance with medication and follow-up is essential for successful posttransplant outcomes. The complex factors related to compliance are both patient centered and treatment centered. Through awareness and understanding of these factors, the transplant team can implement strategies that may assist patients to remain compliant. There is a subset of patients in whom transplantation is not justified on the grounds of noncompliance due to increasing evidence of diminished long-term survival.

REFERENCES

1. Lai MK, Huang CC, Chu SH, et al: Noncompliance in transplant recipients: Experience in Taiwan. Clin Transplant 6:291–293, 1992.
2. Siegal BR, Greenstein S, Schechner R, et al: A multicenter study of patient compliance after renal transplantation. Presented at the American Society of Transplant Physicians, Houston, Texas, May 19, 1993.
3. Schweizer RT, Rovelli M, Palmeri D, et al: Noncompliance in organ transplant recipients. Transplantation 49(2):374–377, 1990.
4. Lanza RP, Cooper DKC: Heart Transplantation: The Present Status of Orthotopic and Heterotopic Heart Transplantation. Boston, MTD Press, 1984.
5. Johnson MR: Transplant coronary disease: Nonimmunologic risk factors. J Heart Lung Transplant 11(3, pt 2):S124–S131, 1992.
6. Winters GL, Kendall TJ, Radio SJ, et al: Post-transplant obesity and hyperlipidemia. Major predictors of severity of coronary arteriopathy in failed human heart allografts. J Heart Transplant 9(4):364–371, 1990.
7. Paris W, Muchmore J, Pribil A, et al: Study of the relative incidences of psychosocial factors before and after heart transplantation and the influence of posttransplantation psychosocial factors on heart transplantation outcome. J Heart Lung Transplant 13(3):424–432, 1994.
8. Olbrisch ME, Levenson JL: Psychosocial evaluation of heart transplant candidates: An international survey of process, criteria and outcomes. J Heart Lung Transplant 10(6):948–955, 1991.

9. Herrick CM, Mealey PC, Tischner LL, Holland CS: Combined heart failure transplant program: Advantages in assessing medical compliance. J Heart Transplant 6(3):141–146, 1987.
10. Cramer JA, Mattson RH, Prevey ML, et al: How often is medication taken as prescribed? A novel assessment technique. JAMA 261:3273–3277, 1989.
11. Rudd P, Ahmed S, Zachary V, et al: Compliance with medication timing: Implications from a medication trial for drug development and clinical practice. Clin Res Pharmacoepidemiol 6:15–27, 1992.
12. Christensen DB: Drug-taking compliance: A review and synthesis. Health Serv Res 13:171–187, 1978.
13. Donovan JL, Blake DR: Patient noncompliance: Deviance or reasoned decision making? Soc Sci Med 34(5):507–513, 1992.
14. Ried LD, Christensen DB: A psychosocial perspective in the explanation of patients' drug-taking behavior. Soc Sci Med 27(3):277–285, 1988.
15. Meichenbaum D, Turk DC: Facilitating Treatment Adherence. A Practitioner's Guidebook. New York, Plenum Press, 1987.
16. Grady KL, Russell KM, Srinivasan S, et al: Patient compliance with annual diagnostic testing after heart transplantation. Transplant Proc 25(5):2978–2980, 1993.
17. Cramer JA, Scheyer RD, Mattson RH: Compliance declines between clinic visits. Arch Intern Med 150:1509–1510, 1990.
18. Stoudemire A, Thompson TL: Medication noncompliance: Systematic approaches to evaluation and intervention. Gen Hosp Psychiatry 5:233–239, 1983.
19. Cromer BA, Tarnowski KJ: Noncompliance in adolescents: A review. J Dev Behav Pediatr 10(4):207–215, 1989.
20. Cramer J: Overview of methods to measure and enhance patient compliance. In Cramer JA, Spilker B (eds): Patient Compliance in Medical Practice and Clinical Trials. New York, Raven Press, 1991, pp 3–10.
21. Cromer BA: Behavioral strategies to increase compliance in adolescents. In Cramer JA, Spilker B (eds): Patient Compliance in Medical Practice and Clinical Trials. New York, Raven Press, 1991, pp 99–107.
22. Rogers KR: Nature of spousal supportive behaviors that influence heart transplant compliance. J Heart Transplant 6(2):90–95, 1987.
23. Tazelaar SL, Prieto M, Lake KD, Emery RW: Heart transplantation in high risk psychosocial patients [abstract]. J Heart Lung Transplant 11:207, 1992.
24. Hanrahan JS, Taylor DO, Eberly C, et al: Cardiac allograft survival in "reformed" substance abusers [abstract]. J Heart Lung Transplant 10(1 pt 2):158, 1991.

Chapter 25

The Adolescent Transplant Patient: Psychosocial Considerations

Wendy Loken, PhD
Gloria Acuña, RN, BSN

Adolescence is an often tumultuous period, marked by a variety of important physical, psychological, and social changes. The "typical" adolescent may experience turmoil surrounding issues of physical growth, physiologic changes, emotional and cognitive maturation, and social pressures which contribute to making the task of developing a healthy sense of identity difficult. Unfortunately, this task is too often impeded by the presence of chronic illness. Chronic illness may be associated with disturbances in body image, changes in family dynamics, and difficult social relationships, which can have a negative impact on the adolescent's emerging self-concept. In addition, life-threatening illnesses add the dimension of confronting personal mortality, which is often difficult in adolescents who may lack the requisite cognitive and emotional maturity.[1]

Given these potential difficulties, it is not surprising that adolescents with chronic illness have been found to exhibit 35% more behavior problems than their healthy counterparts.[2] These problems include social withdrawal, poor peer relations, anxiety, and depression. In addition, adolescents who face heart transplants may experience a host of other difficulties, including worries about inflicting financial strain upon their families, concerns regarding medication, surgery-related changes in personal appearance (e.g., scarring, weight gain), and identity issues associated with cadaveric transplantation. For example, it is not unusual for individuals to experience some difficulty incorporating a new heart into their body image,[3] as was poignantly observed in a 17-year-old woman facing a heart transplant who expressed grave concerns that she would not be "the same person" once she had a new heart.

For the chronically ill adolescent, issues surrounding developing autonomy and independence and the formation of a healthy personal identity apart from one's illness may prove particularly problematic.[2] This difficulty is often illustrated in the tendency of clinicians as well as some parents to label children according to their illnesses and treatments (e.g., as a "cystic" or a "transplant"), which, in addition to the exhaustive attention that is often paid to the child's disease, may limit attention to other aspects of the underlying adolescent. For some children, the illness or accompanying treatments may become their identify.[4] This can prove a particular challenge for the adolescent who is expected to make serious changes (e.g., relocating near the transplant center) while waiting for the organ. In such situations it becomes important to monitor the adolescent's symptoms and to encourage him or her to engage in as many "normal" activities as possible.

Chronic illness often leads to increased dependency, which can have significant impact on the adolescent's natural movement toward independence. For the posttransplant adolescent, the requirements to take daily medications and to engage in regular follow-up visits may intensify feelings of restriction and dependency. Unfortunately, conflicts between dependence and independence may result in potentially dangerous noncompliant behavior, as in the adolescent who becomes increasingly rebellious and appears to engage in frequent "power struggles" with both family and treatment personnel. Often, simply talking with the patient about the desire for greater independence may be beneficial. In addition, the patient should be included in as many treatment decisions as possible and allowed some degree of control over noncritical aspects of compliance.

In addition, compliance can be further complicated by familial factors. For example, as the adolescent regains health, the family may resist relinquishing their role as caretakers, thereby creating further restrictions on the adolescent's growing independence. The transplant team must have a good understanding of the patient's family dynamics and of the typical patterns of familial communication. Should compliance problems arise, the team may then be in a better position to work out possible solutions with the family of the adolescent. Ideally, the transplant team and the family can work together to allow the adolescent as much control in as many situations as possible, so that the patient can feel independent enough to accept the restrictions imposed in compliance.

Understanding noncompliance in the adolescent is often difficult, as it can be complicated by a variety of factors, including depression, self-destructive behavior, denial, or cognitive impairments.[1] Many of these difficulties can be readily treated with subtle changes in medications, psychotherapy, or supportive counseling, or instructing the patient in the use of external memory aids (e.g., using a notebook to record important information). When serious compliance problems arise, both adolescent patient and family must be evaluated to ascertain the appropriate course of action.

Finally, Parmelee makes the important point that illness may actually have beneficial effects on a child's behavioral development.[5] The adolescent facing a heart transplant has been forced to deal with existential issues concerning life and death that may promote an advanced level of maturity and a greater appreciation of life experiences. They have often had to learn to adapt to physical disability, which may lead to greater empathy and increased resourcefulness. In addition, the presence of an ill child can bring together and strengthen family relationships as members more toward the common goal of caring for the child.

PSYCHOLOGICAL EVALUATION

Psychological evaluation is often helpful in gaining an understanding of potential problems that the adolescent facing transplant may encounter. The psychologist is able to assess developmental, cognitive, and personality aspects of the adolescent. In addition, if the patient is experiencing acute distress, the psychologist can use techniques to assist the patient in developing more effective coping strategies.

Test results often present the chronically ill individual as anxious, socially isolated, and having considerable concern about physical matters or death.[1] Although these concerns may be seen as pathologic in healthy individuals, they may, in fact, be quite understandable in the adolescent facing transplant. An important role of the psychological evaluation, then, is in predicting which behaviors or concerns may prove problematic in terms of compliance or in making an effective adjustment to life as a transplant recipient. If serious problems are detected, the psychologist attempts to distinguish those that would likely interfere significantly with outcome from those that may not be sufficiently pathologic to exclude the candidate, but may complicate the postoperative course.

A typical test battery includes tests of general cognitive abilities and personality assessment. These may include subtests of the Wechsler Adult Intelligence Scale-Revised (WAIS-R), subtests of the Wechsler Memory Scale-Revised (WMS-R), Trail-Making Tests A and B, and the Minnesota Multiphasic Personality Inventory (MMPI). Potential areas of difficulty are further explored with other psychological and neuropsychological tests. For example, if the patient exhibits weaknesses in memory or attentional abilities, further neuropsychological testing may be performed.

The most important component of a psychological evaluation is often the clinical interview. Here, the psychologist develops an understanding of the adolescent's level of emotional and cognitive maturity, evaluates the status of the family support system, and identifies any ambivalence that may exist regarding the transplant. In addition, the psychologist evaluates any history of "acting out" behavior in an attempt to distinguish healthy from unhealthy movements toward autonomy that could indicate potential threats to postoperative compliance. Finally, rapport must be established with the adolescent in case further psychotherapeutic intervention is required.

General cognitive screening is important to assess the adolescent's memory, problem-solving, and attentional abilities. This allows a general indication of the patient's strengths and weaknesses and can be important for recommending an individualized approach to teaching important information. If cognitive impairments are suggested, the psychologist can also assist in determining whether they are secondary to emotional (e.g., depression) or medical factors (e.g., poor cerebral perfusion). Personality inventory is conducted to ascertain potential factors that may prove problematic (e.g., strong antisocial tendencies) and to indicate problems with depression or anxiety that the adolescent may otherwise be denying.

Since July 1981, 25 pediatric patients at the University Medical Center have undergone cardiothoracic transplantation (20 heart, 4 heart/lung, and 1 double lung). Of these pediatric patients, 9 are in the age range of 12 to 19 years. Graft survival since the advent of cyclosporine in this pediatric group vs. adult recipients is 35% and 65% respectively (Fig. 1). However, there was no difference in rates of rejection and infection between the age groups (Figs. 2 and 3).

Because of the turmoil of the adolescent years, patients in this age group who have received transplants are often the most challenging. The following approaches may be beneficial in assisting the adolescent patient to deal with the stress of transplantation and achieve successful posttransplant outcomes.

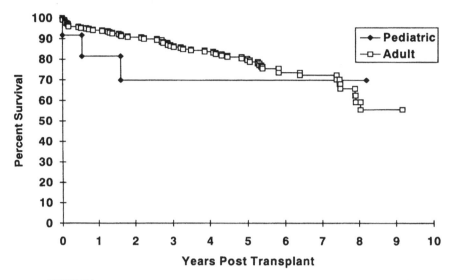

FIGURE 1.   Graft survival in pediatric vs. adult cardiothoracic transplant recipients.

Approaches for Preparation in Adolescent Transplant Recipients

- Allow adolescents to be an integral part of decision-making about their care. This allows for understanding of long-term consequences.
- Start preparation at time of listing to assist with ability to cope, cooperate, and comply.
- Tactfully explore the adolescent's knowledge base with sensitivity to avoid feelings of inadequacy, dependence, and confusion.
- Stress the importance of compliance and cooperation. Be honest about the consequences.
- Stress peer contact; network if possible with other transplant programs.
- Emphasize the "normal."

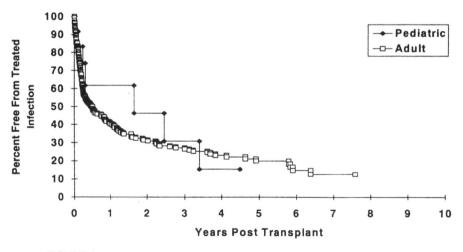

FIGURE 2.   Infection rates in pediatric vs. adult cardiothoracic transplant recipients.

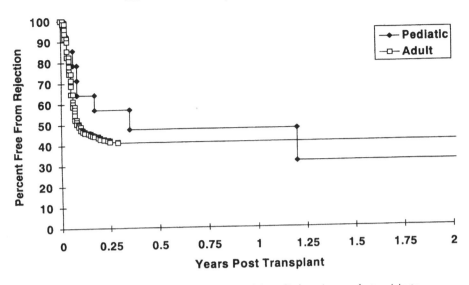

FIGURE 3. Rejection rates in pediatric vs. adult cardiothoracic transplant recipients.

CONCLUSION

The adolescent transplant patient presents a variety of challenges well known to most transplant programs. Establishing a network for peer support may prove helpful in this very important developmental period. Supporting them and meeting their needs requires patience, creativity, and understanding on the part of the transplant team.

REFERENCES

1. Pfefferbaum B: Adolescence and illness. Annu Rev Psychol 5:451–467, 1986.
2. Newachek PW, McManus MA, Fox HB: Prevalence and impact of chronic illness among adolescents. Am J Dis Child 145:1367–1373, 1991.
3. Frierson RL, Lippmann SB: Heart transplant candidates rejected on psychiatric indications. Psychosomatics 28:347–353, 1987.
4. Perrin JM: Adolescents with chronic disease. Am J Dis Child 145:1361–1362, 1986.
5. Parmelee AH: Children's illnesses: Their beneficial effects on behavioral development. Child Dev 57:1–10, 1986.

Biopsy-Negative Graft Dysfunction

Chapter **26**

Mary O'Kane, BA, RN, CCTC

Perhaps the greatest challenge in transplant medicine is the accurate diagnosis and effective treatment of graft rejection. The standard method for diagnosis of rejection in heart transplant patents is endomyocardial biopsy (EMB). Occasionally, patents present with clinical symptoms and echocardiographic evidence of rejection yet have normal biopsies. The difficult dilemma is commonly referred to as nonspecific rejection, or biopsy-negative graft dysfunction (BNGD). In a typical case of BNGD, the patient may present with symptoms of rejection, including fatigue, increased shortness of breath, malaise, weight gain, and atrial arrhythmias with or without hypotension. the echocardiogram subsequently shows LV dysfunction, and yet the biopsy reported Grade O, IA or IB.[1,2]

It has been standard practice to treat only patients whose biopsies show persistent Grade II or Grade III rejection. Standard rejection treatment involves augmentation of immunosuppression or bolus steroids. Thus, it is vital to accurately distinguish rejection from other processes for which other, and perhaps less risky, therapeutic options are appropriate. Experience has shown that the diagnosis of rejection cannot be determined solely by histology shown on EMB. The clinician must also consider the patient's complaints, physical findings, and ventricular function evaluated by echocardiography as well as the known sampling error that occurs with random sample biopsy.

Considerable effort and time has been spent to find a more reliable and early method to diagnose rejection, yet EMB remains the gold standard[3] because it is safe and considered consistently accurate. However, biopsy alone cannot be relied on for the diagnosis of rejection. The patient's complaints, physical assessment, and echocardiographic ventricular

269

function must all be considered. Echocardiography, careful histologic examination, patient assessment and timeliness assist in the early diagnosis of this problem.

ECHOCARDIOGRAPHY

Echocardiography is one of the most valuable tools for assessing heart function. Several echocardiographic indices exist that allow for serial assessment of rejection. Before reviewing the variables in these echocardiographic parameters in transplant rejection, it is useful to define the echocardiographic indices used to assess cardiac function and the echocardiographic difference between the allografted heart and a normal one.

Measurements of blood flow using Doppler echocardiography play an important role in the evaluation of the allografted heart. The four echocardiographic indices used to determine allograft function include the following:[4]

1. *IVRT (Isovolumetric Relaxation Time)* is the interval between aortic valve closure and mitral valve opening. IVRT is prolonged in the transplanted heart compared with the normal heart but is thought to decrease during rejection.

2. *PHT (Pressure Half Time)* is that required for the peak gradient across the mitral valve to be reduced by one-half. It is quantitatively related to the velocity of flow across the mitral valve. The flow is thought to decrease during rejection because of decreased compliance of the left ventricle.

3. *DT (Deceleration Time)* begins at the early peak of acceleration time across the mitral valve and continues to the end of rapid filling.

4. *FS (Fractional Shortening)* measures systolic function.; it is preload and afterload dependent and is defined as the left ventricular end-diastolic end-systolic dimension representing the change in the short axis areas of the left ventricle.

Impact of Change in Indices

Changes in echocardiographic indices are useful in the diagnosis of rejection. Such diagnosis may be sensitive because of the changes in the restrictive physiology of the transplanted heart during rejection. Even though function of the allograft improves over the first several weeks and even months[5] these indices are sensitive enough to detect change when the patient develops rejection. Many researchers have tried to find a specific index that will allow reliable diagnosis of rejection but the indices are neither specific nor sensitive enough to confidently diagnose rejection without EMB.[6–13]

Valentine initially found that the IVRT and the PHT were shortened during rejection. Others felt these changes were not consistent enough. Valentine retested this theory and found the decrease in echocardiographic indices to be significant even when the biopsy was negative because at times restrictive physiology precedes histologic findings of rejection and the patient should either be treated with high-dose steroids or repeat EMB. She predicted that progressive decline in allograft function could be minimized with treatment of these early signs of rejection.[7,8,14,15]

The functional shortening may be the most sensitive index to follow. Olson and colleagues found that the DT and FS were most specific in the diagnoses of rejection. The DT is the easiest index to follow; and the FS, which had not been shown previously to be predictive for rejection, was found to be very indicative of early rejection.[16] Thus, the overall ventricular dysfunction of both systolic and diastolic parameters may be precursors for rejection. All researchers do agree that echocardiography is an important adjunct in the diagnosis of allograft rejection indices and changes in indices studied along a continuum may well be significant enough to warrant treatment of some patients even though the biopsy is not significant for rejection.

In the presence of BNGD an additional means to rule out rejection is of import. With significant decrease in graft function, the patient must be evaluated thoroughly even though the biopsy is negative. Following serial echocardiograms is useful for monitoring cardiac function over time. When a patient is seen with symptoms of rejection and has a negative biopsy, treatment is warranted if graft function confirmed by echocardiography is different from that previously recorded.

Another area of concern is whether histologic mild rejection should be treated. Yeoh suggests that there should be at least two physical findings of rejection in the patient assessment in addition to EMB findings so that treatment is not based entirely on a biopsy report. Some of the signs and symptoms associated with rejection include atrial arrhythmias, a new S3, bilateral rales of the lung bases or congestion on chest radiograph, hypotension, fatigue, and shortness of breath. Importantly, Yeoh also found that a decrease in systolic function found on echocardiography was a strong indicator that symptomatic mild rejection was likely to progress to moderate rejection quickly. Such findings required increased surveillance or treatment.[17]

HISTOLOGIC EVALUATION

The classic findings of cellular rejection on EMB are infiltrating lymphocytes, interstitial edema, and cell necrosis. Vascular rejection is more difficult to diagnose by EMB unless viewed under light microscopy in association with special staining.

Vascular rejection may be one of the causes of BNGD. It is rarer, more difficult to diagnose, and sometimes accompanies by cellular rejection. Vascular rejection may occur in the absence of characteristic histologic findings in spite of documented graft dysfunction and is most likely to happen early in the postoperative period, usually in the first several weeks. The course may be rapid and, in many cases, fatal. Vascular rejection is suspected under light microscopy by identifying endothelial cell swelling and interstitial edema; but the only reliable way to diagnose vascular rejection is with immunofluorescence.[18] Because of this, viewing early biopsies with immunofluorescence under election as well as light microscopy may be useful. Although light microscopy is sufficient to identify vascular infiltrates, cyclosporine itself can also cause interstitial edema and endothelial infiltrates.

Interestingly, the use of cyclosporine may make identifying vascular rejection even more difficult. Cyclosporine causes bands of lymphocytic infiltrates in the endocardium and sometimes even in the myocardium. This so-called *Quilty effect* makes diagnosis of vascular rejection more difficult. Following patients systematically with scheduled biopsies, echocardiography, and clinic visits is vital.[19]

BNGD may also result from focal rejection. As noted, biopsies are done through the same site and the bioptome follows approximately the same path. Thus, areas in the right ventricle are repeatedly biopsied. Biopsy reports frequently note scarring and thrombus from earlier biopsies. This sampling error may be one reason for BNGD; that is, rejection may be focal, but histologically it cannot be confirmed. Most transplant centers now do EMB under echocardiographic guidance, which is cost effective and also allows a better view of the ventricle so the bioptome can be better positioned, decreasing the amount of sampling errors.

The last histologic consideration in BNGD is chronic vascular rejection or transplant arteriopathy. Vascular occlusions of transplant arteriopathy can lead to myocardial infarction, congestive heart failure, arrhythmias, and even sudden death. It is the most important cause of graft failure after the first 6 to 12 months. The only way to diagnose transplant arteriopathy is by angiogram. in order to rule out transplant arteriopathy as a cause for BNGD, an early angiogram may be necessary.

TIMELINESS

Finally, it is important to consider timeliness as a factor for rejection in the transplant patient. Patients are most susceptible to rejection during the first 6 months following transplant, with the first 3 months being even more critical. Other indicators or likely times for rejection include a recent history of noncompliance, when weaning or decreasing steroid dose, and the time after induction therapy, usually 12 weeks after therapy with OKT3, ATG, or ALG. As noted earlier, the assessment of transplant recipients must not rely on diagnoses of rejection by EMB alone but must also consider timeliness, other histologic factors, echocardiographic findings, and patient clinical findings.

In conclusion, there are still immune processes about which little is known and which may contribute to BNGD. The process of BNGD remains undefined and may not be related to any of these theories, but it is important to consider them and to treat the patient when there is strong suspicion because reversal of myocardial dysfunction may occur.

Acknowledgment. Special thanks to Jeanne Olson for her assistance in editing the echo definitions and results.

REFERENCES

1. Billingham ME: Endomyocardial biopsy diagnosis of acute rejection in cardiac allografts. Prog Cardiovasc Dis 33:11–18, 1990.
2. Billingham ME: Dilemma of variety of hostopathologic systems for acute cardiac allograft rejection by endomyocardial biopsy. J Heart Transplant 9:272–276, 1990.
3. Kemkes BM, Schutz A, Engelhardt M: Noninvasive methods of rejection diagnosis after heart transplantation. J Heart Lung Transplant 11(4):S221–S231, 1992.
4. Fiegenbaum H: Echocardiography. Philadelphia, Lea & Febiger, 1994.
5. Seacord EM, Miller LW, Pennington G, et al: Reversal of constrictive/restrictive physiology with treatment of allograft rejection. Am Heart J 120):455–459, 1990.
6. Valentine HA, Yeoh TK, Gibbons R, et al: Sensitivity and specificity of diastolic indexes for rejection surveillance: Temporal correlation with endomyocardial biopsy. J Heart Lung Transplant 10:757–765, 1991.
7. Valentine HA: Rejection surveillance by Doppler echocardiography. J Heart Lung Transplant 12:422–426, 1993.
8. Valentine HA, Fowler MB, Hunt SA, et al: Changes in Doppler echocardiography indexes of left ventricular function as potential markers of acute cardiac rejection. Cardiac Transplant 76(Suppl V):86–92, 1987.
9. Amende I, Simon R, Seegers A, et al: Diastolic dysfunction during acute cardiac allograft rejection. Circulation 81(2):66–69, 1990.
10. Furniss SS, Murray A, Hunter S, et al: Value of echocardiographic determination of isovolumetric relaxation time in the detection of heart transplant rejection. J Heart Lung Transplant 10:1557–1561, 1991.
11. Ciliberto GR, Mascardlo MA, Gronda E, et al: Acute rejection after heart transplantation: Noninvasive echocardiography evaluation. J Am Coll Cardiol 23:1156–1161, 1994.
12. Olson JD, Goldenberg IF, Pritzker M, Emery RW: Doppler echocardiographic indices as markers of acute cardiac rejection. Cardiac Surgery: State of the Art Reviews 3:633–637, 1989.
13. Mannaerts HF, Simoons ML, Balk AH, et al: Pulsed-wave transmitral Doppler doe not diagnose moderate acute rejection after heart transplantation. J Heart Lung Transplant 12:411–421, 1993.
14. Valentine HA, Yeoh TK, Gibbons R, et al: Sensitivity and specificity of diastolic indexes for rejection surveillance: Temporal correlation with endomyocardial biopsy. J Heart Lung Transplant 10:757–765, 1991.
15. Valentine HA, Appleton CP, Hatle LK, et al: Influence of recipient atrial contraction on left ventricular filling dynamics of the transplanted heart assessed by Doppler echocardiography. Am J Cardiol 59:1159–1163, 1987.
16. Yeoh TK, First WH, Eastburn TE, et al: Clinical significance of mild rejection of the cardiac allograft. Circulation 86:267–271, 1992.
17. Hammond EH, Yowell RL, Nunoda S, et al: Vascular (humoral) rejection in heart transplantation: Pathologic observations and clinical implications. J Heart Transplant 8:430–443, 1989.
18. Winters GL: The pathology of heart allograft rejection. Arch Pathol Lab Med 115:266–272, 1991.

Chapter 27

Pregnancy after Heart Transplantation

Linda Ohler, MSN, RN, CCTC, CCRN, CNS
Lisa Klein, MSN, RNC

With improvements in cardiac transplant survival rates and quality of life, new dimensions of transplant health care have evolved which include pregnancy in organ recipients. The literature reports successful pregnancies following renal transplantation; however, the number of reported cases of heart recipients who have conceived and delivered healthy infants is less than 35.[1-7] The National Transplantation Pregnancy Registry was developed at Thomas Jefferson University Hospital in Philadelphia in 1991 with the assistance of Sandoz Pharmaceuticals.[7] This registry, as well as data collected by Wagoner and associates, is providing health care professionals with specific information on the impact of pregnancy on heart transplant recipients.[5-7] The goal of this registry is to determine risk factors for the mother as well as the infant. To date, the most commonly reported risk factor for pregnant transplant recipients is premature births, with 58% of live births occurring 4 or 5 weeks from term.[7] Data are also being collected on pregnancies produced by fathers who are organ transplant recipients.[7]

Before 1991, information about pregnancy in transplant recipients was applied from knowledge gained from case reports of renal transplant recipients. The first reported pregnancy in a renal transplant recipient was in 1958 in a young woman who had received a kidney from an identical twin.[2] Some estimates report more than 2,000 pregnancies in renal transplant recipients, with others estimating that 1 in 50 women renal recipients of childbearing age becomes pregnant.[8,9] Data on the effects of pregnancy on heart transplant recipients are mostly anecdotal at this time because so few cases have been reported. In extracting and applying information on the effects of pregnancy from renal allograft recipients,

TABLE I. Reported Complications for 27 Heart or Heart-Lung Transplant Recipients during Pregnancy

Hypertension	12
Premature delivery	8
Preeclampsia	6
Diabetes	1
Infection	4
Premature rupture of membranes	3
Renal insufficiency	4
Rejection during pregnancy	6

Data from Wagoner LE, Taylor DO, Olsen SL, et al: Immunosuppressive therapy, management, and outcome of heart transplant recipients during pregnancy. J Heart Lung Transplant 12:993–1000, 1993.

heart transplant team members are most concerned about renal function, rejection, infections, and the impact of increased blood volume on the denervated heart. Table 1, listing complications reported in pregnant heart transplant recipients, is based on data reported to Wagoner and associates, which include 32 patients who became pregnant following heart or heart–lung transplantation. There were three therapeutic abortions and two spontaneous abortions for a net total of 27 deliveries and 29 live births, including 2 sets of twins.[6] Table 2 summarizes the methods of delivery. Table 3 lists the reported complications for the 29 infants.

POTENTIAL RENAL PROBLEMS

Pregnancies in normal females increase glomerular filtration rate because of the increased blood volume. Nephrotoxic effects of cyclosporine may elevate serum creatinine levels as well as decrease the rate of creatinine clearance. Because of this, renal function is closely monitored in all transplant recipients, and pregnancy intensifies this concern. When renal function is moderately impaired, pregnancy may accelerate the decline.[4] Therefore, the need to closely monitor renal function in transplant recipients during pregnancy becomes imperative. An increase in the frequency of urinary tract infections has been reported in renal transplant recipients.[10] Wagoner and associates have reported that 41% of pregnant heart recipients required increased cyclosporine doses during their pregnancies to maintain therapeutic levels.[6] However, 22% of the patients had their cyclosporine doses lowered empirically in efforts either to decrease the risk of teratogenicity or to decrease nephrotoxic effects of the drug.[6] Concern with higher dosage of cyclosporine is, of course, the drug's impact on renal function.

TABLE 2. Method of Delivery in 32 Reported Pregnancies

Vaginal	18
Cesarean	9
Intrauterine deaths	0
Therapeutic abortions	3
Spontaneous abortions	2
Multiple births	2 sets of twins

Data from Wagoner LE, Taylor DO, Olsen SL, et al: Immunosuppressive therapy, management, and outcome of heart transplant recipients during pregnancy. J Heart Lung Transplant 12:993–1000, 1993.

TABLE 3.   Reported Complications for Infants Born of Heart Transplant Recipients (n = 29)

Patent ductus arteriosus	2
Respiratory distress	4
Anemia	1
Low birth weight	5
Polycythemia	1
Hypoglycemia	1

Data from Wagoner LE, Taylor DO, Olsen SL, et al: Immunosuppressive therapy, management, and outcome of heart transplant recipients during pregnancy. J Heart Lung Transplant 12:993–1000, 1993.

MONITORING FOR REJECTION DURING PREGNANCY

No increased incidence of rejection has been reported in renal allografts during pregnancy.[8] Because clinical signs or symptoms of heart rejection rarely occur, surveillance biopsies are performed on a regular basis in all patients who have received heart transplants. Although some centers use echocardiography as guidance for endomyocardial biopsies, most biopsies are performed in the cardiac catheterization laboratory under fluoroscopy, which poses a risk of radiation exposure to the fetus, which is greatest in the first two trimesters. The dilemma becomes one of risking exposure to radiation or using diagnostic tools that are considered less than accurate in detecting rejection. Failure to detect and treat a rejection, or initiating rejection treatment unnecessarily, both have obvious consequences.[11]

DENERVATED HEART IN PREGNANCY

The denervated heart presents many concerns and questions to health care professionals. Such concerns increase during pregnancy and, with the ensuing labor and delivery processes, when cardiac output increases 20% with each contraction.[6] The denervated heart responds to these increased demands through an increase in stroke volume in response to the increase in central venous pressure and volume.[11] Changes in heart rate are also affected by denervation. Heart transplant recipients rely on circulating catecholamines for increases in heart rate and contractility because the denervated heart is not influenced by the autonomic nervous system.[11] Potential risks related to these hemodynamic changes occurring during pregnancy, labor, and delivery warrant further investigation.[11]

FAIRFAX HOSPITAL EXPERIENCE

Our institution recently had experience with pregnancy in a 21-year-old female heart recipient, who became pregnant 14 months after transplantation. This case was especially challenging considering the patient's difficult pretransplant course, which included mechanical bridging with intraaortic balloon pump (IABP) and emergency cardiopulmonary bypass after cardiac arrest. Her posttransplant course was complicated by renal failure requiring chronic hemodialysis for a period of 6 months, early grade 3B rejection[12] treated with OKT3, and a prolonged period of in-hospital recovery (47 days).

Throughout the pregnancy a multidisciplinary team approach was used, including obstetricians, neonatologists, transplant surgeons, cardiologists, nephrologists, clinical nurse specialists, transplant coordinators, social workers, a nutritionist, and pharmacists.

During the relatively uncomplicated pregnancy, the patient was treated for several urinary tract infections. Renal function was monitored by serial 24-hour urine collections.

During the third trimester, creatinine clearance dropped to 31 ml/minute, but she did not require dialysis. Heart function was monitored echocardiographically. During the eighth month, atrial dysrhythmias developed and pulse steroid therapy was given for presumed rejection.

At 34 weeks' gestation, the patient had premature rupture of membranes. Intravenous antibiotic prophylaxis and stress steroid coverage were initiated. After 22 hours of labor without cervical dilation, delivery of a five-pound-six-ounce girl was accomplished by cesarean section. Apgar scores were eight and nine. The mother was discharged on the fourth postpartum day and was treated as an outpatient for a urinary tract infection. She was eventually readmitted for treatment of a perirectal abscess. The baby remained in the hospital for 8 days because of feeding problems associated with prematurity but has developed normally and is now 19 months old.

CONCLUSION

To confront and deal with the aforementioned problems involved in the case of a pregnant heart-transplant recipient, a multidisciplinary approach was developed at our institution. Communication between the obstetrics department and transplant staff was excellent. Three team meetings were scheduled during pregnancy, and one following delivery. This multidisciplinary, multidepartmental approach is highly recommended because it promotes communication and provides a learning opportunity for individuals involved in this interesting case. Our experience with pregnancy in a heart-transplant recipient resulted in an excellent outcome for mother and child.

Acknowledgment. Our thanks go to Dr. Lynne Wagoner who provided our teams with much information and support throughout this experience.

REFERENCES

1. Sims CJ: Organ transplantation and immunosuppressive drugs in pregnancy. Clin Obstet Gynecol 34(1):100–111, 1991.
2. Baumgardner GL, Matas AJ: Transplantation and pregnancy. Transplant Rev 6(3):139–162, 1992.
3. Kirk EP: Organ transplantation and pregnancy: A case report and review. Am J Obstet Gynecol 164:1629–1634, 1991.
4. Hou S: Pregnancy in organ transplant recipients. Med Clin North Am 73:667–683, 1989.
5. Scott JR, Wagoner LE, Olsen SL, et al: Pregnancy in heart transplant recipients: Management and outcome. Obstet Gynecol 82(3):324–327.
6. Wagoner LE, Taylor DO, Olsen SL, et al: Immunosuppressive therapy, management, and outcome of heart transplant recipients during pregnancy. J Heart Lung Transplant 12:993–1000, 1993.
7. Armeti VT, Moritz MJ: Parenthood after transplant. Lifetimes 13, 1992.
8. Davison JM: Pregnancy in renal allograft recipients: Prognosis and management. Clin Obstet Gynecol 1:1027, 1987.
9. Davison JM: Dialysis, transplantation and pregnancy. J Kidney Dis 17:127, 1991.
10. O'Connell PJ, Caterson RJ, Stewart JH, et al: Problems associated with pregnancy with renal allograft recipients. Int J Artif Org 12:147, 1989.
11. Hunt SA: Pregnancy in heart transplant recipients: A good idea? J Heart Lung Transplant 10:499–503, 1991.
12. Billingham ME, Cary NRB, Hammond ME, et al: A working formulation for the standardization of nomenclature in the diagnosis of heart and lung rejection: Heart rejection study group. J Heart Lung Transplant 9:587–593, 1990.

Index

Page numbers in **boldface** indicate complete chapters.